PSYCHIATRY - THEORY, APPLICATIONS AND TREATMENTS

THE INTERNATIONAL PSYCHIATRY AND BEHAVIORAL NEUROSCIENCES YEARBOOK

VOLUME II - 2012

PSYCHIATRY - THEORY, APPLICATIONS AND TREATMENTS

Additional books in this series can be found on Nova's website
under the Series tab.

Additional E-books in this series can be found on Nova's website
under the E-book tab.

NEUROSCIENCE RESEARCH PROGRESS

Additional books in this series can be found on Nova's website
under the Series tab.

Additional E-books in this series can be found on Nova's website
under the E-book tab.

PSYCHIATRY - THEORY, APPLICATIONS AND TREATMENTS

THE INTERNATIONAL PSYCHIATRY AND BEHAVIORAL NEUROSCIENCES YEARBOOK

VOLUME II - 2012

NASH BOUTROS
EDITOR IN CHIEF

TOMIKI SUMIYOSHI
ASSOCIATE EDITOR FOR JAPANESE

ARASH JAVANBAKHT
ASSOCIATE EDITOR FOR FARSI

EVGENY M. KRUPITSKY
ASSOCIATE EDITOR FOR RUSSIAN

New York

Library of Congress Cataloging-in-Publication Data

ISBN: 978-1-62257-566-4

ISSN: 2160-1720

Published by Nova Science Publishers, Inc.† New York

Contents

Preface ix

Editorial Board xi

Psychotic Disorders 1

Chapter 1 Epidemiological and Diagnostic Axis I Gender Differences in Dual-Diagnosis Patients 3
Laia Miquel, Carlos Roncero, Cristina López-Ortiz and Miguel Casas

Chapter 2 Schizophrenia and Lateralized Brain Dysfunction: An ERP Study During Monaural and Dichotic Listening 17
A. Vignapiano, E. Merlotti, A. Mucci, A. Brancucci and S. Galderisi

Chapter 3 Observation on the Therapeutic Effect of Electroacupuncture Combined with Small Dose of Clozapine in Clinical Treatment of Refractory Schizophrenia 29
Xiong Dian-Zhang, Yuan Yu-Ru, Leng Xiao-Bing and Liu Lin-Lin

Chapter 4 Brazilian Consensus on Second-Generation Antipsychotics and Metabolic Disorders: Review 35
Helio Elkis, Clarissa Gama, Henrique Suplicy, Marcos Tambascia, Rodrigo Bressan, Ruy Lyra, Saulo Cavalcante and Walter Minicucci

Chapter 5 Severe Catatonic Schizophrenia in a 17-Year-Old Adolescent Female 55
Barbara Sixt, Claas van Aaken, Klaus Hennighausen, Christian Fleischhaker and Eberhard Schulz

Chapter 6 The Effects of Pharmacotherapy in Psychiatry: Impact, Perception and Interpretation 65
Slawomir Murawiec

Chapter 7 The Schizophrenia Cognition Rating Scale Japanese Version (Scors-J) **75**
Yasuhiro Kaneda, Yoshinori Ueoka, Tomiki Sumiyoshi, Norio Yasui-Furukori, Toru Ito, Yuko Higuchi, Ichiro Kawamura and Michio Suzuki, Tetsuro Ohmori

Mood Disorders **85**

Chapter 8 Formalized Consensus Guidelines (FCG) Screening and Management of Bipolar Disorder **87**
Pierre-Michel Llorca, Philippe Courtet, Patrick Martin, Mocrane Abbar, Christian Gay, Jean-Albert Meynard, Franck Baylé, Michel Hamon, Christophe Lançon, Florence Thibaut, Sylvie Lancrenon, Sébastien Guillaume and Ludovic Samalin

Chapter 9 The Study of Effects of 20-Hz Repetitive Transcranial Magnetic Stimulation (rTMS) in Patients with Medication Resistant Major Depressive Disorder **115**
Sanaz Khomami, Reza Rostami, Reza Kazemi and Abbas Rahiminezhad

Neuropsychiatry **125**

Chapter 10 Advocacy of Elderly Persons with Dementia and Evaluation of Their Mental Capacity: Consistency between Results of Intelligent and Cognitive Tests and Capacity to Perform Financial and Everyday Activities **127**
Osamu Matsuda and Masahiko Saito

Chapter 11 Linguistic Validation of the Japanese Version of the Quality of Life in Epilepsy Inventory (QOLIE-31-P) **145**
Yushi Inoue, Dai Inayoshi, Yoshinobu Kasai, Teiichi Onuma, Mutsuo Sasagawa, Kazuichi Yagi and Joyce A. Cramer

Chapter 12 Cotard's Syndrome **161**
Hans Debruyne, Michael Portzky, Kathelijne Peremans and Kurt Audenaert

Child and Adolescent **175**

Chapter 13 Child Abuse and Its Long-Term Consequences: An Exploratory Study on Egyptian University Students **177**
Khalid Mansour, Eman Roshdy, Peter E. Langdon, Omaima A. Daoud, Mahmood El-Saadawy, Ali Al-Zahrani and Abdulshafi Khashaba

Chapter 14 The Effect of Puppet Play Therapy Intervention on the Communicative Skills of Autistic Children **199**
Seyyed Mohsen Asghari Nekah, Gholam-Ali Afrooz, Abbas Bazargan and Mohsen Shokoohi Yekta

Substance Use **217**

Chapter 15 The Association Study of the Relationship between Fourteen Candidate Gene Polymorphisms and Dispositions to Alcoholism **219**
Omar Šerý, Jan Lochman, Kateřina Gláslová, Radim Štaif, Miroslav Novotný, Vladimír Kmoch and Petr Zvolský

Chapter 16 A Double-Blind, Placebo-Controlled, Randomized Clinical Trial of Escitalopram for the Treatment of Affective Disorders in Alcohol Dependent Patients in Early Remission **239**
E. M. Krupitsky, S. M. Yerish, A. S. Kiselev, V. A. Berntsev, N. A. Alexandrovsky, M. N. Torban, S. P. Eroshin and O. F. Eryshev

Chapter 17 Comparative Study of Beer and Hard Liquor Use – Related Alcohol Dependency in Saint Petersburg, Russia **257**
R. D. Ilyuk, K. V. Rybakova, A. S Kiselev and E. M. Krupitsky

Chapter 18 Treatment of Family Codependency As a Factor Promoting Remission in Opiate Addicts **275**
Natalia Baranok

Violence **281**

Chapter 19 The Psychosocial Impact of Political Violence on Palestinian and Jewish Adolescents **283**
Alean Al-Krenawi

Chapter 20 The Frequency of Law Breaking and Compulsory Hospitalization among Mentally Ill People in Katowice, Poland **305**
Eliza Górniak, Karolina Furczyk and Krzysztof Krysta

Index **311**

PREFACE

The idea of the International Psychiatry and Behavioral Neurosciences (IPBN) was born as a result of the many occasions where, in the course of working on review articles or meta-analyses (MA) I frequently encountered papers that needed to be included but were never translated into English. Usually an English abstract is available but this is never sufficient for the purposes of a detailed critical review or a close examination of the data as in meta-analyses. Most researchers simply ignore the published work and is commonly observed the review or the MA uses English as a limiting term in the initial searches for relevant literature thus weeding out all works done allover the world in and published in other languages. While this is unfortunate, it is understandable as it is usually very expensive to accurately translate such data papers. Furthermore, while working on reviews or MAs one rapidly discovers the very many important works that were not published in English.

Once I began discussing the idea with publishers and indeed some authors whose native tongue is not English, I was faced with the assertion that if a paper was not published in English it was not worth translating. I simply could not agree with this notion. The International Editorial Board's work on putting volumes one and two together has indeed proven this assertion to be wrong. One of the major obstacles in securing papers for either volumes was the difficulty in getting authors to translate their papers. Many of the authors I personally contacted spoke very little English. This was particularly prominent with far Asian authors. This also was a significant source of distress to me as I became aware of very many top quality and strong papers with much data that could have substantial impact on the conduct of research or even clinical practice in the English speaking world.

Research performed and published in local regions and in local publications (at time in English) tends not to get wide dissemination. Much of this work reflects special aspects of the disorder or the local population. It is paramount for the understanding of the illness to know what is common to all cultures and what varies between communities.

The number of journals related to Psychiatry and Behavioral Neurosciences that are published in languages other than English is simply huge. With each journal publishing 4 12 issues every year the number of publications rapidly adds up well beyond the capacity of any one volume to do it justice. The table below includes rough estimates (obtained from PubMed) of papers published in certain areas of psychiatry in a number of Languages where a number of journals publish psychiatry-related papers. The totals included in the table are by definition gross under estimations as they did not include publications in Arabic, Farsi, Portuguese, Thai, Korean, Turkish, Czech, etc... Also the topics searched (e.g., schizophrenia, bipolar, etc...) do not comprehensively cover the entire fields of Psychiatry and behavioral neurosciences.

	Russian	German	French	Japanese	Chinese	Spanish	Polish	Turkish	Total Disorder
Schizoph	26	62	59	48	18	22	20	6	261
Bipolar	0	18	46	11	4	13	5	7	104
ADHD	5	21	15	7	6	21	7	1	83
Autism	4	10	33	6	3	10	4	1	71
Depression	95	215	164	104	118	132	50	17	897
OCD	1	5	3	1	1	2	0	2	15
Personality AXIS-II	7	92	52	6	1	29	8	2	197
Addiction	17	28	45	11	8	28	15	0	137
total	155	451	417	194	149	257	109	36	1732

The format of the translated papers was kept as close to the original format of publication as possible. A number of papers were modified enough that they were no longer simple translations of prior papers. These papers do not have a reference to an original publication. The accuracy of translation was the sole responsibility of the authors. In a very small number of papers some difficulty was encountered with language. These papers were not rejected as they were considered important. All efforts were made to provide the important message of the paper and provide the contact information for the investigators so interested readers can contact them for additional information or even for exploring possible collaborations.

A new feature was included in Volume II, namely providing brief synopses about the journals represented in the volume. In as much as possible the scope of the journal, publisher and a website were provided.

It is the hope of the Editor and the editorial board that the International Psychiatry and behavioral Neurosciences year Book will rapidly become a forum for influential publications from around the world to have wider dissemination and be more readily accessible to all researchers and clinicians with interest in Psychiatry and Behavioral Neurosciences.

EDITORIAL BOARD

tel: +420-224965345, 5220
Email: martin.anders@vfn.cz

Pavel Mohr, Ph.D., Associate Professor MUDr.
Third Medical School, Charles University and Prague Psychiatric Center Ustavni 91 Praha 8 - Bohnice Czech Republic
e-mai: mohr@pcp.lf3.cuni.cz

Flemish Team:

Associate Editor: Professor Georges Otte. MD
labo Neuro-Fysiologie
P.C. Dr. Guislain
Ferrerlaan 88 a te 9000 Gent
georges.otte@fracarita.org

German Team:

Associate Editor: Oliver Pogarell. MD
Dr. med, Ludwig-Maximilians-Universität München
Oliver.Pogarell@med.uni-muenchen.de
PD Dr. med. Christine Norra
Dept of Psychiatriy, University of Bochum
Alexandrinenstr. 1
D-44791 Bochum, Germany
Tel: +49-234-5077-163
Fax: +49-234-5077-204
E-Mail: Christine.Norra@rub.de

Italian Team:

Associate Editor: Silvana Galderisi, MD. Professor, Italy.
University of Naples, SUN, Italy.
sgalderi@tin.it

Armida Mucci, MD, PhD. Assistant Professor of Psychiatry
University of Naples, SUN, Italy.
Armida.mucci@gmail.com

Japanese Team:

Associate Editor: Tomiki Sumiyoshi, M.D., Ph.D.
Associate Professor, Department of Neuropsychiatry
University of Toyama Graduate School of Medicine
and Pharmaceutical Sciences, 2630 Sugitani, Toyama
930-0194 Japan
Phone: +81-76-434-7321(7323)
Fax: +81-76-434-5030
tomikisumiyoshi840@hotmail.com

Turkish Team:

Associate Editor: Prof. Dr. Kemal Arikan, MD, PhD.
Head of the Academic Psychiatry and Psychoterapy Center-Istanbul"
mkarikan@istanbul.edu.tr
Prof. Dr. Nevzat Tarhan, MD
NPI Hospital Istanbul
ntarhan@mcaturk.com

PSYCHOTIC DISORDERS

In: The International Psychiatry and Behavioral ...
Editor: Nash Boutros
ISBN: 978-1-62257-566-4

Chapter 1

EPIDEMIOLOGICAL AND DIAGNOSTIC AXIS I GENDER DIFFERENCES IN DUAL-DIAGNOSIS PATIENTS

Laia Miquel*[1,2,*]*, Carlos Roncero*[1,2,3]*,
***Cristina López-Ortiz*[2] *and Miguel Casas*[2,3]**
[1]Outpatients drug clinic, CAS Vall d'Hebron, Hospital Vall d'Hebron, Agencia de Salut Pública de Barcelona, Spain
[2]Department of Psychiatry, Hospital Universitari Vall d'Hebron, Barcelona, Spain
[3]Department of psychiatry and legal medicine, Universidad Autónoma de Barcelona, Cerdanyola del Vallès, Spain

ABSTRACT

Introduction: Dual-diagnosis is the co-occurrence of a substance abuse disorder and a psychiatric condition. Gender has been found to be associated with differences in prevalence of mental disorders as well as outcome, prognosis and treatment seeking.

Material and Methods: Articles published in Medline, Web of Science and Journal Citation Report until December 2009 that examined gender, prevalence and clinical characteristics of Dual-diagnosis patients over 18 years old were reviewed.

Conclusions: The distribution of Axis I disorders in dually-diagnosed patients and single disorder patients, by gender, is similar. The prevalence of psychotic and bipolar disorders is higher in men, whereas anxiety and affective disorders is higher in women. Dually-diagnosed females with psychotic disorders do not show the better prognosis in relation to men found in women with a singular psychotic disorder. Polydrug use is more prevalent in dual-diagnosis males.

* Corresponding author:Laia Miquel (Medical Doctor). CAS Vall d'Hebron; University Hospital Vall d'Hebron. Department of Psychiatry. Passeig Vall d'Hebron, 119-129; 08035; Barcelona, Spain, TEL: 934 893 880; FAX: 934 894 587. Email: lamiquel@vhebron.net

Keywords: gender, dual-diagnosis, women, addiction, substance use disorder, severe mental disorders

INTRODUCTION

Dual-diagnosis (DD) is the coexistence of a mental disorder and a substance use disorder (SUD). The etiopathogenesis is still unknown, though various biopsychosocial factors are believed to be involved. Epidemiological studies have objectified that the prevalence of this pathology is high (Regier et al., 1990). Some studies found that 21% of psychotic patients, 37% of patients with first psychotic episodes and 24% of patients admitted to psychiatric departments, presented one or more diagnoses for alcohol or illegal drug use (Cantwell et al., 1999; Claassen et al., 1997; Rodriguez-Jimenez et al., 2008). Studies done on patients with dual-diagnosis showed that psychotic disorders were the most frequent diagnosis (53.1% schizophreniform disorder, 28.1% schizophrenia) (Rodriguez-Jimenez et al., 2008). However, in patients diagnosed with SUD, affective disorders were the most prevalent psychiatric pathology (DiNitto, Webb and Rubin, 2002; Sanabria, Díaz, Varela and Brana, 2002). Nevertheless, not all studies coincide on this point. In one study, anxiety disorders were the most frequent (65%), followed by affective disorders (33%) and antisocial personality disorder (28%) (Tomasson and Vaglum, 1995). In Spain, affective disorders were the most frequent in drug-dependent patients (21.6%), followed by anxiety disorders (11.7%) and schizophrenia (3.1%) (Gual, 2007).

Gender has been said to influence the prevalence of mental illnesses, the pathoplasty, the way symptoms are expressed, the duration, the prognosis and the demand for and response to treatment (Gearon, Nidecker, Bellack, and Bennett, 2003; Seedat et al., 2009). In recent years, interest around gender influence on mental illnesses and SUD has been growing. The majority of studies have evaluated differences between sexes in patient samples with mental diagnoses and with SUD separately, with the number of studies on patients with dual-diagnosis being very few. Even now, data discrepancies exist, due to the variability of results that could be related to the heterogeneity of the populations studied, the diagnostic instruments and the evaluation of consumption, and psychopathological state. Although it is believed that dual-diagnosis is more frequent in men, women are considered to be proportionally at more risk of developing both disorders.

The objective of this study is to review the aforementioned gender differences at an epidemiological, psychopathalogical and diagnostic level in dual-diagnosis patients with an axis I disorder.

METHODOLOGY

Published articles were reviewed in the MEDLINE, Web of Science and Journal Citation Reports databases up until 2009. The following combinations of search terms were used: ("dual diagnosis", "gender", "gender differences", "substance", "mental disorders", "mental illness", "psychosis", "depression", "bipolar disorder", "obsessive-compulsive disorder", "post-traumatic stress disorder", "anxiety", "generalized anxiety disorder"). The review was limited to articles in Spanish, English and French on subjects of over 18 years of age. Bibliographic references in the aforementioned articles were also reviewed. The articles studying population samples of patients admitted to or under outpatient treatment in mental health networks and those referring to dual-diagnosis were included.

The articles which analyzed gender differences in socio-demographic variables (race, marital status, level of education, work activity and social functioning), and in clinical variables (psychiatric prevalence, age at onset of the axis I disorder, type of substance consumed, number of substances consumed, type of diagnosis and clinical severity) were reviewed. Articles with a sample composed exclusively of SUD patients with a comorbid personality disorder, and those which did not specify the percentage of patients with a dual-diagnosis were excluded.

Also excluded were articles which only compared patients with or without DD, without considering gender. Studies with result variables on adherence to treatment, use of health care resources, cognitive level, and those that did not use either DSM or CIE criteria were also not analyzed. From 218 related articles, 40 fulfilled the selection criteria.

Gender Differences

Studies on patients with dual-diagnosis have found that schizophrenia is more frequent among men (57.7% vs. 38%, $p<0.01$) (Comtois and Ries, 1995; Westreich, Guedj, Galanter, and Baird, 1997) and affective disorders are more so among women; principally major depressive disorder (MDD) (16.55% vs. 10.2%; $p<0.01$) (Comtois and Ries, 1995).

In general psychiatric units there are more dual-diagnosis men than women (87.5% males vs. 12.5% females, $p<0.001$) (Rodriguez-Jimenez et al., 2008). However, when patient samples in detoxification units or in outpatient clinics for addictions are studied, the relationship is the inverse, with a higher percentage of DD women than men (table 1).

In Spain, a study done mainly on patients who attended drug-dependence units, found that 47.5% of the women had a dual diagnosis, while only 30.3% of the men did so; $p=0.000$) (Gual, 2007). Although in absolute numbers there are more DD men than women, data suggest, coinciding with other authors, that female drug-users have a greater co-occurring psychopathology than males (Brady, Grice, Dustan and Randall, 1993; Denier, Thevos, Latham, and Randall, 1991). Also, women with a mental disorder are at an odds of 1.9-2.4 of having a SUD, in respect to not having one ($p<0.01$) (Abram, Teplin, and McClelland, 2003). It can be concluded that women are at a higher risk of having both disorders at the same time (Chiang et al., 2007).

Gender differences at a socio-demographic level among dual-diagnosis patients are small. No significant differences have been found with regard to age, race or place of residence, in patients with a diagnosis for schizophrenia, schizoaffective disorder, bipolar disorder or double major depressive disorder (Comtois and Ries, 1995; Westreich et al., 1997). Level of education among DD patients with schizophrenia and schizoaffective disorder also did not differ (Brunette and Drake, 1997; Gearon and Bellack, 2000; Gearon, Nidecker et al., 2003).

Concerning work or occupation, studies don't coincide in their results. A single study found that women receive significantly more welfare than men (61% vs. 17%) (DiNitto et al., 2002).

Table 1. Gender differences in the prevalence of dual diagnosis

Author	Year	Sample	Instruments	Drug	Results
Brady KT	*1993*	100 (50 M, 50 W) inpatients DTX U.	SCID	Cocaine Alcohol	70% women vs. 48% men; $p<0.005$.
Chiang SC	*2007*	155 (123 M, 32 W) Outpatients	MINI	Heroin	62.5% women vs. 58.5% men; $p<0.05$.
Landheim AS	*2003*	260 inpatients and outpatients with SUD	CIDI MCMI-II	Illegal and legal drugs	96% women vs. 82% men; $p<0.01$.
Tomasson K	*1995*	351 inpatients DTX U. (71% M)	DIS MMSE DSM-III-R	Alcohol Other drugs.	82% women vs. 74% men, $p<0.0001$.
Zlotnick C	*2008*	272 patients in prison with SUD (66% M)	CJDATS SCID	Illegal and legal drugs	64.1% women vs. 35% men; $p<0.0001$, adjusted for sociodemographic variables. Throughout the course of life 46.7% of the women presented one or more disorder compared with 24.7% of the men (OR 2.7).

M: Men; W: Women: DTX U: detoxification unit.

Another study found that significantly more men than women work full or part time (67.7% vs. 44.0%, $\chi^2 = 18.89$; $p<0.000$). Men reported a greater number of days of employment problems in the previous month (average number of days = 13.23 vs. 8.33; $F = 13.02$; $p<0.000$) (Mowbray, Ribisl, Solomon, Luke, and Kewson, 1997).

Women, as in studies on patients with a SUD or a non dual psychiatric diagnosis, have on average more children (2.13 vs. 1.46; $F=10.19$; $p<0.002$) of which more were dependent on the mother (average = 0.71 vs. 0.30; $F=18.15$; $p<0.000$) (Mowbray et al., 1997). 72% of women vs. 41% of men have their own home ($p<0.05$) (Westreich et al., 1997).

The percentage of women living with a drug consuming partner (40%) was higher than that of men (20%), (phi 0.25) which could be a factor in maintaining the consumption (29% vs. 0% of men; $p<0.01$) (DiNitto et al., 2002). Men have more legal problems than women (DiNitto et al., 2002) with more arrests (68.2% vs. 44.47%; $\chi^2 =22.06$; $p<0.000$) than among women, and the same goes for the severity of the legal problems ($M=3.53$ vs. 2.69; $F=9.73$; $p<0.002$) (Mowbray et al., 1997). 32% of women and 12% of men have been victims of crime ($p<0.05$) (Westreich et al., 1997).

Differences in the consumption of cannabis in dual-diagnosis patients are not consistent in the different relevant studies. This is also the case for consumption of opiates. Some studies detected only a slight tendency in men towards greater marihuana consumption ($\chi^2 = 3.46$; $p<0.10$) (Comtois and Ries, 1995) (Mueser, Yarnold, and Bellack, 1992), while others detected a significantly greater addiction to marihuana among men (54% vs. 18%; $p<0.02$) (Gearon, Nidecker et al., 2003). However, in one study, heroin consumption in women was greater (22% vs. 0%; $p<0.02$) (Gearon, Nidecker et al., 2003) whereas in another, consumption of opiates was greater in men (Mueser et al., 1992).

The consumption of alcohol in DD males is greater and that of stimulants is only greater in women diagnosed with schizoaffective disorder. No significant differences were found either in sedative abuse (Mueser et al., 1992), or in cocaine consumption (Westreich et al., 1997). Again, no differences were found in the reasons for which men and women consume (Gearon, Nidecker et al., 2003) or in the severity of the addiction evaluated on the Addiction Severity Index (ASI) (Gearon, Nidecker et al., 2003).

Many studies coincide in that men are polydrug users to a higher degree than women (66.5% men vs. 47.1% women $p<0.002$) (Comtois and Ries, 1995) (13% of men and 9% of women) (Gearon, Nidecker et al., 2003). It still is not clear whether women acquire a dual-diagnosis sooner or later than men. Some studies done on DD patients didn't find any significant differences between sexes in the age of beginning drug consumption (Brunette and Drake, 1997; Gearon, Nidecker et al., 2003). A study on a sample of 467 hospitalized patients (28% schizophrenia and schizoaffective disorder, 14% major depressive disorder, 15% minor depressive disorder, 26% adjustment disorders or personality disorders, 21% organic mood disorders) found that the greater proportion of women (62.9% vs. 48.8%, $\chi^2 = 8.30$, $p<0.004$) were in the under 34 year-old group (Mowbray et al., 1997).

DD men's social functioning was worse than that of women ($t=-2.84$; $p<0.001$), possibly due to men having a more frequent diagnosis of schizophrenia (Comtois and Reis, 1995).

DD women are 3.8 times more likely than men to have a sexually transmitted disease, such as HIV possibly due to the fact that women more frequently use prostitution to acquire drugs (26% vs. 0% $p<0.02$) (Gearon, Nidecker et al., 2003). The ASI results on medical problems were contradictory. Some authors didn't find any gender differences (DiNitto et al., 2002), while others observed more problems among women (M=3.55 vs. 2.84; F=7.87; $p<0.005$) (Mowbray et al., 1997).

Psychosis

Dual-diagnosis is very frequent. 47% of patients diagnosed with schizophrenia or schizophreniform disorder develop a SUD in the course of their lives, with the most frequent being alcohol consumption. The odds of a schizophrenic developing a SUD are 4.6 times greater than that of the average person (Regier et al., 1990). In a sample of 67 patients diagnosed with schizophrenia and schizoaffective disorder, of whom 34 were dual-diagnosis cases, no gender differences were observed in the age of onset of the dual-diagnosis between the sexes, with the effect size being small (d=0.2) (Gearon and Ballack, 2000). Although in both sexes the age at onset of psychosis was earlier in DD patients than in non DD patients (F (1.66)=5.17, $p<0.02$).

Males diagnosed with schizophrenia are more likely than females to consume alcohol and cannabis (F=13.9; R=0.18; $p<0.05$) (Mueser et al., 1990). 26.2% of men had a cannabis addiction, compared to 8% of women (p=0.008) (Brunette y Drake, 1997). Substance consumption in schizophrenia affects both men and women in a similar way (earlier onset, greater clinical severity, worse prognosis, etc) (Mueser et al., 1990). Gender differences haven't been found either in number of days of consumption or in its severity measured on the ASI (Gearon and Ballack, 2000). Although the clinical course is similar, there exist a greater number of married women (48.5% vs. 21.4%); (58.8% vs. 41.2% p=0.0006), with a greater number of dependent children (Brunette and Drake, 1998; Brunette and Drake, 1997). The consumption of cannabis has been associated with an earlier onset of schizophrenia in both sexes. In women, the daily use of cannabis (z=-1.92; p=0.05), represents a greater risk of developing the disorder (hazard ratio=5.154) than in men (hazard ratio 3.36). No differences were found for other degrees of cannabis consumption (Compton et al., 2009). Women are more at risk of developing psychotic symptoms more rapidly than men (Gearon and Bellack, 2000). Being a female stops being a good prognostic factor when schizophrenia is combined with a SUD (Gearon and Bellack, 2000). They suffer a greater number of hospitalizations, more positive symptoms and lower level of overall functioning (Gearon and Bellack, 2000). DD males committed a higher average number of crimes than females (13.9 vs. 42.6; df=2; p=0.01) (Brunette and Drake, 1998). Women suffered more assaults (32.4% vs. 16.8%; df= 1; p=0.04) and had a greater history of both physical and/or sexual abuse (Brunette and Drake, 1998). DD females suffered more medical problems (40.5% vs. 23.7%; df=1; p=0.04) (Brunette and Drake, 1997).

Affective Disorders

Affective disorders in drug and alcohol users are very prevalent. Around 30-50% have a depressive disorder (Regier et al., 1990). Double affective disorders, as in the general population, continue to be more frequent in women, except for bipolar disorder type I (Cornelius et al., 1995; Kessler et al., 1997). The majority of studies coincide in that affective disorders are more frequent in women than in men, independently of the sample type analyzed (Table 2). Women problem drinkers drink in a more compulsive way in relation to men, demonstrating premorbid anxiety and primary depression (Dunne, Galatopoulos, and Schipperheijn, 1993). The risk and rate of suicide is also higher in DD women with clinical depression (Rounsaville, 2007), the risk being of 4.4 (1.9-10.2); p=0.001 (Chiang et al., 2007).

It has been proposed that the SUD in women with a dual-diagnosis is secondary to the mental disorder and could appear as a possible method of self-medication aimed at alleviating the emotional stress. Hanna et al. (1997) performed an analysis on gender differences among three groups of patients: one with primary depression; the second with a SUD and concurrent depression; the third with secondary depression. They found that the proportion of women in the group with primary depression was greater (54% women vs. 46% men) than in the group with secondary depression (57% men vs. 43% women) and that the differences were statistically significant (Hanna and Grant, 1997). In males, as the depression is secondary to the consumption, it is considered more refractory (Brady et al., 1993).

A relationship has been established between anxiety symptoms concurrent with a depressive disorder and the consumption of alcohol according to gender. In men a linear relationship can be established in that the greater the anxiety, the greater is the consumption of alcohol. This is not the same in women, where the level of alcohol consumption descends when the level of anxiety is very high (Fischer and Goethe, 1998).

Table 2. Distribution of affective disorders by gender

Author	Year	Sample	Instruments	Results
Chiang SC	*2007*	155 (123 M, 32 W). Abuse/addiction heroin outpatients	MINI	OR=4.7 (1.9-11.6); $p=0.001$ (excluding bipolar disorder)
Conner, KR	*2009*	60 studies were analyzed. Patients were cocaine users	BDI, SCID, PRISM, BSI, HRSD, HSCLE	A higher degree of clinical depression was found in the women who were cocaine addicts (K=13. r=0.14 (0.11-0.16), Z=10.04; $p<0.001$).
Cornelius JR	*1995*	604 alcoholics in hospital psychiatric treatment	DSM-IV	The women alcoholics demonstrated more depression than the men ($F=4.28$, $df=1.596$, $p=0.039$).
Kessler RC	*1997*	8098 interviewed in general population	CIDI	34.5% of women alcohol abusers vs. 10.2% of men ($p<0.05$) and 53.5% women with an alcohol addiction vs. 28.1% of men ($p<0.05$) demonstrated clinical depression.
Schutte KK	*1997*	219 W, 220 M outpatients SUD		The women referred more clinical depression at baseline than the men (Average=17.78 ± 6.36 vs. 14.32 ± 7.23; $p<0.05$).
Tomasson K	*1995*	351 inpatients DTX U. (71% men)	MMSE DSM-III-R	26.9% men vs. 49% women; $p<0.0001$.

M: Men; W: Women: DTX U: deintoxification.

Table. 3 Characteristics of women with a Dual-diagnosis

History	History of physical / sexual abuse	GREATER DIFICULTY IN HANDLING
	Polydrug using	
	Family history of alcoholism	
	Previous depressive episodes	
	Social phobia	
Symptoms	Higher rates of mixed symptoms	WORSE CLINICAL OUTCOME
	Increased risk of rapid cycling	
	More suicide attempts	
	Fewer acts of violence	
	Fewer legal problems	

According to experts polled in a Spanish study, more than 20% of bipolar patients consumed some kind of substances (Casas et al., 2008). A dual-diagnosis bipolar disorder is more frequent in men than in women (56% vs. 43%)(Frye et al., 2003), although the prevalence of bipolar disorder type I in non consumers is equal in both genders (Baldassano et al., 2005). 29.1% of bipolar women have a history of alcohol consumption, compared to 49% of men (p=0.001).

However, compared with the general population there are significant differences. Bipolar women are at a 7.35 times greater risk of alcoholism, whereas men are only at a 2.77 times greater risk compared with women and men of the general population (Frye et al., 2003). The clinical handling of bipolar patients with a dual-diagnosis is more complex given that they have a worse clinical course (Casas et al., 2008) (Table 3). Women presented more depressive episodes than men (93.4% vs. 54%; p=0.000) and their average number of depressive symptoms was also significantly higher (16.76±6.43 vs. 11.88±7.48; t=2.79; df=1.63; p=0.007) (Salloum et al., 2001).

Anxiety Disorders

Anxiety disorders are strongly associated with the consumption of legal and illegal substances and the abuse of analgesic drugs in women (Tucker and Westermeyer, 1995).

Various studies coincide in that dual anxiety disorders are more frequent in women than men (53% of women vs. 47% men, p<0.05) and (73.5% women vs. 62.2% men, p<0.05) (Tucker and Westermeyer, 1995; Tomasson and Vaglum, 1995). Gender differences are found in the presence of clinical anxiety, especially when combined with alcohol (48.8% women abusers vs. 22.7% men, and 60.7% women with an alcohol dependence vs. 35.8% men) (Kessler et al., 1997).

Also, the proportion of women to men with a dual-diagnosis (53%) was greater than the proportion of women in the non dual group (35%) (Westermeyer, Tucker and Nugent, 1995). The same as with depressive disorder, the onset of anxiety disorders is usually earlier than SUD in women (Hesselbrock, Meyer, y Keener, 1985).

Although there have been few studies done on patients with obsessive-compulsive disorder (OCD), gender differences have been detected in one type. In women hoarders, higher rates of substance use have been shown ($F = 12.03$, $p < = 0.001$) than in non hoarders, and also for alcohol abuse ($F = 4.64$, $p < 0.03$) (Wheaton, Timpano, Lasalle-Ricci, and Murphy, 2008).

A history of traumatic events in patients with a psychiatric disorder is high and predominantly so in women. The number of women with a history of traumatic events is similar in dual and non-dual diagnosis women. However, DD women presented a higher number of traumas than those who only presented with a SUD (Reynolds et al., 2005).

Gearon et al. (2003) observed that in a sample of 54 patients with schizophrenia and schizoaffective disorder, the majority being cocaine-addicts, 96% had a history of traumatic events, although only 46% of the sample was diagnosed with PTSD, with women being twice as prevalent as men. Among the traumas causing the PTSD, women had a higher rate of sexual and/or physical abuse and men experienced more crimes and natural disasters (Gearon, Kaltman, Brown and Bellack, 2003). Women are more likely to develop a PTSD (beta = 2.106; $p<0.05$) (Montoya, Covarrubias, Patek, and Graves, 2003). In drug-dependent women with PTSD there is a higher level of social, laboral and family disability (Gearon et al., 2003).

The prevalence of generalized anxiety disorder (GAD) in women is greater than in men (5.3% vs. 2.8% respectively). However, the presence of GAD in men increases the risk of comorbidity with a substance or alcohol use disorder (OR=2.7(1.7-4.1)).

Women with GAD have a significantly higher comorbidity with other affective disorders except for bipolar disorder, and other anxiety disorders except for social phobia. Furthermore, DD women presented a greater number of somatic complaints, with the degree of impairment being greater for women with GAD, than for men (Vesga-Lopez et al., 2008).

Conclusion

The study of the epidemiological, diagnostic and clinical differences according to gender in dual-diagnosis patients can be done from two perspectives. Firstly, by means of the evaluation of the differences between men and women with a dual diagnosis, and secondly, by comparing dual and non dual diagnosis patients in line with gender. Both perspectives on the study are complex as there are few systematic studies and the samples are in most cases reduced and heterogeneous, which would explain the difficulty in drawing conclusions.

Controversy exists around whether dual-diagnosis is more frequent in men or in women as there are differences in the studies depending on treatment settings. In general, in psychiatric units there are more DD men than women, whereas in drug dependency units the proportion of women suffering for dual-diagnosis is higher. General epidemiological data according to diagnosis doesn't offer large variations between dual and non dual patients. DD men have a higher prevalence of schizophrenia and women of affective disorders and anxiety, as is true for people in general. Sociodemographically, large differences between DD men and women don't exist, except in that women have more dependent children, more risk of victimization and fewer legal problems than men. All the studies coincide in that male dual patients demonstrate a greater tendency towards polydrug use. However, conclusions cannot be drawn around the differences in substance use by gender in DD patients due to sampling variability. The prognosis of psychotic women with a dual-diagnosis is similar to that of DD men and notably worse than that of women without a SUD. They also have a greater family burden and a greater history of assault and medical problems.

In relation to patients with an affective disorder who consume drugs or alcohol, it is known that consumption in women is related to anxiety and that women are at a greater risk of suicide or attempted suicide and more frequently have a pattern of compulsive self-medication and consumption. It could be hypothesized that the etiopathogenic origin is different from that of the SUD, in relation to gender. The majority of studies show that the affective disorders in women are primary disorders, whereas in men, they are predominantly secondary to the SUD and more difficult to treat. From a psychopathologic point of view, the risk of demonstrating a SUD changes by gender. For example, bipolar women have a higher risk of having a SUD compared with the general population, in relation to men.

Concerning anxiety disorders, it can be said that DD women have a similar prevalence of PTSD to that of patients with only a single mental disorder, but higher than that of those with a SUD. Other disorders such as GAD, more common in women, are also more prevalent in DD men. For all these reasons mentioned above, gender differences in dual-diagnosis patients should be studied more thoroughly, as variations do exist that can influence the diagnosis, the treatment and the planning of services.

ACKNOWLEDGMENTS AND CONFLICTS OF INTEREST

None of the authors has any conflict of interest.

REFERENCES

Abram, K. M., Teplin, L. A., y McClelland, G. M. (2003). Comorbidity of severe psychiatric disorders and substance use disorders among women in jail. *American Journal of Psychiatry, 160*, 1007-1010.

Baldassano, C. F., Marangell, L. B., Gyulai, L., Ghaemi, S. N., Joffe, H., Kim, D. R. Cohen, L. S. (2005). Gender differences in bipolar disorder: Retrospective data from the first 500 STEP-BD participants. *Bipolar Disorders, 7*, 465-470.

Brady, K. T., Grice, D. E., Dustan, L., y Randall, C. (1993). Gender differences in substance use disorders. *The American Journal of Psychiatry, 150*, 1707-1711.

Brunette, M., y Drake, R. E. (1998). Gender differences in homeless persons with schizophrenia and substance abuse. *Community Mental Health Journal, 34*, 627-642.

Brunette, M. F., y Drake, R. E. (1997). Gender differences in patients with schizophrenia and substance abuse. *Comprehensive Psychiatry, 38*, 109-116.

Cantwell, R., Brewin, J., Glazebrook, C., Dalkin, T., Fox, R., Medley, I., y Harrison, G. (1999). Prevalence of substance misuse in first-episode psychosis. *The British Journal of Psychiatry : The Journal of Mental Science, 174*, 150-153.

Casas, M., Franco, M. D., Goikolea, J. M., Jimenez-Arriero, M. A., Martinez-Raga, J., Roncero, C., Szerman, N. (2008). Bipolar disorder associated to substance use disorders (dual diagnosis). Systematic review of the scientific evidence and expert consensus. *Actas Espanolas De Psiquiatria, 36*, 350-361.

Chiang, S. C., Chan, H. Y., Chang, Y. Y., Sun, H. J., Chen, W. J., y Chen, C. K. (2007). Psychiatric comorbidity and gender difference among treatment-seeking heroin abusers in taiwan. *Psychiatry and Clinical Neurosciences, 61*, 105-111.

Claassen, C. A., Gilfillan, S., Orsulak, P., Carmody, T. J., Battaglia, J., y Rush, A. J. (1997). Substance use among patients with a psychotic disorder in a psychiatric emergency room. *Psychiatric Services (Washington, D.C.), 48*, 353-358.

Compton, M. T., Kelley, M. E., Ramsay, C. E., Pringle, M., Goulding, S. M., Esterberg, M. L.,Walker, E. F. (2009). Association of pre-onset cannabis, alcohol, and tobacco use with age at onset of prodrome and age at onset of psychosis in first-episode patients. *The American Journal of Psychiatry, 166*, 1251-1257.

Comtois, K. A., y Ries, R. K. (1995). Sex differences in dually diagnosed severely mentally ill clients in dual-diagnosis outpatient treatment. *Am.J.Addict., 4*, 245-253.

Cornelius, J. R., Jarrett, P. J., Thase, M. E., Fabrega, H.,Jr, Haas, G. L., Jones-Barlock, A.,...Ulrich, R. F. (1995). Gender effects on the clinical presentation of alcoholics at a psychiatric hospital. *Comprehensive Psychiatry, 36*, 435-440.

Denier, C. A., Thevos, A. K., Latham, P. K., y Randall, C. L. (1991). Psychosocial and psychopathology differences in hospitalized male and female cocaine abusers: A retrospective chart review. *Addictive Behaviors, 16*, 489-496.

DiNitto, D. M., Webb, D. K., y Rubin, A. (2002). Gender differences in dually-diagnosed clients receiving chemical dependency treatment. *Journal of Psychoactive Drugs, 34*, 105-117.

Dunne, F. J., Galatopoulos, C., y Schipperheijn, J. M. (1993). Gender differences in psychiatric morbidity among alcohol misusers. *Comprehensive Psychiatry, 34*, 95-101.

Fischer, E. H., y Goethe, J. W. (1998). Anxiety and alcohol abuse in patients in treatment for depression. *The American Journal of Drug and Alcohol Abuse, 24*, 453-463.

Frye, M. A., Altshuler, L. L., McElroy, S. L., Suppes, T., Keck, P. E., Denicoff, K.,...Post, R. M. (2003). Gender differences in prevalence, risk, and clinical correlates of alcoholism comorbidity in bipolar disorder. *The American Journal of Psychiatry, 160*, 883-889.

Gearon, J. S., y Bellack, A. S. (2000). Sex differences in illness presentation, course, and level of functioning in substance-abusing schizophrenia patients. *Schizophrenia Research, 43*, 65-70.

Gearon, J. S., Kaltman, S. I., Brown, C., y Bellack, A. S. (2003). Traumatic life events and PTSD among women with substance use disorders and schizophrenia. *Psychiatric Services (Washington, D.C.), 54*, 523-528.

Gearon, J. S., Nidecker, M., Bellack, A., y Bennett, M. (2003). Gender differences in drug use behavior in people with serious mental illnesses. *The American Journal on Addictions / American Academy of Psychiatrists in Alcoholism and Addictions, 12*, 229-241.

Gual, A. (2007). Dual-diagnosisin Spain. *Drug and Alcohol Review, 26*, 65-71.

Hanna, E. Z., y Grant, B. F. (1997). Gender differences in DSM-IV alcohol use disorders and major depression as distributed in the general population: Clinical implications. *Comprehensive Psychiatry, 38*, 202-212.

Hesselbrock, M. N., Meyer, R. E., y Keener, J. J. (1985). Psychopathology in hospitalized alcoholics. *Archives of General Psychiatry, 42*, 1050-1055.

Kessler, R. C., Crum, R. M., Warner, L. A., Nelson, C. B., Schulenberg, J., y Anthony, J. C. (1997). Lifetime co-occurrence of DSM-III-R alcohol abuse and dependence with other psychiatric disorders in the national comorbidity survey. *Archives of General Psychiatry, 54*, 313-321.

Montoya, I. D., Covarrubias, L. D., Patek, J. A., y Graves, J. A. (2003). Posttraumatic stress disorder among hispanic and african-american drug users. *The American Journal of Drug and Alcohol Abuse, 29*, 729-741.

Mowbray, C. T., Ribisl, K. M., Solomon, M., Luke, D. A., y Kewson, T. P. (1997). Characteristics of Dual-diagnosispatients admitted to an urban, public psychiatric hospital: An examination of individual, social, and community domains. *The American Journal of Drug and Alcohol Abuse, 23*, 309-326.

Mueser, K. T., Yarnold, P. R., y Bellack, A. S. (1992). Diagnostic and demographic correlates of substance-abuse in schizophrenia and major affective-disorder. *Acta Psychiatrica Scandinavica, 85*, 48-55.

Mueser, K. T., Yarnold, P. R., Levinson, D. F., Singh, H., Bellack, A. S., Kee, K., Yadalam, K. G. (1990). Prevalence of substance abuse in schizophrenia: Demographic and clinical correlates. *Schizophrenia Bulletin, 16*, 31-56.

Regier, D. A., Farmer, M. E., Rae, D. S., Locke, B. Z., Keith, S. J., Judd, L. L., y Goodwin, F. K. (1990). Comorbidity of mental disorders with alcohol and other drug abuse. results from the epidemiologic catchment area (ECA) study. *JAMA : The Journal of the American Medical Association, 264*, 2511-2518.

Reynolds, M., Mezey, G., Chapman, M., Wheeler, M., Drummond, C., y Baldacchino, A. (2005). Co-morbid post-traumatic stress disorder in a substance misusing clinical population. *Drug and Alcohol Dependence, 77*, 251-258.

Rodriguez-Jimenez, R., Aragues, M., Jimenez-Arriero, M. A., Ponce, G., Munoz, A., Bagney, A.,Palomo, T. (2008). Dual-diagnosisin psychiatric inpatients: Prevalence and general characteristics. [Patologia dual en pacientes psiquiatricos hospitalizados: prevalencia y caracteristicas generales] *Investigacion Clinica, 49*, 195-205.

Rounsaville, B. J. (2007). DSM-V research agenda: Substance abuse/psychosis comorbidity. *Schizophrenia Bulletin, 33*, 947-952.

Salloum, I. M., Cornelius, J. R., Mezzich, J. E., Kirisci, L., Daley, D. C., Spotts, C. R., y Zuckoff, A. (2001). Characterizing female bipolar alcoholic patients presenting for initial evaluation. *Addictive Behaviors, 26*, 341-348.

Sanabria, M. A., Díaz, O., Varela, J., y Brana, T. (2002). Relevancia para el tratamiento de la sintomatología depresiva de los pacientes adictos. *Adicciones, 14*, 25-31.

Seedat, S., Scott, K. M., Angermeyer, M. C., Berglund, P., Bromet, E. J., Brugha, T. S.,...Kessler, R. C. (2009). Cross-national associations between gender and mental disorders in the world health organization world mental health surveys. *Archives of General Psychiatry, 66*, 785-795.

Tomasson, K., y Vaglum, P. (1995). A nationwide representative sample of treatment-seeking alcoholics - a study of psychiatric comorbidity. *Acta Psychiatrica Scandinavica, 92*, 378-385.

Tucker, P., y Westermeyer, J. (1995). Substance abuse in patients with comorbid anxiety disorder. *Am.J.Addict., 4*, 226-233.

Vesga-Lopez, O., Schneier, F. R., Wang, S., Heimberg, R. G., Liu, S. M., Hasin, D. S., y Blanco, C. (2008). Gender differences in generalized anxiety disorder: Results from the national epidemiologic survey on alcohol and related conditions (NESARC). *The Journal of Clinical Psychiatry, 69*, 1606-1616.

Westermeyer, J., Tucker, P., y Nugent, S. (1995). Comorbid anxiety disorder among patients with substance abuse disorders. risk factors on initial evaluation. *Am.J.Addict., 4*, 97-106.

Westreich, L., Guedj, P., Galanter, M., y Baird, D. (1997). Differences between men and women in dual-diagnosis treatment. *The American Journal on Addictions / American Academy of Psychiatrists in Alcoholism and Addictions, 6*, 311-317.

Wheaton, M., Timpano, K. R., Lasalle-Ricci, V. H., y Murphy, D. (2008). Characterizing the hoarding phenotype in individuals with OCD: Associations with comorbidity, severity and gender. *Journal of Anxiety Disorders, 22*, 243-252.

In: The International Psychiatry and Behavioral ...
Editor: Nash Boutros
ISBN: 978-1-62257-566-4

Chapter 2

SCHIZOPHRENIA AND LATERALIZED BRAIN DYSFUNCTION: AN ERP STUDY DURING MONAURAL AND DICHOTIC LISTENING

A. Vignapiano**[*,1], **E. Merlotti**[1], **A. Mucci**[1], **A. Brancucci**[2] and **S. Galderisi**[1]

[1]Department of Psychiatry, University of Naples SUN Italy
[2]ITAB- University "G. d'Annunizio" Chieti, Italy

ABSTRACT

Structural and functional abnormalities of the brain left hemisphere, were frequently observed in patients with schizophrenia. However, negative and discrepant findings were also reported. Our study was aimed to investigate the presence of lateralized brain dysfunction in patients with schizophrenia by using event-related potentials recorded during a monaural and dichotic presentation of tones. The ERP component N100, related to sensory processing of stimuli and generated in the temporal lobe cortex, was analyzed. In both patients and healthy subjects, dichotic listening inhibited the augmenting pattern of N100 amplitude with increasing tone intensity. In both groups a positive relationship between the intensity of the stimulation and the amplitude of the N100 over the right central sites in the monaural condition was found; over the left central lead, instead, while healthy subjects exhibited the augmenting pattern, patients failed to do so. This abnormality did not correlate with the severity of psychopathology. Our results suggest a state of functional inhibition of the left auditory cortex, akin to that induced by dichotic listening, in subjects with schizophrenia, independent of psychopathology or drug therapy.

Keywords: Schizophrenia; Hemispheric asymmetry; dichotic listening; ERPs; N100

[*] Corresponding Author: A. Vignapiano Department of Psychiatry, University of Naples SUN Italy. vignapiano2004@libero.it

INTRODUCTION

Several studies investigated the possibility that functional and/or structural hemispheric asymmetries may represent a neurobiological substrate of schizophrenia [1-5]. An important development within this field was provided by the application of brain imaging techniques that allow more detailed insights on brain structure. Some authors have reported a volume reduction in the dorsolateral prefrontal, orbitofrontal and hippocampal cortex only in the left hemisphere of subjects with schizophrenia [6-8], whereas others have found a bilateral reduction of the same structures [9,10]. A meta-analysis of studies, using the voxel-based morphometry approach, reported the presence of abnormalities in the left superior temporal gyrus and in the medial area of left temporal lobe [11]. Moreover, using functional imaging techniques, such as PET and SPECT, some authors found a hypoactivation of the left dorsolateral prefrontal cortex in subjects with acute schizophrenia, as compared with healthy controls [12]; this abnormality was more evident in subjects with higher scores on the Positive And Negative Syndrome Scale (PANSS) [13].

The low temporal resolution of these brain imaging techniques may represent a limitation in the study of the functional basis of mental activity, characterized by the rapid succession of complex events. A significant contribution to the study of the neurobiology of schizophrenia may be provided by studies using techniques characterized by a high temporal resolution such as event-related potentials (ERPs). Some studies have investigated the abnormalities of the ERP component N100 [14,15]. Results showed an amplitude reduction in patients with schizophrenia. According to some authors, this abnormality might be related to the severity of the clinical features and illness duration [15,16]. In patients with chronic schizophrenia, a negative correlation of the N100 amplitude with both positive and negative symptoms was found [16]. Brockhaus-Dumke et al. [17] observed that the N100 amplitude reduction, already present in the early stages of schizophrenia, becomes more evident in the chronic stages of the disease. A recent study has reported that the N100 amplitude reduction is present only in patients with schizophrenia who have primary and persistent negative symptoms [18]. The previously reviewed studies did not examine whether the decrease of N100 amplitude had an asymmetric hemispheric distribution. A study by Hubl et al. [19] on subjects with chronic hallucinations showed a lower N100 amplitude on the left hemisphere regions, during passive listening of complex tones. The majority of studies did not find any change of the N100 latency in patients with schizophrenia [20, 21]. The presence of anatomical and functional asymmetries in the organization of the central nervous system, especially in the neocortex, is a well-known phenomenon in humans. These asymmetries become apparent when processing complex stimuli, such as sounds or words.

The dichotic listening technique has been successfully used in the study of hemispheric functional asymmetries [22, 23]. The technique involves the presentation of two different simultaneous auditory stimuli to either ear. By using this technique, the left and right auditory cortices can be separately tested. According to the ''structural theory'' proposed by Kimura [24], during dichotic listening the ipsilateral pathways are inhibited by the contralateral ones; this mechanism represents the basis of the contralateral ear "advantage effects", usually observed in dichotic listening tasks. Brancucci et al. [25] tested neurophysiologically the Kimura's structural theory in a magnetoencephalografy study conducted in healthy controls during monotic and dichotic listening. Their results showed that the M100 amplitude (an auditory evoked magnetic field component similar to N100) over the right auditory cortex increased progressively when tones of increasing intensity were monotically presented to the right ear. This effect on M100 was abolished when a concurrent tone of constant intensity was dichotically delivered to the left controlateral ear, suggesting that the controlateral pathway inhibited the ipsilateral one.

Other studies used the dichotic listening technique to investigate the functional integrity of the left hemisphere during auditory stimuli processing and the interaction between stimuli processing and attention, in patients with schizophrenia. The results showed deficits in the processing of the dichotic stimuli and an inability to change the ear advantage by shifting selective attention [22-26]; this may indicate a "double" laterality dysfunction involving both automatic and controlled processing deficits in schizophrenia [27]. However, Oie et al. [28] in a group of patients with early-onset schizophrenia did not find any left hemisphere impairment.

The authors hypothesized that chronicity, drug treatment or psychopathological characteristics may play a role in the left hemisphere deficit found in chronic schizophrenia. Connolly et al. [29] examined the contralateral amplitude predominance of N100 during passive listening to monaural tones, in patients with clinically stable schizophrenia and healthy controls.

Patients were characterized by a smaller N100 amplitude with respect to controls, an effect that was slightly more pronounced at temporal sites. Patients did not show the normal N100 contralateral dominance effect, particularly at the right hemisphere temporal leads. These data suggest that the disturbance in schizophrenia of the normal pattern of controlateral dominance is due more to left than right auditory pathways and may thus indicate an abnormally reduced right hemisphere response to left ear stimulation or an ipsilateral dominance in the left auditory pathway. However, other studies [1-5, 11, 19] did not confirm this evidence and the neurobiological basis of dichotic listening deficits in schizophrenia still remains unclear.

Our study aimed to investigate hemispheric asymmetries through the analysis of event-related potentials recorded during listening to monaural and dichotic complex stimuli, in a group of patients with schizophrenia and healthy controls and to identify the possible influence of clinical features on the neurophysiological response in the patient group.

Materials and Methods

Subjects

Patients included in this study were recruited among those who were regularly attending the outpatient units and day-care programs of the University Psychiatric Department of Naples. Those who had a clinical diagnosis of schizophrenia and were reported to be clinically stable were tested to verify that they met the following inclusion criteria: 1) age between 18 and 60 years; 2) a DSM-IV diagnosis of schizophrenia, confirmed by the Structured Clinical Interview for DSM-IV (SCID-I); 3) no significant change in the clinical state or in drug treatment during the preceding 3 months; 4) a negative neurological examination; 5) a negative history of severe mental retardation, neurological illness, head injury, alcoholism or drug abuse or dependence in the last 12 months; 6) no previous insulin coma, leucotomy or electroconvulsive therapy.

Healthy volunteers, matched with patients for age (±3 years), gender and handedness were recruited among the Department personnel and medical students. Controls were selected according to the following criteria, verified by clinical interview: 1) absence of psychiatric disorders in both personal and family history; 2) negative neurological examination; negative history for all the conditions mentioned at point 5 for patients. The study was approved by the Ethics Committee of the Medical Hospital of the Second University of Naples and all subjects expressed their willingness to participate in the study procedures, providing a written informed consent, after a complete description of the study.

None of the subjects had auditory impairments, as shown by auditory functional assessment. All subjects were right-handed as assessed by the Edinburgh inventory (Oldfield, 1971). According to the above-mentioned inclusion criteria, 19 patients with schizophrenia e 26 healthy controls were recruited. A neurophysiological evaluation was carried out in all enrolled subjects. A psychopathological evaluation was also carried out in patients.

Psychopathological Evaluation

Psychopathological evaluation was carried out by using the Positive And Negative Syndrome Scale (PANSS). In our study, we used the five-factor model of schizophrenic symptoms [30]. The five factors are the negative, excitement, depression, positive and cognitive impairment ones. The negative component included: blunted affect, emotional withdrawal, poor rapport, passive/apathetic withdrawal, lack of spontaneity, motor retardation. The excitement component included five symptoms, two of which were extracted from the positive subscale and the other three from the general psychopathology PANSS subscale (excitement, hostility, tension, uncooperativeness and poor impulse control). The depression component included: anxiety, guilt feelings and depression. The positive component included delusions, hallucinations, grandiosity, suspiciousness and unusual thought content.

The cognitive impairment included five symptoms: conceptual disorganization, difficulty in abstract thinking, stereotyped thinking, disorientation and poor attention.

Electrophysiological Evaluation

ERPs were recorded during passive listening to three types of auditory stimuli, delivered through earphones: monaural (the stimuli were delivered to the right ear), monotic (two different and concurrent stimuli are delivered at one ear) and dichotic (two different and concurrent stimuli are delivered at left and right ear). Twenty auditory stimuli were built using eight basic tones: A1=261 Hz, 70 dB; A2 =261 Hz, 80 dB; B1=293 Hz, 60 dB; B2=293 Hz, 70 dB; B3=293Hz, 80dB; E1=391 Hz, 60 dB; E2=391 Hz, 70 dB; E3=391 Hz, 80 dB. The "A" tones were used as masking tones and delivered to the left ear. "B" tones (test tone 1) are comparable to tones "E" (test tone 2) in terms of pitch height. The test tone were delivered to the right ear. In order to support the working hypothesis that the response of the primary auditory cortex to ipsilateral stimulation are inhibited, each test tone was delivered with a masking tone during dichotic listening. Monaural presentation of test tones with masking tone at intensity of 70 dB (A1) and 80 dB (A2), and monaural presentations of test tones were used as general control conditions. According to Brancucci et al. [25] the eight basic tones are delivered in different combination to left and/or right ear to constitute the twenty stimuli.

Subjects listened passively to a randomized sequence of the twenty stimuli. No task was required. The recording session was segmented in 6 blocks of 102 stimuli (5 minutes inter-block pause). Subjects were instructed to relax but not to sleep, maintaining a constant level of attention throughout the whole session, and to avoid movements during the recording. The whole experiment lasted about 1 hour.

Scalp electrical activity was recorded from 30 unipolar leads (Fpz, Fz, Cz, CPz, Pz, Oz, F3, F4, C3, C4, FC5, FC6, P3, P4, CP5, CP6, O1, O2, Fp1, Fp2, F7, F8, T3, T4, T5, T6, AF3, AF4, PO7, PO8), following the 10-20 System (American Electroencephalographic Society, 1994), referred to the linked earlobes (a resistor of 10 kΩ was interposed between the earlobe leads). The forehead was used for grounding. Two electrooculogram leads (Fp1-A1 for vertical and Pg1-Pg2 for horizontal eye movements) were added for artifact monitoring. The impedance of the electrodes was maintained below 5 kΩ. Light gauze pads were placed over the closed eyelids to reduce blink artifacts. Scalp electrical activity was recorded using the 32 channel digital EEG system EASYS2 (Brainscope, Prague), with a time constant of 0.03 (high-pass filter of 0.50 Hz) and a low-pass filter of 70 Hz; the amplification of the signal was 25,000 times and the sampling rate was 256 Hz. A calibration was performed for all channels, using a 50 μV sine wave, before each recording session. ERP data were digitally filtered with a 0.5-30 Hz bandpass. For each set of data epochs with artifacts were manually identified and excluded from further analysis. The computer software identified the stimuli off-line and selected epochs of electrical activity starting 120 ms before stimulus presentation and ending 1250 ms after it. The 120 ms activity preceding the stimuli was averaged, for each channel, across all time points and epochs, to calculate a single baseline value that was subtracted from the post-stimulus average.

The latency and amplitude of each ERP component were measured using the Vision Analyser software (Brain Products Gmbh, Germany). The program contains a "peak-finder" function which enables automatic peak detection and markers labelling. The latency range of the N100 was predetermined on the group grand-mean waveforms and was set at 50-200 msec in the patients group and 80-200 msec in the control group. As other studies[31,32] found the N100 peak reduction in patients with schizophrenia at the paramedian/central leads (C3 and C4), measurements were made on these leads.

Data Analysis

Independent one-way analyses of variance (ANOVAs) were used to test group differences between patients with schizophrenia and healthy controls on demographic variables and education. ANOVAs with diagnosis as the between factor and stimulus type (monaural or dichotic), leads (C3, C4) and tones intensity (60, 70, 80 dB) as within-factors were carried out on the N1 latency and amplitude measures. The Greenhouse–Geisser correction for the inflation of degrees of freedom was used, when appropriate. In case of group differences on age and education, these variables were entered as covariates. Tukey's HSD procedure was used for post hoc comparisons only when a significant main effect or interaction was found. Correlations between N100 amplitude, scores on PANSS factors, duration of illness and age at illness onset were explored by means of Pearson's correlation coefficient. Significance level for all statistical tests was set at $p \leq 0.05$.

Results

Demographic and Clinical Features

Demographic data and psychopathological features of the sample are described in Table I. One-way repeated measures ANOVAs showed a significant difference on education ($F_{1,43}=11.76$; $p<0.001$) between patients and controls. Patients were slightly older than controls, but this difference only approached statistical significance ($F_{1,43}=3.59$; $p<0.06$). Both variables were used as covariates for the subsequent analyses of variance.

Table I. Demographic data of patients with schizophrenia and healthy controls; clinical features of subjects with schizophrenia

	Patients with schizophrenia N=19; males=17	Healthy Controls N=26; males=24
Age (years)	39.7±6.9	34.7±3.4
Education (years)	11.4±3.2*	15.1±3.7
Age at illness onset (years)	22.5±5.1	
Duration of illness (years)	16.7±8.5	
PANSS		
Negative factor	15.42±4.82	
Excitement factor	7.52±2.90	
Depression factor	7.00±2.00	
Positive factor	10.42±3.98	
Cognitive impairment factor	11.37±4.66	

All data are means±SD.
* Significant difference between patients and healthy controls: p<0.001.
Age and education were used as a covariate for all successive analyses.

Electrophysiological Variables

ANOVA on N100 amplitude showed a significant interaction lead x stimulus type x tones intensity x diagnosis ($F_{2,82}=3.35$ $p<0.04$). Simple effects investigated by the Tukey's post-hoc analyses revealed the following.

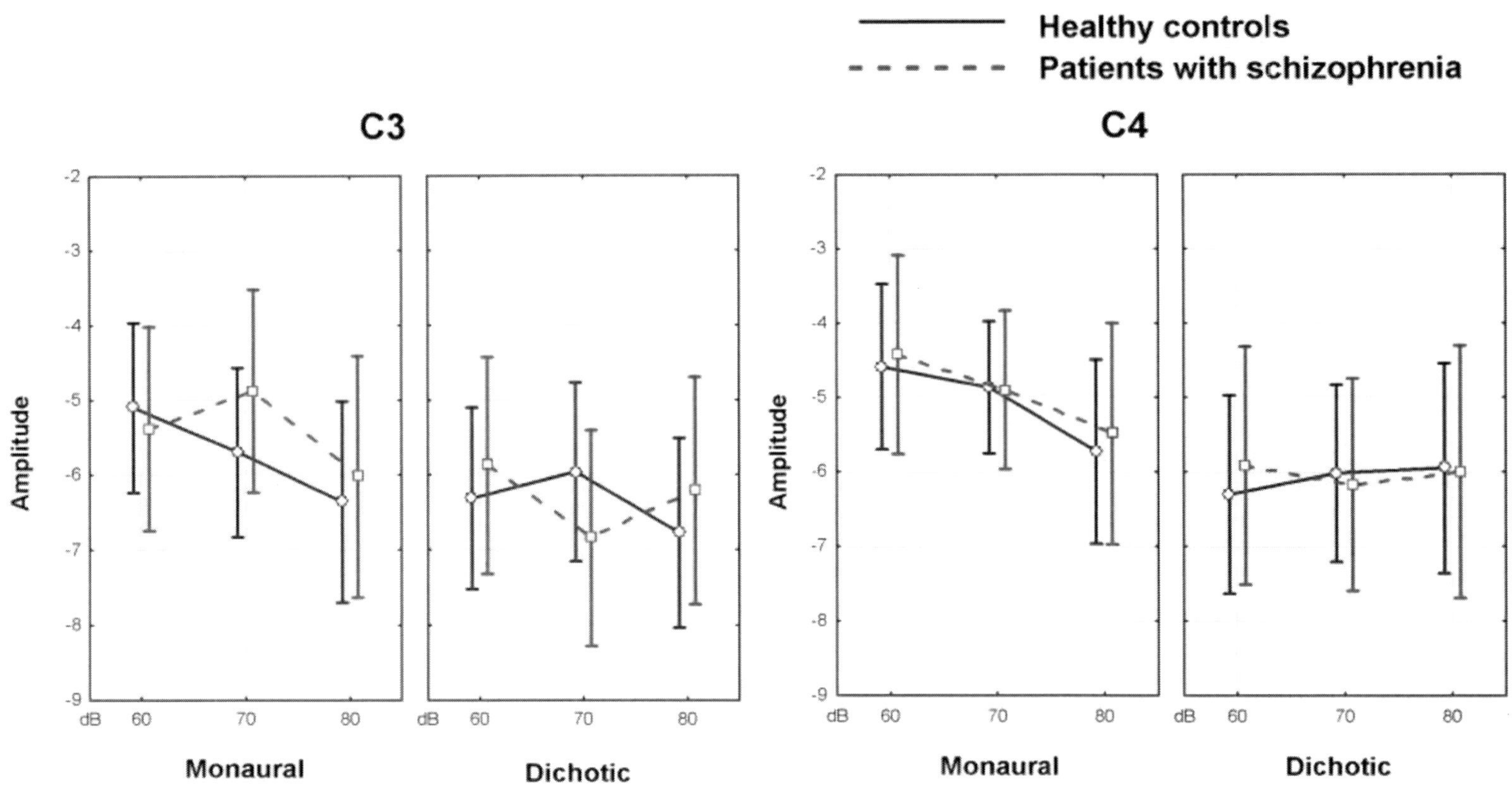

Figure 1. N100 amplitude in patients with schizophrenia and healthy subjects at C3 (left) and C4 (right) during monaural and dichotic conditions. ANOVA showed Lead x Stimulus type x Tones Intesity x Diagnosis interaction: $F(2,82)=3.35$, $p<0.03$. Vertical lines indicate 95% confidence intervals.

In the monaural condition, a positive relationship between tones intensity and N100 amplitude was found in healthy subjects (80 dB vs 60 dB, $p<0.0007$) but not in patients (80 dB vs 60 dB $p=0.95$), over the left central lead (C3) (Figure 1), and in both groups over the right central lead (C4) ($p<0.02$ and $p<0.03$, respectively). The relationship between N100 amplitude and tones intensity was abolished in the dichotic condition in both groups.

The latency of N100 component did not differ between groups.

Correlation between Electrophysiological and Clinical Features

There was no significant relationship between any N100 measure and any clinical variable. In order to obtain a synthetic index of the intensity-related N100 amplitude variations the difference between the N100 amplitude elicited by 80 dB stimulation and that elicited by 60 dB stimulation was calculated. No significant correlation was observed between this index and any clinical variable.

Discussion

The main results of our study are the following: 1) the replication of the neurophysiological pattern of response to both monaural and dichotic stimulation in healthy subjects; 2) in the patients group, the absence of a positive relationship between the intensity of stimulation and the amplitude of the N100 over the left central lead in the monaural condition; 3) the absence of electrophysiological anomalies during dichotic stimulation in the patient group.

In the healthy subject group, our results are similar to those previously reported in the literature concerning the characteristics of the N100 component elicited by monaural and dichotic listening [25, 34]. Our results showed that the N100 amplitude is contingent on the intensity of auditory stimulation of the sensory receptors, showing an increase for stimuli of increasing intensity in the monaural condition, as reported by other studies [35, 36]. These results, in healthy subjects, confirm the adequacy of our experimental paradigm. The effect on N100 was abolished when a concurrent tone of constant intensity was dichotically presented at the controlateral ear. These results might be explained as an inhibition of the ipsilateral auditory pathway by the controlateral one during dichotic listening [25, 34]. The effect of dichotic stimulation was observed in both patients and controls over both the right and left central leads.

In the monaural condition, a positive relationship between the intensity of the stimulation and the amplitude of N100 was observed in both groups, over the right central site, while the same relationship was absent only in the patient group, over the left central lead. These results suggest a state of functional inhibition of the left auditory cortex, akin to that induced by dichotic listening, in the patient group.

Our experiment did not include any task for the subjects, therefore we cannot attribute the reported abnormality to complex cognitive factors, such as impaired attention. Several authors have reported, in patients with schizophrenia, both functional and structural abnormalities of the superior temporal gyrus of the left hemisphere which includes the left auditory cortex [9, 11, 19]. These abnormalities seem to be independent of the drug therapy [37]. In addition, previous studies on patients with schizophrenia with chronic, treatment-resistant auditory hallucinations showed an impaired connectivity in the left fronto-temporal cortex. This abnormality could have a developmental origin and may contribute to explain how internally generated language is perceived as externally generated [38]. This hypothesis is supported by functional brain imaging data that provided direct evidence of the involvement of primary auditory areas in auditory hallucinations [39]. A previous electrophysiological study showed that subjects with chronic hallucinations presented a reduced N100 amplitude over the left hemispheric regions during passive listening to tones [19].

Our study demonstrated an impairment of the N100, a component with generators in the left auditory cortex, which was not related to attention or positive symptoms, in treated clinically stable patients with schizophrenia. This abnormality consists in a reduced response of the N100 amplitude recorded over the left temporal cortex to the intensity of the stimulation when non-attended tones were presented to the contralateral ear. Our results suggest that functional abnormalities of the left auditory cortex are present during a clinically stable phase, in which positive symptoms (such as hallucinations and delusions) are significantly reduced. Alterations of the long-range connectivity of the auditory pathways might be hypothesized in patients with schizophrenia, as recently reported in subjects with early-onset schizophrenia [40]. In our study, there was no significant correlation between N100 latency/amplitude and any clinical feature (as assessed by PANSS factors: negative, excitement, depression, positive and cognitive impairment) [30].

As for the right hemisphere the relationship between amplitude and tone intensity is maintained, our results suggest an altered hemispheric asymmetry with hypoactivation of the left hemisphere temporal regions; these findings are generally consistent with several previous report [1-5] that have investigated the abnormalities of hemispheric asymmetry in schizophrenia. Furthermore, in line with other studies using dichotic listening paradigms, our results show no abnormalities of the N100 during the dichotic presentation of complex tones [41, 42].

Our results cannot be attributed to pharmacological factors both for the increase of N100 amplitude for monaural stimuli on the right lead and for the absence of electrophysiological abnormalities during dichotic listening of complex tones. Indeed, if the N100 amplitude abnormality would be related to drug therapy, the same abnormality would have been detected in both conditions (monaural and dichotic) and on both leads (C3 and C4). The reported abnormality in the left hemispheric regions supports the evidence that in schizophrenia there may be an altered regulation of the sensory information flow with a decreased ability to retain relevant stimuli and a difficulty in sensory integration. This defect, found also in subjects at the first episode of illness, with or without use of antipsychotic drugs, represents, therefore, a primary deficit of the disorder and not a consequence of drug therapy [43].

In conclusion, we could demonstrate, in line with previous study, that the left auditory cortex has a reduced ability to adapt its response to changes of external stimuli, probably due to an alteration of long-range connectivity in the auditory pathways in schizophrenia.

References

[1] Gruzelier JH. Hemispheric imbalances in schizophrenia. *Int. J. Psychophysiol.* 1984;1:227-40.

[2] Galderisi S, Maj M, Mucci A, Monteleone P, Kemali D. Lateralization patterns of verbal stimuli processing assessed by reaction time and event-related potentials in schizophrenic patients. *Int. J. Psychophysiol.* 1988;6:167-76.

[3] Kemali D, Galderisi S, Maj M, Mucci A, Di Gregorio M. Lateralization patterns of event-related potential and performance indices in schizophrenia: relationship to clinical state and neuroleptic treatment. *Int. J. Psychophysiol.* 1991;10:225-30.

[4] Crow TJ. Schizophrenia as failure of hemispheric dominance for language. *Trends Neurosci.* 1997;20:339-43.

[5] Sumich A, Chitnis XA, Fannon DG, O'Ceallaigh S, Doku VC, Falrowicz A, et al. Temporal lobe abnormalities in first-episode psychosis. *Am. J. Psychiatry.* 2002;159:1232-5.

[6] Hirayasu Y, Tanaka S, Shenton ME, Salisbury DF, De Santis MA, Levitt JJ, et al. Prefrontal gray matter volume reduction in first episode schizophrenia. *Cereb. Cortex* 2001;11:374-81.

[7] Premkumar P, Fannon D, Kuipers E, Cooke MA, Simmons A, Kumari V. Association between a longer duration of illness, age and lower frontal lobe grey matter volume in schizophrenia. *Behav. Brain Res.* 2008;193:132-9.

[8] Schobel SA, Kelly MA, Corcoran CM, Van Heertum K, Seckinger R, Goetz R, et al. Anterior hippocampal and orbitofrontal cortical structural brain abnormalities in association with cognitive deficits in schizophrenia. *Schizophr. Res.* 2009;114:110-8.

[9] Shenton ME, Kikinis R, Jolesz FA, Pollak SD, LeMay M, Wible CG, et al. Abnormalities of the left temporal lobe and thought disorder in schizophrenia. A quantitative magnetic resonance imaging study. *N. Engl. J. Med.* 1992;327:604-12.

[10] Galderisi S, Quarantelli M, Volpe U, Mucci A, Cassano GB, Invernizzi G, et al. Patterns of structural MRI abnormalities in deficit and nondeficit schizophrenia. *Schizophr. Bull* 2008;34:393-401.

[11] Honea R, Crow TJ, Passingham D, Mackay CE. Regional deficits in brain volume in schizophrenia: a meta-analysis of voxel-based morphometry studies. *Am. J. Psychiatry* 2005;162:2233-45.

[12] Spence SA, Hirsch SR, Brooks DJ, Grasby PM. Prefrontal cortex activity in people with schizophrenia and control subjects. Evidence from positron emission tomography for remission of 'hypofrontality' with recovery from acute schizophrenia. *Am. J. Psychiatry* 2005;162:2233-45.

[13] Novak B, Milcinski M, Grmek M, Kocmur M. Early effects of treatment on regional cerebral blood flow in first episodi schizophrenia patients evaluated with ^{99}Tc-ECD-SPECT. *Neuro Endocrinol Lett.* 2005;26:685-9.

[14] Ford JM, Mathalon DH, White PM, Pfefferbaum A. Left temporal deficit of P300 in patients with schizophrenia: effects of task. *Int. J. Psychophysiol.* 2000;38:71-9.

[15] Brown KJ, Gonsalvez CJ, Harris AW, Williams LM, Gordon E. Target and non-target ERP disturbances in first episode vs. chronic schizophrenia. *Clin. Neurophysiol.* 2002;113:1754-63.

[16] Sumich A, Kumari V, Gordon E, Tunstall N, Brammer M. Event-related potential correlates of paranormal ideation and unusual experiences. *Cortex* 2008;44:1342-52
[17] Brockhaus-Dumke A, Schultze-Lutter F, Mueller R, Tendolkar I, Bechdolf A, Pukrop R, et al. Sensory gating in schizophrenia: P50 and N100 gating in antipsychotic-free subjects at risk, first-episode, and chronic patients. *Biol. Psychiatry* 2008;64:376-84.
[18] Mucci A, Galderisi S, Kirkpatrick B, Bucci P, Volpe U, Merlotti E, et al. Double dissociation of N1 and P3 abnormalities in deficit and nondeficit schizophrenia. *Schizophr. Res.* 2007;92:252-61.
[19] Hubl D, Koenig T, Strik WK, Garcia LM, Dierks T. Competition for neuronal resources: how hallucinations make themselves heard. *Br. J. Psychiatry* 2007;190: 57-62.
[20] Pfefferbaum A, Ford JM, White PM, Roth WT. P3 in schizophrenia is affected by stimulus modality, response requirements, medication status, and negative symptoms. *Arch. Gen. Psychiatry* 1989;46:1035-44.
[21] Ogura C, Nageishi Y, Matsubayashi M, Omura F, Kishimoto A, Shimokochi M. Abnormalities in event-related potentials, N100, P200, P300 and slow wave in schizophrenia. *Jpn J. Psychiatry Neurol.* 1991;45:57-65.
[22] Bryden MP. Correlates of the dichotic right-ear effect. *Cortex* 1988;24:313-9.
[23] Hugdahl K, Law I, Kyllingsbaek S, Brønnick K, Gade A, Paulson OB. Effects of attention on dichotic listening: an ^{15}O-PET study. *Hum. Brain Mapp.* 2000;10:87-97.
[24] Kimura D. Functional asymmetry of the brain in dichotic listening. *Cortex* 1967;3:163–168.
[25] Brancucci A, Babiloni C, Babiloni F, Galderisi S, Mucci A, Tecchio F, et al. Inhibition of auditory cortical responses to ipsilateral stimuli during dichotic listening: evidence from magnetoencephalography. *Eur. J. Neurosci.* 2004;19:2329-36.
[26] Hugdahl K, Helland T, Faerevaag MK, Lyssand ET, Asbjørnsen A. Absence of ear advantage on the consonant-vowel dichotic listening test in adolescent and adult dyslexics: specific auditory-phonetic dysfunction. *J. Clin. Exp. Neuropsychol.* 1995;17:833-40.
[27] O'Leary DS, Andreasen NC, Hurtig RR, Kesler ML, Rogers M, Arndt S, et al. Auditory attentional deficits in patients with schizophrenia. A positron emission tomography study. *Arch. Gen. Psychiatry* 1996;53:633-41.
[28] Oie M, Rund BR, Sundet K, Bryhn G. Auditory laterality and selective attention: normal performance in patients with early-onset schizophrenia. *Schizophr. Bull* 1998;24:643-52.
[29] Connolly JF, Manchanda R, Gruzelier JH, Hirsch SR. Pathway and hemispheric differences in the event-related potential (ERP) to monaural stimulation: a comparison of schizophrenic patients with normal controls. *Biol. Psychiatry* 1985;20:293-303.
[30] Lykouras L, Oulis P, Psarros K, Daskalopoulou E, Botsis A, Christodoulou GN, et al. Five-factor model of schizophrenic psychopathology: how valid is it? *Eur. Arch. Psychiatry Clin. Neurosci.* 2000;250:93-100.
[31] Boutros NN, Trautner P, Korzyukov O, Grunwald T, Burroughs S, Elger CE, et al. Mid-latency auditory-evoked responses and sensory gating in focal epilepsy: a preliminary exploration. *J. Neuropsychiatry Clin. Neurosci.* 2006;18:409-16.

[32] Lijffijt M, Lane SD, Meier SL, Boutros NN, Burroughs S, Steinberg JL, et al. P50, N100, and P200 sensory gating: relationships with behavioral inhibition,attention, and working memory. *Psychophysiology* 2009;46:1059-68.

[33] Wioland N, Rudolf G, Metz-Lutz MN, Mutschler V, Marescaux C. Cerebral correlates of hemispheric lateralization during a pitch discrimination task: an ERP study in dichotic situation. *Clin. Neurophysiol.* 1999;110:516-23.

[34] Jäncke L, Peters M, Schlaug G, Posse S, Steinmetz H, Müller-Gärtner H. Differential magnetic resonance signal change in human sensorimotor cortex to finger movements of different rate of the dominant and subdominant hand. *Brain Res. Cogn. Brain Res.* 1998;6:279-84.

[35] Eichele T, Nordby H, Rimol LM, Hugdahl K. Asymmetry of evoked potential latency to speech sounds predicts the ear advantage in dichotic listening. *Brain Res. Cogn Brain Res.* 2005;24:405-12.

[36] Sandmann P, Eichele T, Specht K, Jäncke L, Rimol LM, Nordby H, et al. Hemispheric asymmetries in the processing of temporal acoustic cues inconsonant-vowel syllables. *Restor. Neurol. Neurosci.* 2007;25:227-40.

[37] Sweet RA, Henteleff RA, Zhang W, Sampson AR, Lewis DA. Reduced Dendritic Spine Density in Auditory Cortex of Subjects with Schizophrenia. *Neuropsychopharmacology* 2009;34:374-89.

[38] Hubl D, Koenig T, Strik W, Federspiel A, Kreis R, Boesch C, et al. Pathways that make voices: white matter changes in auditory hallucinations. *Arch. Gen. Psychiatry* 2004;61:658-68.

[39] Dierks T, Linden DE, Jandl M, Formisano E, Goebel R, Lanfermann H, et al. Activation of Heschl's gyrus during auditory hallucinations. *Neuron* 1999;22(3):615-21.

[40] Wilson TW, Hernandez OO, Asherin RM, Teale PD, Reite ML, Rojas DC. Cortical gamma generators suggest abnormal auditory circuitry in early-onset psychosis. *Cereb. Cortex* 2008;18:371-8.

[41] Wexler BE, Giller EL Jr, Southwick S. Cerebral laterality, symptoms, and diagnosis in psychotic patients. *Biol. Psychiatry* 1991;29:103-16.

[42] Bruder G, Kayser J, Tenke C, Amador X, Friedman M, Sharif Z, et al. Left temporal lobe dysfunction in schizophrenia: event-related potential and behavioral evidence from phonetic and tonal dichotic listening tasks. *Arch. Gen. Psychiatry*. 1999;56:267-76.

[43] Hong X, Chan R., Zhuang X., Jiang T., Wan X., Wan J., et al. Neuroleptic effect on P50 sensory gating in patients with first-episode never medicated schizophrenia. *Schizophr. Res.* 2008;108:151-57.

In: The International Psychiatry and Behavioral ...
Editor: Nash Boutros

ISBN: 978-1-62257-566-4

Chapter 3

Observation on the Therapeutic Effect of Electroacupuncture Combined with Small Dose of Clozapine in Clinical Treatment of Refractory Schizophrenia

Xiong Dian-Zhang*, Yuan Yu-Ru, Leng Xiao-Bing and Liu Lin-Lin

The Third People's Hospital of Yichun,
Yichun, Jiangxi Province, China

Abstract

Objective: To observe the effect of electroacupuncture(EA) in combination with small dose of clozapine on clinical symptoms of refractory schizophrenia patients so as to evaluate its validity and safety. *Methods:* Eighty schizophrenia patients were randomized into medication group and EA+medication group (n=40/group). Patients in the medication group were treated with conventional oral administration of clozapine (50-100 mg/d to 200-500 mg/d,for 8 weeks) and those of EA+ medication group treated by EA of Baihui (GV 20) and bilateral Taiyang (EX-HN5) and oral administration of clozapine (50mg/d to 100-150mg/d). EA was given to patients, 3 times a week for 8 weeks. Scores of the Positive and Negative Symptom Scale (PANSS) and the Untoward Effect Symptom Scale (TESS) were used to assess the therapeutic effect. *Results:* Following treatment PANSS scores for positive symptoms and common psychiatric symptom of the medication and EA+medication groups all significantly decreased from the 2rd week on ($P<0.05$,$P<0.01$), and those of the negative symptoms were also significantly reduced from the 4th week on ($P<0.05$). Comparison between two groups showed no significant differences in any PANSS scores ($P>0.05$). On the other hand TESS score of EA +medication group was significantly lower than that of medication group ($P<0.01$), suggesting an apparently fewer untoward effects in EA+medcation group. Of the two 40 cases in medication groups, 6(15%) and 5 (12.5%) went into remission, 8 and 8 (20%) experienced marked improvement in their symptoms,

* Corresponding Author: XIONG Dian-zhang, 563349081@qq.com

17(42.5%) and 16(40%) had an improvement, 9 (22.5%) and 11(27.5%) failed, with the effective rates being 77.5% and 72.5% separately. *Conclusion:* Both medication and EA+medication can improve refractory schizophrenia patients' clinical symptoms, but the later has fewer untoward effects.

Keywords: Refractory schizophrenia; Electroacupuncture; Clozapine; PANSS score; TESS score

Introduction

Some schizophrenia patients are unresponsive to antipsychotic medications even after multiple trials of different medications from different chemical families and including electro convulsive therapy (ECT). It remains difficult to treat refractory schizophrenia (they are also called treatment-resistant patients). It has been reported that clozapine and valproate were of some efficacy for refractory schizophrenia in china and abroad, but with high dosages increasing the risk and rate of adverse reactions. A number of articles reported combining Chinese and Western medicine treatments of refractory schizophrenia patients. The purpose of the current experiment was to compare the safety and efficacy of clozapine alone and clozapine plus EA in a group of Chinese refractory schizophrenia patients.

1. Material and Method

From 2006 to 2008 we enrolled 40 refractory schizophrenia cases into treatment with combined electro-acupuncture therapy (EA) + medication with small dose of clozapine and an equal number of similar patients as a control group under treatment with conventional dose of clozapine.

1.1. Inclusion Criteria

1) Schizophrenia diagnosis based on clinical evaluation;
2) PANSS score>60 (condition considered serious or severe);
3) The patients were not sensitive to the full-dose-full-period usage of more than two categories of antipsychotics. Refractory schizophrenia was defined based upon standard in the Chinese <dysphrenia classification and diagnosis standard> (the 3rd Edition);
4) The patients were not sensitive to a complete course of electroconvulsive therapy after 7-12 treatments. Patients' ages were14-60 and the sex was not limited.

Patients who were being treated with antipsychotics were given a one-week wash out period before enrolling into one of the groups. Any patient with cardiac, hepatic or renal disorders was excluded. Informed agreements were obtained from all patients.

1.2. Common Material

Two groups were divided stochastically to the hospital order; the even number entered in the group under the treatment with conventional dose of clozapine (medication group) and the odd numbers was assigned to the EA+medication with small dose of clozapine group (EA+medication group) with 40/group. Table 1 provides a comparison of common material between the patients from the two groups.

Table 1. Comparis on of general cinilcal of schizoprenia patients between mediation and EA+ mediation groups

Groups	male	female	average age	course	PANSS score
Medication	24	16	28.1±12.2	36.3±13.2	82.8±13.6
EA+med	22	18	29.4±11.3	35.2±12.2	82.6±13.7

1.3. Therapy Method

(1) Medication group: clozapine initial dose50-100mg/d, after 7days, 200-500mg/d for maintenance therapy. The period of treatment was 8 weeks.
(2) EA+medication group: main acupoint Baihui supporting acupoint Taiyang (patient supine), the partial conventional skin disinfected, holding a 0.35mm acupunture needle (range from 5 to 10 cm long) and delivering in skin with (range from 2 to 3 cm depth), then connect an electric stimulator (made in quanzhou,fujian province model 7010-Z, 10V) outputs the electrode carries on the stimulation by the arterues electric current, with the frequency40-60A/second.

The limit of the strength of current appears at the neck/face muscle contraction by the patient, bate breath, the oxygen deficit sign. Strong stimulation should last 3-4sec, then the power output is turned down. The patient's breath and facial color restores normally after 30-60sec, then repeat the second stimulation. Do this operation continuously 8-10 times with treatments 3 times a week. Clozapine initial dose50-100mg/d, after 7 days, 100-150mg/d for maintenance therapy. The period of treatment was 8 weeks.

1.4. Therapeutic Effects Observation

(1) *Evaluation of efficacy and safety*: PANSS scores were used to assess the efficacy. PANSS scores were evaluated in 2 weeks/4 weeks /8 weeks, by two independent doctors who were assigned out of study groups and unaware of the treatment. Untoward Effect Symptom Scale (TESS) scores were used to assess the side effects. The time and the method were the same as PANSS. Patients had routine physical examinations every day, blood analysis, hepatic function, blood glucose, blood lipid, ECG examination were also required at the same time.
(2) *Therapeutic effects standards*: Efficacy was assessed by reducing scores of PANSS. A PANSS score reduction >80% was needed for remission, >50% for significant

improvement, >30% for improvement, <30% for lack of effect. The reducing score rate= the score when entering the group - the score at the end of the therapy)/the score when entering the group] ×100%.

(3) *Statistical processing:* using SPSS10.0 to carry out the data analysis. Data of measurement are adapted to the t-test counting material are adapted to the x2 test, the group efficacy effects comparison with x2 examination. Statistical significance was set to $p<0.05$.

2. RESULTS

2.1. Dose of the Western Medicin

The average dose of clozapine in the medication group was 302.45+36.43mg/d, the average dose of clozapine in the EA+ medication group was121.62+16.34mg/d, the average dose of clozapine between the two groups was significantly different.

2.2. Therapeutic Effect

The results of the therapeutic responses from the two groups is listed in Table 2.

Table 2. Comparison of the therapeutic effects between the two groups (%)

Groups	remission	significantly effective	effectual	NR
Medication	6 15%	8 20%	17 42.5%	9 22.5%
EA+med	5 12.5%	8 20%	16 40%	11 27.5%

Table 3. PANSS scores in the two groups

Group	pretreatment	2W	4W	8W
EA+medication				
PS	28.2±4.3	23.6±4.3*	19.4±3.7**	15.7±4.2**
NS	22.9±5.6	20.3±5.1	17.9±5.2*	16.6±4*
GPS	34.8±6.8	31.8±5.9*	28.5±5.2*	22.4±4.6**
TS	82.6±13.7	74.2±12.6*	63.8±12.6**	46.3±11.1**
Medication				
PS	28.5±4.5	23.7±4.4*	19.7±3.6*	15.6±11.5**
NS	22.8±5.7	19.4±5.2	17.4±5.3*	15.6±4.2*
GPS	33.7±6.7	29.9±5.7*	27.2±5*	22.3±4.7**
TS	82.8±13.6	73.8±12.4*	63.7±12.4**	45.2±11.4**

*=p<0.05, **p<0.01, vs pre treatment; PS=positive symptoms, NS=negative symptoms, TS=total scores, GPS=general psychiatric symptoms.

As can be seen from Table 2, the medication group had a remission rate of 35%, and effective rate was 77.5% and the EA+medication group, the remission rate of 32.5%, and effective rate of 72.5%.The difference between the two groups had not statistically significant. PANSS scores of the two groups are listed in table 3. Table 3 shows that both groups had definitive therapeutic effects for the positive symptom, negative symptom, and the General Psychopathology symptom scales in treatment–resistant schizophrenia patients. Each general score between pre and post treatment was statistically significant ($p<0.01$). Comparison between the two groups none of the general scores reached statistical significance between pre treatment and post treatment at any time point.

2.4. Side Effects

TESS average score of EA+ medication group was (5.08+4.56), TESS average score of medication group was (10.38+6.52). Comparison between the two groups was statistically significant ($x=12.38, p<0.01$) with side effects reported less in the combined treatment group.

The common adverse effect of EA+ medication group were salivation, constipation, blurred vision, hypodynamia, palpitation, and sleepiness. When the adverse effect had a slight degree and tolerated by the patient, it was ignored. When the adverse effect was significant or not tolerated by the patient it was treated as necessary.

The main adverse effects of the medication group were salivation, constipation, blurred vision, hypodynamia, palpitation, longing for sleep, tachycardia, ecg changes, abnormal liver function, and leukopenia.

DISCUSSION

Baihui attrition Duchannel is used for epilepsy therapy (need reference here). Modern studies suggest that there are abundant vascular and nerves around Baihui superficial area such as greater occipital nerve, the branches of the nervus frontalis, there are cortical motor area and paracentral lobule around Baihui deep–seated area. Acupuncture Baihui Qubin,the former god-chung, sun and other points, enabling the various indicators of hemorheology in patients with improvement in brain function. Trials using electro-acupuncture stimulation Baihui with temples treatment of refractory schizophrenia combination with small dose of clozapine, could help reduce the necessary dose clozapine. The average dose of clozapine between the groups were compared. The difference was statistically significant despite the comparable clinical efficacy. The results of control group consistent the clozapine effective therapeutic window reported by LinZhiGuang.ect.in 2001. We conclude that electro-acupuncturc combination with small dosc of clozapinc cffcct is significant and is dcscrving of further examination in larger studies. Clinicians with access and training in the methodology should consider that electro-acupuncture stimulation Baihui with the temple in the treatment of refractory schizophrenia patients.

The incidence of adverse reactions, of the EA+medication group was lower than the group with conventional dose of clozapine. Moreover, the severity of adverse reactions was less, according to our assessments in the EA+midication. It is possible that the combined treatment will enhance the patients confidence in the therapy and improve compliance. Thus we conclude that the treatment of the refractory schizophrenia with combined electro-acupuncture stimulation Baihui with the temple and low dose clozapine is a safe and effective treatment worthy of further investigation.

REFERENCES

Chen H D, Yin G L, Jiang B, et al.Studying effect of acupuncture Baihui point for brain function with fMRI method[J]. Zhejiang Zhong Yi Yao Da Xue Xue Bao (*J. Zhejiang. Coll Trad. Chin. Med. ,Chin.*) ,2006,30 (6) :656-659.

Huang H F, Du B G, Zhang C F,et al.Analysis on the curative effect of non-convulsive electric shock treatment of refractory schizophrenia analysis[J]. Zhongguo Xian Dai Yao Wu Ying Yong(*Chin. J. Mod. Drug Appl., Chin.*), 2009,3 (11) :97-98.

Hung W X, Fan F J, Song J L.General situation on point Baihui (GV 20)[J], Shanghai Zhen Jiu Za Zhi (*Shanghai J. Acu-moxi. Chin.*), 2006:25 (2) :111-112.

LI Y C, LI C C, wang D P, et al. The study of clozapine combined with magnesium valproate in the treatment of refractory schizophrenia[J].zhongguo Jian Kang Xin Li Xue Za Zhi (*Chin. J. Health Psychol., Chin.*), 2007,15(5):430-432.

Li Z,Li W D.Refractory schizophrenia diagnosis and treatment[J].Xian Dai Zhong Xi Yi Jie He Za Zhi(M*od. J. Integr. Trad. Chin. Med. West Med.Chin.*), 2009,18(11):1320-1322.

Lin Z G. Weng Y R. Zhang D M.et al. Analysis on the plasma concentraion of clozaine and its related factors[J].Shanghai jig Shen Yi Xue (*Shanghai Arch. Psychistry, Chin.*),2001,13(4):210-213.

Liu P, Xiong D Z. Schizophrenia Clinical Examination and the Best Treatment Option [M]

Psychiatry Branch of the Chinese Medical Association. Chinese Classification and Diagnostic Criteria of Mental Disorders[M] (Chin).3rd ed.Jinan:Shandong Science and Technology Publishing House, 2001:74-78.

Shen Y C. Psychiatry[M] (Chin).4th ed.Beijing: People's Medical Publishing House,2001:730-740.

Yao Y F. Preliminary studies on the Treatment Mechanism of different syndromes treated with Baihui point[J]. Zhen Ci Yin Jiu (*Acupunct Res., Chin.*), 2000.25 (2) :153-155.

Zhong H W.Development of acupuncture treatment mental illness current situation [J]. Zhongguo Zhen Jiu (*Chin. Acumoxi, Chin.*), 2000:20 (1): 59-60.

In: The International Psychiatry and Behavioral ...
Editor: Nash Boutros
ISBN: 978-1-62257-566-4

Chapter 4

BRAZILIAN CONSENSUS ON SECOND-GENERATION ANTIPSYCHOTICS AND METABOLIC DISORDERS: REVIEW*

***Helio Elkis* [1], *Clarissa Gama* [2], *Henrique Suplicy* [3], *Marcos Tambascia* [4], *Rodrigo Bressan* [5], *Ruy Lyra* [6], *Saulo Cavalcante* [6] and *Walter Minicucci* [4]**

1- Schizophrenia Program (PROJESQ)- Institute of Psychiatry- University of São Paulo (USP), São Paulo (SP)- Brazil
2- Schizophrenia Program (PRODESQ)- Psychiatric Service, Porto Alegre Clinical Hospital, Porto Alegre (RS)- Brazil
3- Brazilian Association for the Study of Obesity and Metabolic Syndrome (ABESO)
4- Brazilian Diabetes Society (SBD)
5- Schizophrenia Program (PROESQ)- Federal University of São Paulo (UNIFESP), São Paulo (SP), Brazil
6- Brazilian Society of Endocrinology and Metabology (SBEM)

ABSTRACT

Objective: To discuss current aspects of use of antipsychotics considering their metabolic side effects profile, including weight gain, dyslipidemias, diabetes and metabolic syndrome Such metabolic effects increase the risk of mortality by cardiovascular disease, which is the leading cause of death among patients with schizophrenia.

Method: A consensus meeting was held, with the participation of endocrinologists and psychiatrists specializing in schizophrenia and, based on a literature review, a paper was prepared emphasizing practical and helpful recommendations to clinicians.

---

* Original Publication: Consenso Brasileiro sobre antipsicóticos de segunda geração e distúrbios metabólicos. Rev Bras Psiquiatr 2008:30(1): 77-85

Results and conclusions: Monitoring metabolic side effects is essential to patients taking antipsychotics, particularly in the case of second generation antipsychotics. Efficacy and tolerability should be carefully balanced in all phases of treatment.

Descriptors: Schizophrenia; Antipsychotic agents; metabolic syndrome X; Cardiovascular Diseases; Diabetes Mellitus, Type 2

1. *Projeto Esquizofrenia* (Schizophrenia Program) (PROJESQ), Departament and Institute of Psychiatry, University of São Paulo (USP), São Paulo (SP), Brazil
2. *Programa de Esquizofrenia* (Schizophrenia Program)(PRODESQ), Psychiatry Service, Porto Alegre Clínicas Hospital, Porto Alegre (RS), Brazil
3. *Associação Brasileira para o Estudo da Obesidade e da Síndrome Metabólica* (Brazilian Association for the Study of Obesity and Metabolic Syndrome) (ABESO)
4. *Sociedade Brasileira de Diabetes* (Brazilian Diabetes Society) (SBD)
5. *Programa de Esquizofrenia* (Schizophrenia Program) (PROESQ), São Paulo Federal University (UNIFESP), São Paulo (SP), Brazil
6. Brazilian Endocrinology and Metabology Society (SBEM)

The name of the consensus meeting participants can be found at the end of this paper.

Funding: This consensus was organized by Editora Prous Science, and full educational support was provided by Bristol-Myers Squibb do Brasil.

Conflict of interests: The authors' conflict of interests statements can be found at the end of this paper.

This is an expert consensus and, as such, there was no need to send it to the ethics committee.

INTRODUCTION

Second-generation antipsychotics (SGA) were a major step forward in the drug treatment of schizophrenia in the last decades. If compared to first-generation antipsychotics (FGA), they have the advantage of causing fewer extrapyramidal side effects, such as Parkinsonism, dystonia, akathisia and tardive dyskinesia, as well being more effective against the negative symptoms of schizophrenia (A). SGAs are currently recommended as a first-line treatment for schizophrenia[1-4] (A) and bipolar disorder (A) [5-6]

However, despite their advantages over FGAs, the use of SGAs has been associated to considerable weight gain and metabolic abnormalities, such as dyslipidemia, metabolic syndrome (MS) and diabetes (A). These metabolic abnormalities result in an increased risk of death by cardiovascular disease (CVD), already the leading cause of death among patients with schizophrenia[7] . Therefore, SGA-related metabolic disorders are a current challenge to psychiatrists. In the United States, the American Diabetes Association (ADA), the American Psychiatric Association (APA), the American Endocrinology Association and the American Society for the Study of Obesity convened a consensus development conference on the subject, in November 2003[8] .

There has been a significant increase in the use of SGAs in Brazil over the last few years , hence, the impact of metabolic disorders has become a pressing issue both in the everyday use of antipsychotics, as well as the public health system, since some SGAs are part of the high-cost medications program implemented by the Ministry of Health. Moreover, the algorithm published in 2000, and currently adopted by the Ministry of Health, is not consistent with scientific evidence published in the last few years.

Another peculiarity in the Brazilian scenario is that psychiatric practice in primary care is almost solely concerned with the remission of psychotic symptoms, neglecting other important aspects of the treatment, such as cardiovascular safety, negative symptoms and metabolic disorders, which lead to an increase in clinical morbidity and a deterioration of the quality of life of patients with schizophrenia.

In light of this situation, a Brazilian Consensus development meeting on Second-Generation Antipsychotics and Metabolic Disorders was convened in São Paulo, in March 2007. Experts from the Brazilian Association for the Study of Obesity and Metabolic Syndrome (ABESO), the Brazilian Diabetes Association (SBD), the Brazilian Endocrinology and Metabology Society (SBEM), the Schizophrenia Project from the São Paulo University Clínicas Hospital (PROJESQ), the São Paulo Federal University Schizophrenia Program (UNIFESP) and the Porto Alegre Clínicas Hospital Psychiatric Service Schizophrenia Program (PRODESQ) attended.

An independent psychiatrist was hired to act as moderator and each participant prepared a topic in advance and presented it at the meeting, followed by a group discussion. This paper is based on the presentations and texts submitted by the authors. Each author was requested to write their part based on the best evidence available. The authors used MedLine to review the literature.

The purpose of this consensus is to provide information with practical application, which is why endocrinology and psychiatry experts with vast clinical experience in their areas of sub-expertise took part in the meeting. All endocrinologists had ample experience in working with obese patients or patients with metabolic syndrome or diabetes. The psychiatrists were all experts on psychosis and schizophrenia.

The Agency for Health Care Research and Quality (AHRQ)[9] criteria were used. They define the following evidence grading levels:

- A: randomized, double-blind, placebo-controlled clinical trials.
- B: open, controlled trials and/or large case series.
- C: small case series and case reports.
- D: expert consensus.

The full list of participants and the ‘conflict of interests’ statement can be found at the end of this paper. Bristol-Myers Squibb do Brasil S/A provided full educational support to the logistic organization of the consensus meeting. Prous Science, an international publishing company specializing in further medical education programs, was responsible for the scientific coordination.

No representatives or employees of the sponsoring company had access to the consensus development meeting room or anything to do with its writing.

AN OVERVIEW OF OBESITY, DIABETES AND METABOLIC SYNDROME

The prevalence of excessive weight and obesity has reached epidemic levels, and there should be a 50% increase in the number of cases by 2015, reaching 1.5 billion people, according to the World Health Organization (WHO)[10.] Obesity is closely related to diabetes, type 2: more than 80% of people with type 2 diabetes are overweight or obese, and the risk of developing diabetes is positively associated to the increase in body mass index (BMI) [11]. Data from the Ministry of Health shows that, in Brazil, 32% of people are overweight and 8% obese[12]. Once individuals are overweight or obese, those with higher concentrations of visceral adipose tissue will be more prone to insulin resistance, favoring not only the development of diabetes, but also other comorbidities, such as arterial hypertension and dyslipidemia[13].

The combination of these conditions is known as metabolic syndrome (MS), defined by a set of clinical symptoms that include abdominal adiposity, dylipidemia, hypertension and insulin resistance with deteriorating glucose metabolism. The definition set out by the Adult Treatment Panel III (ATP-III) is one of the most commonly used. It includes the following three of the following abnormalities:

- Abdominal circumference = 102 cm for males and = 88 cm for females,
- HDL < 40 mg/dL for males and HDL < 50 for females,
- Diastolic blood pressure = 85 mmHg or systolic blood pressure = 130 mmHg,
- Fasting triglycerides = 150 mg/dL and fasting glycemia = 110 mmHg.

Dyslipidemia, another component of MS, is determined by high concentrations of very low density lipoproteins (VLDL) and low serum HDL concentration, as well as the presence of small and dense particles (LDL) and postprandial lipemia[13].

MS prevalence depends directly on the diagnosis criteria used. Data from the US National Health and Nutrition Examination Survey, 1999-2000, which used ATP III criteria, showed MS prevalence in 26.7% of the American adult population[14]. Recently, the ARIC study used the same criteria, but with fasting glycemia > 100 mg/dl, and found a 32% prevalence among American adults[15]. MS prevalence has also risen among children and teenagers and, along with obesity, leads to an increase in type 2 diabetes rates in these age groups[16].

Recently, many epidemiologic studies have been carried out in a wide variety of populations so as to understand the actual and independent prognostic impact MS might have on the development of diabetes or cardiovascular disease, i.e., whether MS adds to traditional risks, such as LDL, age, gender and smoking status[17-24]. Blonde et al conducted a systematic review of all relevant papers published as of the release of the NCEP-III guidelines (May 2001) until March 2005[25]. These studies showed that MS patients run twice the risk of cardiovascular events and three times the risk of developing diabetes, and that exacerbated MS is an additional risk. The review shows that MS is an independent risk factor and clinically relevant to diabetes and cardiovascular disease and, therefore, useful for screenings.

MS in itself can explain a large part of the morbidity and the high mortality rates in this population[26], especially as a result of cardiovascular diseases (CVD).

Diabetes is a chronic disease that currently affects approximately 171 million people all over the world, and is estimated to reach 366 million people by 2030, increasing prevalence from 2.8%, in 2000, to 4.4%[27].

According to WHO figures, 987.000 people died as a result of diabetes in 2002, 1.7% of total deaths in the world[28]. This situation will become increasingly worse as projections show there will be a significant increase in the number of those suffering from the disease. Genetic susceptibility cannot be seen to be the sole cause for the considerable increase in the number of those with type 2 diabetes, since there is no doubt that environmental aspects play a key role in this scenario. Diabetes also has a major economic impact on nations. In the United States alone, for instance, 132 billion dollars are estimated to have been spent, directly and indirectly, on the disease in 2002[29]. Despite the introduction of new drugs and a better understanding of this clinical entity in the last few years, the control of this disease continues to be unsatisfactory among most of the population.

To reduce the impact of type 2 diabetes means, before anything else, to reduce the disease's incidence, taking preventive measures to act before it appears, especially among high risk patients. Behavioral and pharmacological interventions have been studied and implemented to that end. Lifestyle changes, such as a controlled diet and physical exercise, as well as oral medication, have shown to be very effective.

The Impact of Metabolic Disorders on Patients with Schizophrenia

The growing obesity epidemic among the general population is a matter of great concern among health professionals. It is clearly associated to the increased risk of development of diabetes, hypertension, hyperlipidemia and osteoarthritis, among other morbidity and mortality causes[30].

The reported prevalence of obesity in patients treated for schizophrenia is approximately 40 to 75%[30,31], a higher rate than the prevalence found in the general population, which ranges from 20 to 30% in the United States. Data from the Ministry of Health shows the prevalence of overweight and obesity to be 32% and 8%, respectively, in Brazil[12].

MS characteristics are very frequent in patients with schizophrenia [32] (A). Studies have shown that the mortality rate among in this population it is twice as high as that of the general population, due to a higher prevalence and severity of clinical conditions, and life expectancy is 20% lower[33].

Although the literature has been focusing on suicide in connection with psychiatric treatment-related deaths, patients with schizophrenia also die of common causes, such as respiratory diseases, myocardial infarction and cerebral vascular accident[33,34] (B). Suicide and cardiovascular diseases are the two most common causes of death in patients with schizophrenia, the latter being twice as frequent as in the general population[30] (B). These conditions occur prematurely and can be exacerbated by the type of lifestyle, smoking, sedentarism and social deprivation. Current evidence suggests that schizophrenia *per se* and/or antipsychotics, especially newer ones, are associated with Cardio Vascular Diseases[8] (B).

Antipsychotics in general are the most effective treatment for schizophrenia, and SGAs, or atypical antipsychotics, are better tolerated and more effective than FGAs, or typical, in controlling the negative symptoms of psychosis, in addition to having fewer extrapyramidal effects[8,35] (A).

Both SGAs and FGAs have been associated with significant problems, including weight gain, increased lipid concentrations, carbohydrate changes and the resulting metabolic and cardiovascular risk[36-38] (B). However, these metabolic changes are not the same among the different antipsychotic agents (A). Four American organizations recently published a consensus report on the metabolic risk profile of the different antipsychotics. They recognized that the risk of weight gain, diabetes and dyslipidemia was not the same across all antipsychotics[8]. Two of them, clozapine and olanzapine, were associated with a higher risk of weight gain, diabetes and dyslipidemia than two others, introduced more recently: ziprasidone and aripiprazole[39]. The other two representatives of this class of antipsychotics, risperidone and quetiapine, presented an average risk of weight gain and inconsistent results for the diabetes and dyslipidemia evaluation[8,39] (B). In any case, less than 50% of patients with schizophrenia being treated with antipsychotics in general gain weight[40] (A). Evidence have shown that the average weight gain in 10 weeks' treatment with different second-generation antipsychotics was greater than with first-generation antipsychotics, and the average weight gain was 4.45 kg, 4.15 kg, 2.10 kg and 0.04 kg for clozapine, olanzapine, risperidone and ziprasidone, respectively[36] (A). Overweight and obesity are currently very common in these patients[31,41] and it has been shown that they have a significantly higher BMI than psychiatric patients who have not been diagnosed schizophrenic and the general population[37] (B). Coupled with these facts, in addition to lowering patients' self-esteem – which encourages them to stop treatment[42], overweight, in this specific psychiatric population, is growing at epidemic rates and leading to an increased risk of comorbities among the general population, both in developed and developing countries[43].

In addition to overweight, hyperlipidemia, hypertension and diabetes have also been recognized as significant complications in these patients[44] (B). The number of these reports has increased as the use of antipsychotics also increases, although it is difficult to determine if the prevalence of these changes in these populations has increased regardless of the treatment.

Although most available studies only address patients with schizophrenia, the data obtained is difficult to be interpreted due to there being little methodological rigor in the diagnosis criteria and anthropometric measures, and to the lack of studies with control groups for the use of antipsychotic and MS[8,30,45] .

Moreover, the increase in lack of physical activity, smoking and inappropriate eating habits, common characteristics in patients with schizophrenia, can also contribute to a higher prevalence of metabolic abnormalities. Environmental aspects involving patients' lifestyles can make them prone to CVDs and endocrine disorders. Smoking, drinking alcohol, inappropriate eating habits and sedentarism increase mortality in the general population and 50 to 90% of patients with schizophrenia are nicotine-dependent (B). Sedentarism, a characteristic commonly found in these patients, can be partly due to the negative symptoms of the disease, as well as the sedating effects of the antipsychotics, added to the long periods of time patients spend in hospitals admittions[32].

Thus, it is difficult to determine whether metabolic disorders are associated with the disease alone, or also an effect of the medications. However, although there is limited data on the metabolic profile and the risk of diabetes in patients with schizophrenia who have never been treated, some studies suggest that these problems may be present in patients before any treatment has been ministered[8] (C). Some studies show that when the first episode of schizophrenia occurs, never medicated patients have three times as much visceral adiposity[45-46], less glucose tolerance and higher insulin resistance than controls who are disease-free[47].

Therefore, it was only recently that physicians and researchers started to assess the relationship between the use of medication and schizophrenia in the MS context[44].

Recent studies suggest that, when compared to the general population, patients with schizophrenia have a high prevalence of MS components, and the prevalence of this condition ranges from, approximately, 37 to 63% [48-51].

Thus, the need for controlled prospective studies is relevant with a view to verifying the magnitude of these associations. The current clinical dilemma regarding obese patients with schizophrenia and those with MS is to determine the best strategy to promote weight loss and limit adverse effects for the long run. However, in order to recommend more specific interventions, the impact of MS on the population with schizophrenia and its association/interaction with individual factors and environmental exposure would have to be more precisely identified[52].

Patients with schizophrenia are particularly more vulnerable to MS because of their more sedentary lifestyle, high prevalence of smoking and inappropriate eating habits[53]. In order to conduct a better assessment of the frequency of MS in patients with schizophrenia, CATIE[54] study researchers analyzed MS prevalences at baseline, as defined by NCEP-III, and compared them to the NHANES III database (the third National Health and Nutrition Examination Survey on the health and nutrition status of the population in the United States)[55]. A much higher MS prevalence was found among patients (40.9%, with a higher prevalence among females); CATIE males were 85% more likely to have MS than NHANES controls, and CATIE females were 137% more likely to have MS than their NHANES counterparts[55]. This data shows that careful attention should be paid to the periodic assessment of this syndrome so as to minimize any risks associated with antipsychotic treatment.

Authors such as L'Italien et al., in a recent systematic review, showed that MS age-adjusted prevalence in patients with schizophrenia is 39.5%; twice as high as the prevalence in the general population[56].

Patient Initial Screening for Metabolic Risks

The lifestyle of an individual with psychotic disorders, as well as his or her antipsychotic treatment, can contribute to the development of metabolic changes or make them more severe (A).

Increased evidence of the effects of antipsychotic treatment on these risk factors and of health implications in a vulnerable population are indicative of the need for careful screening and monitoring of these patients. Patients should be screened before beginning treatment with antipsychotics, they should be weighed and have their height measured (to calculate their

BMI), and their abdominal circumference (at the umbilical scar level), blood pressure, glycemia, total cholesterol, HDL cholesterol and fasting triglycerides should also be measured (D). Additionally the patients' personal and family history of obesity, diabetes, dyslipidemia, arterial hypertension and cardiovascular disease should also be obtained.

This screening should determine if the patient is overweight (BMI between 25 and 30) or obese (BMI > 30), if he or she has visceral obesity (abdominal circumference > 102 cm for males and > 88 cm for females), diabetes (fasting glycemia > 126 mg/dl), arterial hypertension (arterial blood pressure >140/90 mmHg), or dyslipidemia (total cholesterol > 200 mg/dl, HDL cholesterol < 40 mg/dl, triglycerides > 150 mg/dl), or is glucose-intolerant (fasting glycemia between 100 and 125 mg/dl).

If any of these conditions are identified, suitable treatment should be started and the psychiatrist should not hesitate to refer the patient to a specialist (D). Overweight or obese patients should be advised on their diet and physical exercise (A). Patients and their relatives should be warned about the fact that antipsychotic medication may contribute to weight gain and increase the risk of diabetes and dyslipidemia (D).

Antipsychotics with lower risk of weight gain, diabetes and dyslipidemia should be considered for patients likely to develop these pathologies (C). By making this initial screening a routine, it is possible to detect these important risk factors early (C).

Monitoring and Management of Patients who Develop Metabolic Disorders

These pathologies are closely related to each other, therefore, when one of them is identified in a patient, it is essential to conduct a propaedeutic assessment of correlated diseases, since, when present simultaneously, their morbidities are amplified[57] (B).

As soon as these pathologies are diagnosed, individual or simultaneous treatments should be started, since their association with cardiovascular disorders, as well as other morbidities, are well established[57] (A).

Table 1. Medication used in the treatment of Diabetes Mellitus, Type 2

Medication	Mechanism of Action
Insulin sensitizers (i.e.: metformin, thyazolidinedione and glitazones)	Reduce insulin resistance
Sulphonylureas and meglitinides	Act on insulin secretion
Gliptins and exenatide	Act on beta cells and gastrointestinal hormone disorders
Acarbose	Acts on the intestinal absorption of glucose
Rimonabant	Acts on the endocannabinoid system
Insulin	Similar to endogenous insulin. May act quickly, slowly or both

Treatments targets are relieving symptoms and avoiding chronic and acute complications and, as a result, improving the patient's quality of life and increasing expectancy[58] (B). Given the high health risks, these patients should be submitted to an initial screening and uninterrupted monitoring, which should not be suspended even if the control is meeting expectations. At the same time, patients and their relatives should be given basic information about the pathology and advised on how to conduct the treatment, as well as told what the goals, costs and advantages of this procedure (D).

1. Overweight Guidelines

Obesity is a chronic disease that is difficult to control, with high incidence and morbidity rates. It requires constant treatment for the rest of the patient's life[59] (D). Obesity can be treated by as well as other measures (A). For example treatment of obesity includes a change in lifestyle, including a diet that must be adapted to the patient's social and economic situation and the practice of physical exercise. With regard to physical activities, there must be a balance between aerobic and anaerobic exercises, but aerobic exercises should be predominant: approximately five times a week for 30 minutes, respecting each patient's physical condition (D). Amphetamine-based drugs are not recommended for the treatment of obesity in psychotic patients (C), with sibutramine being an occasional exception, when patients are adequately monitored by a psychiatrist. However, its effectiveness with patients using antipsychotics has not been proven. Although sibutramine has effectively helped patients with schizophrenia being treated with olanzapine to loose weight, it has not been effective in doing the same for patients being treated with clozapine [61] (A). Moreover, possible sibutramine-induced cases of psychosis have been reported, confirming the need for caution when using this drug [62] (C). The consensus group did not come to a unanimous decision concerning the use of sibutramine in psychotic patients, and some participants were by no meansagainst the use of this substance. Apparently, orlistat is not contraindicated for use with patients being treated with antipsychotics (D). Weight control goals: although there is an increase in morbidity in cases where the BMI is higher than 25, a 5 to 10% weight loss leads to an improvement in metabolic disorders (B).

2. Diabetes Mellitus Type 2 Guidelines

Non-drug treatment is based on the education of patients with regard to diabetes, as well as a change in lifestyle, trying to follow the guidelines set out in the previous topic concerning overweight, since approximately 80 to 90% of type 2 diabetes cases are overweight. However, food and nutrition education must be very specific when it comes to diabetic patients, and carbohydrate counting also plays an important part. Unfortunately, less than 10% of patients manage to achieve effective levels of control with this type of treatment alone, even though it must be conducted concurrently with the recommended drug therapy(C). Drug treatment for diabetes type 2 is based on various types of drugs, which act in different areas and have different mechanisms of action, as well as indications and combinations.

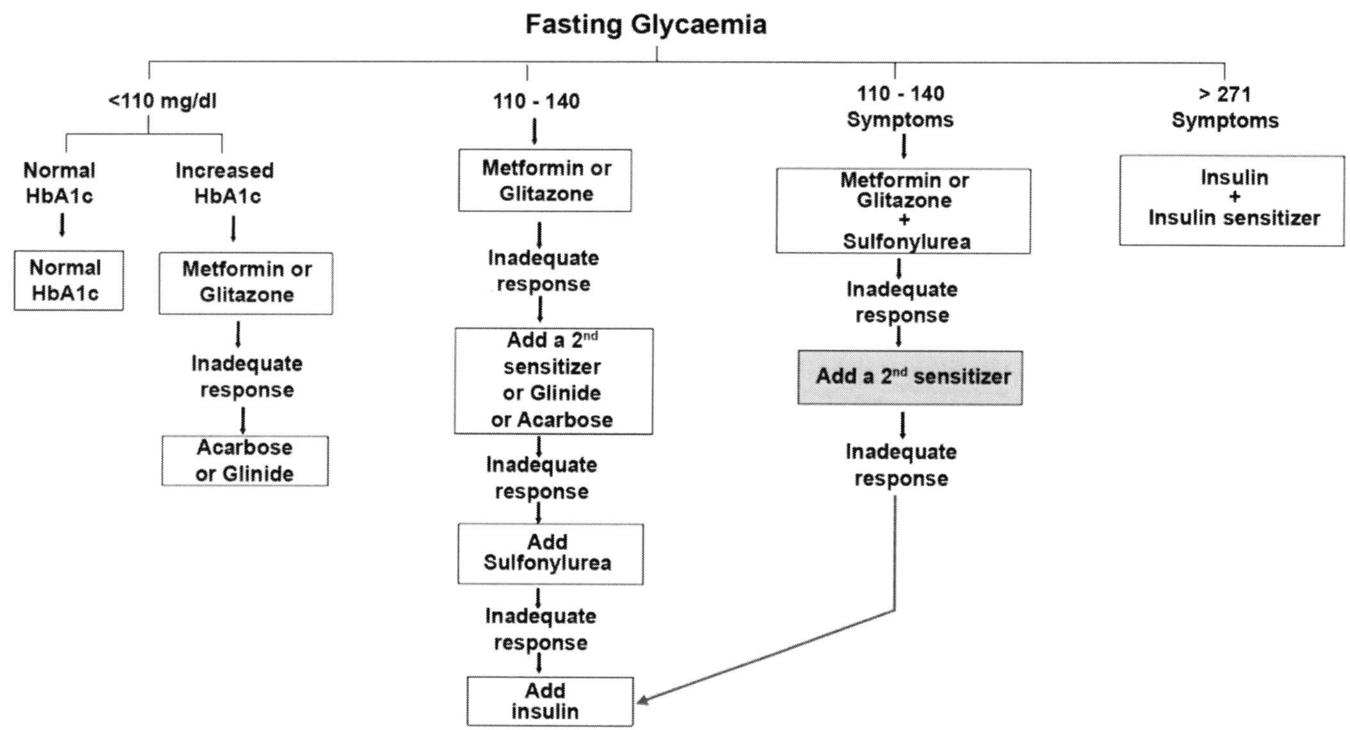

Figure 1. Algorithm for the treatment of diabetes (Brazilian Diabetes Society).

We usually start with one of them, but soon others must be associated due to secondary failure. Table 1 shows a list of drugs used in the treatment of type 2 diabetes. The Brazilian Diabetes Society suggests an algorithm for the treatment of diabetes (Figure 1).

The desired glycemic control goals varies according to the guidelines as follows. Table 2 shows the goals according to different institutions.

Table 2. Glycemic control goals

Parameter	ADA	IDF	SBD
Fasting glycemia (mg/dl)	90 to 130	110 to 140	110
Postprandial glycemia	<180	145 to 180	140
HbA 1c (%)	<1.70	<6.5	NSLT

ADA- American Diabetes Association
IDF-International Diabetes Federation
SBD- Brazilian Diabetes Society
NSLT- Normal Superior Limit Threshold

3. Dyslipidemia Guidelines

The Framingham Risk Score should be used to stratify patients and, following that, goals should be established for each type of risk (low, average or high) and a change in lifestyle implemented, either alone or in association with a specific drug for each type of dyslipidemia [63-65] (A).

Table 3. Goals for lipid control

	Goals		
Level of Risk	LDLC	HDLC	TG
High Patients with CAD, PVD, CA or Risk for CAD in 10 years ≥20% Patients with Diabetes	 < 100mg/dL < 100mg/dL	 >40mg/dL >45mg/dL	 < 150mg/dL < 150mg/dL
Medium Risk for DAC in 10 years > 10% and < 20%	< 130mg/dL	>40mg/dL	< 150mg/dL
Low Risk for CAD in 10 years ≤ 10%	< 130mg/dL*	>40mg/dL	< 150mg/dL

CAD- Coronary Artery Disease.
PVD- Peripheral Vascular Disease.
CA- CarotidAtherosclerosis.
LDL- Low Density Lipoprotein Cholesterol.
HDL- High Density Lipoprotein Cholesterol.
TG- Triglycerides.
*Levels of <160mg/dL are also acceptable.

Non-drug therapy for the treatment of dyslipidemia includes a change in lifestyle of overweight patients and a specific diet established according to the individual aspects of each type of dyslipidemia. Only 6 to 15% of patients reach the goals by means of this treatment alone [64] (C). A drug treatment is recommended when lifestyle changes are not enough to achieve the desired goals [63-65]. Statins are the most commonly used drugs in the treatment of hypercholesterolemia, but other drugs can be added to a combination therapy, such as: nicotinic acid, bile acid sequestrant resin and ezetimibe[63-65] (A).

Fibrates are more commonly used to treat hyperglyceridemia, but nicotinic acids and statins can be used in certain cases[65] (A).

Table 3 shows lipid control goals according to the Brazilian Dyslipidemia and Atherosclerosis Prevention Guidelines[66] (B).

Monitoring

When prescribing SGAs, psychiatrists should evaluate the patient's height and waist circumference, as well as his weight Blood glucose levels above 99 mg/dl are considered abnormal, and patients presenting such levels should be investigated with a glucose tolerance test; patients with fasting glycemia above 126mg/dl (after two measurements) or with a random measurement equal to or above 200mg/dl, and presenting polydipsia and polyuria, should be treated for diabetes (B). Table 4 shows our recommended monitoring scheme (D).

More frequent evaluations may be necessary, depending on the clinical picture. Differently from the American consensus[8] we recommend that the lipid control should be performed annually, as set out in the NCEP ATP3 (D) (the ADA/APA[8] consensus recommends lipid profile monitoring every five years). In addition to fasting glycemia, the Brazilian Diabetes Society also advises that postprandial glycemia (2 hours) and Glycosylated Haemoglobin (HbA1c) should also be evaluated.

Risk-Benefit Analysis of Second Generation Antipsychotics

We present bellow some evidence found in the literature that should be taken into account for the evaluation of the risk-benefit analysis of the use of antipsychotics and weight gain/metabolic disorders:

1. Before treatments for schizophrenia were available, authors such as Kraepelin and Bleuler had already observed changes in the weight of patients (C).
2. Schizophrenia is a chronic psychiatric disorder and has sometimes a deterioration course, thus resulting in a lack of physical activity which favors weight gain.
3. The inner nature of the disorder can lead to changes in eating habits, impacting both weight gain and loss, in particular as it becomes more severe and especially during psychotic episodes.
4. The association between mental illnesses and diabetes was described by Maudsley already in the 19th century, and cases of diabetes in patients with schizophrenia were

described in the pre-neuroleptic era, when many studies showed glucose intolerance and diabetes occur twice or three times as frequently in the population with schizophrenia than in the general population [67] (C)

5. Cases of diabetes and changes in glucose tolerance with first generation antipsychotics have been observed since the introduction of chlorpromazine in clinical practice, in the mid-20th century[68] (C).
6. Recent evidence clearly shows that, when compared to conventional antipsychotics, second generation antipsychotics are also associated to weight gain and changes in glucose and lipid metabolism (A). However, the mechanism behind those changes is yet to be completely elucidated[30].
7. Some studies show that there is a correlation between psychopathological improvement and weight gain in patients being treated with second generation anti-psychotics [69.]
8. The weight gain mechanism associated to antipsychotic response also appears to be regulated genetically[70].

In light of this evidence, in cases where weight gain or metabolic changes associated to the use of antipsychotics is observed, the level of compromise caused by the disease should be checked, as well as the response history to previous antipsychotics, the level of adherence to the treatment, medical or psychiatric comorbidities, among others[8].

Such aspects should be considered within the context of the treatment phase

1. Phases of the Treatment for Schizophrenia, Weight Gain and Glycemic/Metabolic Changes: Management

Most guidelines, such as those set out by the American Psychiatric Association[3] or the World Federations of Societies of Biological Psychiatry[1], or treatment algorithms, such as the Texas Medication Algorithm Project (TMAP)[2] or the algorithm for the treatment of schizophrenia of the International Psychopharmacology Algorithm Project (IPAP)[4], recommend that the treatment for schizophrenia be divided in two phases: in phase 1, the patient can receive an initial monotherapy regime treatment, preferably with second generation antipsychotics, for no less than six weeks (phase 1a). If the response is satisfactory, the antipsychotic should be used as maintenance medication. If the patient does not respond to the first treatment it recommended as second one, preferably with a second generation antipsychotic in monotherapy, in adequate dosages for no less than six weeks (phase 1b).

Again, if the response is positive, the patient should continue taking the respective antipsychotic. If not, some algorithms, such as TMAP2suggest a third attempt, this time with a first generation antipsychotic (phase 1c).

All guidelines and algorithms mentioned above are unanimous in stating that patients who do not respond to phase 1 should be considered refractory and eligible for treatment with clozapine (A), the antipsychotic proven to be the most effective in these cases. Thus, the second phase of schizophrenia treatment is reserved for refractory cases and the chosen antipsychotic for such a treatment is clozapine (A).

In this situation, the physician should consider carefully three factors: the phase of the treatment, the response and the side effects (in this case, weight gain and glycemic/metabolic changes).

We would, then, have the following situations: for patients who have not responded to treatment phases 1a, 1b, 1c, a change of antipsychotics should be considered as a result of their lack of efficacy. At this point, an important issue arises if the patient is responding well to a specific medication, but is gaining weight and presenting metabolic changes. In this case, it would be desirable if the antipsychotic should be switched for another one, with less impact on weight gain/metabolic changes. However such new antipsychotic should have comparable efficacy as the previous antipsychotic, to which the patient had previously responded. If this is not possible, or some doubts remain regarding the efficacy of the new antipsychotic, the physician should not switch the antipsychotic and, instead, implement measures such as dieting or correction of the metabolic parameters (such as using oral antidiabetic drugs or statins).

If the patient is responding to clozapine, but gaining weight or presenting glycemic/metabolic changes, clozapine should not be suspended, as there is no evidence that other antipsychotics are as effective in this stage of the disease. In this case, measures such as weight loss, changes in eating habits and lifestyle, physical exercise or the use of substances that can improve glycidic and lipid metabolism should be implemented.

Therefore, if the patient presents weight gain and/or glycemic/metabolic changes, the psychiatrist should carefully consider whether the medication should be replaced or maintained, always taking into account the treatment phase and the efficacy previously obtained in relation to the adverse side effects.

ACKNOWLEDGMENTS

The authors would like to thank Professor Paulo Belmonte Abreu and Dr. Carmen Leitão Azevedo, from the Porto Alegre Clínicas Hospital, for their help.

They would also like to thank Dr. John Newcomer, from Washington University School of Medicine, for his comments during the meeting.

The participants in the consensus meeting were:

Clarissa Gama (PRODESQ), Helio Elkis (PROJESQ), Henrique Suplicy (ABESO), Marcos Tambascia (SBD), Rodrigo Bressan (PROESQ), Ruy Lyra (SBEM), Saulo Cavalcante (SBEM), Walter Minicucci (SBD). Dr. John Newcomer (Washington University School of Medicine) was briefly present (30 minutes) during the beginning of the meeting, but did not take part in the consensus discussions.

Moderator: Dr. Mônica Kayo (Independent Consultant hired by Prous Science).

CONFLICT OF INTERESTS STATEMENT

Dr. Helio Elkis stated he has given lectures for Astra-Zeneca and worked as a consultant for Janssen-Cilag and Bristol-Myers Squibb. He stated he has received direct and indirect research support from the following companies: Pfizer, Eli-Lilly, Acadia Pharmaceuticals and Janssen-Cilag.

Dr. Clarissa Gama stated she has no potential conflict of interests.

Dr. Henrique Suplicy stated he has received direct and indirect research support from Roche, Merck, Novartis, Abbott, Sanofi-Aventis, Jansen-Cilag and Pfizer. He has also worked as a consultant for Roche.

Dr. Marcos Tambascia stated he has given lectures for NovoNordisk, Sanofi-Aventis, Eli-Lilly, Merck-Sharp-Dohme, Pfizer, Glaxo-Smithkline and Novartis. He was a member of the board of consultants at Pfizer and Glaxo-Smithkline and has received direct and indirect research support from Pfizer, Sanofi-Aventis, NovoNordisk, Eli-Lilly and Roche.

Dr. Rodrigo Bressan is a level 2 researcher for CNPQ. He has given lectures for Astra-Zeneca and Eli-Lilly. He is a member of the board at Janssen-Cilag and has received direct and indirect research support from the following companies: Astra-Zeneca, Bristol-Myers Squibb, Eli-Lilly, Novartis and Janssen-Cilag.

Dr. Ruy Lira stated he has given lectures for Glaxo-Smithkline, Sanofi-Aventis, AstraZeneca, Novartis, Pfizer, Merck-Sharp-Dohme and Eli Lilly. He was a member of the board of consultants at Glaxo-Smithkline, Sanofi Aventis, Astra Zeneca, Novartis and Pfizer.

Dr. Saulo Cavalcante stated he has given lectures for Eli-Lilly, Merck-Sharp-Dohme, Pfizer, Merck SA, Glaxo-Smithkline, Novartis and Bristol-Myers Squibb Brasil. He was a member of the board of consultants at Pfizer, Glaxo-Smithkline and Novartis and has received direct and indirect research support from Eli-Lilly.

Dr. Walter J. Minicucci stated he has given lectures for NovoNordisk, Sanofi-Aventis, Eli-Lilly, Merck-Sharp-Dohme, Pfizer and Medtronic.

Dr. Mônica Kayo has worked as a consultant for Acadia Pharmaceuticals, Janssen-Cilag, Sandoz, Abbott and Bristol-Myers Squibb.

None of the speakers holds shares or has investments in pharmaceutical companies.

REFERENCES

[1] Falkai P, Wobrock T, Lieberman J, Glenthoj B, Gattaz WF, Möller HJ. Força-tarefa da WFSBP para diretrizes para o tratamento biológico da esquizofrenia. Parte 1: Tratamento agudo e Parte 2: Tratamento de longo prazo. *Rev. Psiq. Clin.* 2006;33(Supl 1): 7-64.

[2] Miller AL, Hall CS, Buchanan RW, Buckley PF, Chiles JA, Conley RR, Crismon ML, Ereshefsky L, Essock SM, Finnerty M, Marder SR, Miller DD, McEvoy JP, Rush AJ, Saeed SA, Schooler NR, Shon SP, Stroup S, Tarin-Godoy B. The Texas Medication Algorithm Project Antipsychotic Algorithm for Schizophrenia: 2003 Update. *J. Clin. Psychiatry*. 2004;65(4):500-8.

[3] American Psychiatric Association. Practice guideline for the treatment of patient with schizophrenia. 2nd edition. *Am. J. Psychiatry.*, February 2004.

[4] IPAP. International Pharmacological Algorithm Project. Available at: www.ipap.org

[5] Chou JC-Y. Review and Update of the American Psychiatric Association Practice Guideline for Bipolar Disorder. *Prim. Psychiatry.* 2004;11(9):73-84.

[6] Suppes T, Dennehy EB, Hirschfeld RM, Altshuler LL, Bowden CL, Calabrese JR, Crismon ML, Ketter TA, Sachs GS, Swann AC; Texas Consensus Conference Panel on Medication Treatment of Bipolar Disorder. The Texas implementation of medication algorithms: update to the algorithms for treatment of bipolar I disorder. *J. Clin. Psychiatry*. 2005;66(7):870-86.

[7] Colton CW, Manderscheid RW. Prev Chronic Dis [serial online] 2006 Apr [date cited]. Available at URL: http://www.cdc.gov/pcd/ issues/2006/apr/05_0180.htm

[8] American Diabetes Association; American Psychiatric Association; American Association of Clinical Endocrinologists; North American Association for the Study of Obesity. Consensus development conference on antipsychotic drugs and obesity (Consensus Statement). *Diabetes Care*. 2004;27(2):596-601.

[9] Agency for Healthcare Research and Quality. Systems to rate the strength of scientific evidence. Evidence report/technology assessment; 47. AHRQ publication no.02-E015;2002. Available at: www.ahrq. gov/clinic/epcsums/strengthsum.htm

[10] World Health Organization. Preventing chronic diseases -a vital investment. *Obesity newsletter*. 2005;8(2):3-28.

[11] Willett WC, Dietz WH, Colditz GA. Guidelines for healthy weight. *N. Engl. J. Med.* 1999;341(6):427-34.

[12] Diretrizes para Cardiologistas sobre Excesso de Peso e Doença Cardiovascular dos Departamentos de Aterosclerose, Cardiologia Clínica e FUNCOR da Sociedade Brasileira de Cardiologia. *Arq. Bras.* Cardiol. 2002;78(Suppl 1):1-13.

[13] Kissebah AH, Krakower GR. Regional adiposity and morbidity. Physiol Rev. 1994;74(4):761-811.

[14] Ford ES, Giles WH, Mokdad AH, Increasing prevalence of the metabolic syndrome among U.S. Adults. *Diabetes Care*. 2004;27(10):2444-9.

[15] McNeil AM, Rosamond WD, Girman CJ, Golden SH, Schmidt MI, East HE, Ballantyne CM, Heiss G. The metabolic syndrome and 11-year risk of incident cardiovascular disease in the atherosclerosis risk in communities study. *Diabetes Care*. 2005;28(2):385-90.

[16] Rosenbloom AL, Joe JR, Young RS, Winter WE. Emerging epidemic of type 2 diabetes in youth. *Diabetes Care* 1999;22(2):345-54.

[17] L'Italien GJ, Ford I, Shepherd J. The metabolic syndrome is an independent predictor of cardiac events in WOSCOPS males. Presented at: 52nd Annual Meeting of the American College of Cardiology; March 30–April 2, 2003; Chicago, Ill.

[18] McNeill AM, Rosamond WD, Girman CJ, Ballantyne CM. A new definition of the metabolic syndrome predicts incident coronary heart disease and stroke [abstract]. *Circulation*. 2002;106(Suppl II):765.

[19] Lakka HM, Laaksonen DE, Lakka TA, Niskanen LK, Kumpusalo E, Tuomilehto J, Salonen JT. The metabolic syndrome and total and cardiovascular disease mortality in middle-aged men. *JAMA*. 2002;288(21):2709-16.

[20] Sattar N, Gaw A, Scherbakova O, Ford I, O'Reilly DS, Haffner SM, Isles C, Macfarlane PW, Packard CJ, Cobbe SM, Shepherd J. Metabolic syndrome with and without CRP as a predictor of coronary heart disease and diabetes in the West of Scotland Coronary Prevention Study. *Circulation*. 2003;108(4):414-9.

[21] Lorenzo C, Okoloise M, Williams K, Stern MP, Haffner SM; San Antonio Heart Study. The metabolic syndrome as a predictor of type 2 diabetes. *Diabetes Care.* 2003;26(11):3153-9.

[22] Ninomiya JK, L'Italien G, Criqui MH, Whyte JL, Gamst A, Chen RS. Association of the metabolic syndrome with history of myocardial infarction and stroke in the Third National Health and Nutrition Examination Survey. *Circulation.* 2004;109(1):42-6.

[23] Malik S, Wong ND, Franklin SS, Kamath TV, L'Italien GJ, Williams RJ. The impact of the metabolic syndrome and diabetes on mortality from coronary heart disease, cardiovascular disease and all causes in United States adults. *Circulation.* 2004;110(10):1239-44.

[24] Hu G, Qiao Q, Tuomilehto J, Balkau B, Borch-Johnsen K, Pyorala K; ECODE Study Group. Prevalence of the metabolic syndrome and its relation to all cause and cardiovascular mortality in non-diabetic European men and women. *Arch. Int. Med..* 2004;164(10):1066-76.

[25] Blonde L, Ray S, Carson W, L'Italien GJ. Metabolic Syndrome is an Important Predictor of Cardiovascular Disease and New onset Diabetes – A Systematic Review of the Literature. Pôster apresentado na 158a. Reunião Anual da Associação Psiquiátrica Americana, Atlanta, GA, maio de 2005.

[26] Isomaa B, Almgren P, Tuomi T, Forsén B, Lahti K, Nissén M, Taskinen MR, Groop L. Cardiovascular morbidity and mortality associated with the metabolic syndrome. *Diabetes Care.* 2001;24(4):683-9.

[27] Wild S, Roglic G, Green A, Sicree S, King H. Global Prevalence Of Diabetes – Estimates For The Year 2000 And Projections For 2030. *Diabetes Care.* 2004;27(5):1047-53.

[28] World Health Organization: The World Health Report 2003. Geneva, *World Health Organization*, 2003.

[29] Hogan P, Dall T, Nikolov P; American Diabetes Association. Economics costs of diabetes in U.S. in 2002. *Diabetes Care.* 2003;26(3):917-32.

[30] Wirshing D. Schizophrenia and obesity: impact of antipsychotic medications. *J. Clin. Psychiatry.* 2004;65(Suppl 18):13-26.

[31] Leitão-Azevedo CL, Abreu MG, Guimaraes LR, Moreno D, Lobato MI, Gama CS, Belmonte-de-Abreu PS. Sobrepeso e obesidade em pacientes esquizofrênicos em uso de clozapina comparado com o uso de outros antipsicóticos. *Rev. Psiquiatr. Rio. Gd. Sul.* 2006;2:120-8.

[32] Ryan MC, Thakore JH. Physical consequences of schizophrenia and its treatment: the metabolic syndrome. *Life Sci.* 2002;71(3): 239-57.

[33] Newman SC, Bland RC. Mortality in a cohort of patients with schizophrenia: a record linkage study. Can. J. Psychiatry. 1991;36(4):239-45.

[34] Brown S, Inskip H, Barraclough B. Causes of the excess mortality of Schizophrenia. *Brit. J. Psychiatry.* 2000;177:212-7.

[35] Newcomer JW. Metabolic disturbances associated with antipsychotic use. *J. Clin. Psychiatry.* 2001;62(Suppl 27) :3-4.

[36] Allison DB, Mentore JL, Heo M, Chandler LP, Cappelleri JC, Infante MC, Weiden PJ. Antipsychotic-induced weight gain: a comprehensive research synthesis. *Am. J. Psychiatry.* 1999;156(11):1686-96.

[37] Allison DB, Fontaine KR, Heo M, Mentore JL, Cappelleri JC, handler LP, Weiden PJ, Cheskin LJ. The distribution of body mass index among individuals with and without schizophrenia. *J. Clin. Psychiatry*. 1999;60(4):215-20.
[38] Casey DE, Haupt DW, Newcomer JW, Henderson DC, Sernyak MJ, Davidson M, Lindenmayer JP, Manoukian SV, Banerji MA, Lebovitz HE, Hennekens CH. Antipsychotic-induced weight gain and metabolic abnormalities: implications for increased mortality in patients with schizophrenia. *J. Clin. Psychiatry*. 2004;65 Suppl 7:4-18; quiz 19-20.
[39] Newcomer JW. Metabolic considerations in the use of antipsychotic medications: a review of recent evidence. *J. Clin. Psychiatry*. 2007;68(Suppl 1):20-7.
[40] Baptista T. Body weight gain induced by antipsychotic drug: mechanisms and management. Acta Psychiatr Scand. 1999;100(1):3-16.
[41] 41. Leitão-Azevedo CL, Guimaraes LR, Abreu MG, Gama CS, Lobato MI, Belmonte-de-Abreu PS. Increased dyslipidemia in schizophrenic outpatients using new generation antipsychotics. *Rev. Bras. Psiquiatr*. 2006;28(4):301-4.
[42] Henderson DC, Cagliero E, Gray C, Nasrallah RA, Hayden DL, Schoenfeld DA, Goff DC. Clozapine: diabetes mellitus, weight gain, and lipid abnormalities: a five-year naturalistic study. *Am. J. Psychiatry*. 2000;157(6):975-1.
[43] National Heart, Lung, and Blood Institute Expert Panel on the Identification, Evaluation, and Treatment of Overweight and Obesity in Adults. Clinical guidelines on the identification, evaluation, and treatment of overweight and obesity in adults: the evidence report. *Obes. Res*. 1998;6(Suppl 2):51S-209S.
[44] Toalson P, Ahmed S, Hardy T, Kabinoff G. The metabolic syndrome in patients with severe mental illnesses. *Prim Care Companion J. Clin*. Psychiatry. 2004;6(4):152-8.
[45] Nasrallah HA, Newcomer JW. Atypical antipsychotics and metabolic dysregulation. *J. Clin. Psychopharmacol*. 2004;24(5 Suppl 1):S7-14.
[46] Thakore JH, Mann JN, Vlahos I, Martin A, Reznek R. Increased visceral fat distribution in drug-naïve and drug-free patients with schizophrenia. *Int. J. Obes. Relat. Metab. Disord*. 2002;26(1):137-41.
[47] Ryan MC, Collins P, Thakore JH. Impaired fasting glucose tolerance in first-episode, drug-naïve patients with schizophrenia. *Am. J. Psychiatry*. 2003;160(2):284-9.
[48] Heiskanen T, Niskanen L, Lyytikainen R, Saarinen PI, Hintikka J. Metabolic syndrome in patients with schizophrenia. *J. Clin. Psychiatry*. 2003;64(5):575-9.
[49] Basu R, Brar JS, Chengappa KN, John V, Parepally H, Gershon S, Schlicht P, Kupfer DJ. The prevalence of the metabolic syndrome in patients with schizoaffective disorder - bipolar subtype. *Bipolar. Disord*. 2004;6(4):314-8.
[50] Cohn T, Prud'homme D, Streiner D, Kameh H, Remington G. Characterizing coronary heart disease risk in chronic schizophrenia: high prevalence of the metabolic syndrome. *Can. J. Psychiatry*. 2004;49(11):753-60.
[51] Kato MM, Currier MB, Gomez CM, Hall L, Gonzalez-Blanco M. Prevalence of metabolic syndrome in hispanic and non-hispanic patients with schizophrenia. *Prim. Care Companion J. Clin. Psychiatry*. 2004;6(2):74-7.
[52] Meyer JM. Schizophrenia and the metabolic syndrome. Medscape Psychiatry & Mental Health 2005;8(1):2005 Medscape. Available at: http://www.medscape.com/viewarticle/506136

[53] Enger C, Weatherby L, Reynolds R, Glasser D, Walker A. Serious cardiovascular events and mortality among patients with schizophrenia. *J. Nerv. Ment. Dis.* 2004;192(1):19-27.

[54] Lieberman JA, Stroup TS, McEvoy JP, Swartz MS, Rosenheck RA, Perkins DO, Keefe RS, Davis SM, Davis CE, Lebowitz BD, Severe J, Hsiao JK; Clinical Antipsychotic Trials of Intervention Effectiveness (CATIE) Investigators. Effectiveness of antipsychotic drugs in patients with chronic schizophrenia. *N. Engl. J. Med.* 2005;353(12):1209-23.

[55] McEvoy JP, Meyer JM, Goff DC, Nasrallah HA, Davis SM, Sullivan , Meltzer HY, Hsiao J, Scott Stroup T, Lieberman JA. Prevalence of the metabolic syndrome in patients with schizophrenia: baseline results from the Clinical Antipsychotic Trials of Intervention Effectiveness (CATIE) schizophrenia trial and comparison with national estimates from NHANES III. *Schizophr. Res.* 2005;80(1):19-32.

[56] L'Italien GJ, Meyer J, Koro CE. The prevalence of metabolic syndrome among schizophrenia patients is double that of the general population. Presented at: Annual Meeting of the American Diabetes Association; June 3-8, San Diego, CA.

[57] Bonora E, Targher G, Formentini G, Calcaterra F, Lombardi S, Marini F, Zenari L, Saggiani F, Poli M, Perbellini S, Raffaelli A, Gemma L, Santi L, Bonadonna RC, Muggeo M. The Metabolic Syndrome is an independent predictor of cardiovascular disease in Type 2 diabetic subjects. Prospective data from the Verona Diabetes Complications Study. *Diabet Med.* 2004;21(1):52-8.

[58] Guedes EP. Tratamento do Diabetes Mellitus tipo 2 na Síndrome Metabólica. In: Godoy-Matos AF, organizador. Síndrome Metabólica. São Paulo: Atheneu; 2006. p.177-86.

[59] Mancini MC. Obesidade: da Etiologia ao Diagnóstico. In: Lyra R, Cavalcanti N, organizador. Diabetes Mellitus. Rio de Janeiro: *Diagraphic Editora;* 2006. p. 139-44.

[60] Henderson DC, Copeland PM, Daley TB, Borba CP, Cather C, Nguyen DD, Louie PM, Evins AE, Freudenreich O, Hayden D, Goff DC. A double-blind, placebo-controlled trial of sibutramine forn olanzapineassociated weight gain. *Am. J. Psychiatry.* 2005;162(5):
954-62.

[61] Henderson DC, Fan X, Copeland PM, Borba CP, Daley TB, Nguyen DD, Zhang H, Hayden D, Freudenreich O, Cather C, Evins AE, Goff DC. A double-blind, placebo-controlled trial of sibutramine for clozapine-associated weight gain. *Acta Psychiatr. Scand.* 2007;115(2):101-5.

[62] Taflinski T, Chojnacka J. Sibutramine-associated psychotic episode. Am *J. Psychiatry.* 2000;157(12):2057-8.

[63] Third Report of the National Cholesterol Education Program (NCEP) Expert Panel on Detection, Evaluation, and Treatment of High Blood Cholesterol in Adults (Adult Treatment Panel III). *Circulation.* 2002;106(25):3143-421.

[64] Kraus RM, Eckel RH, Howard B, Appel LJ, Daniels SR, Deckelbaum RJ, Erdman JW Jr, Kris-Etherton P, Goldberg IJ, Kotchen TA, Lichtenstein AH, Mitch WE, Mullis R, Robinson K, Wylie-Rosett J, St Jeor S, Suttie J, Tribble DL, Bazzarre TL. Dietary Guidelines revision 2000. A statement for healthcare professionals from the Nutrition Committee of the American Heart Association. *Circulation.* 2000;102(18):2884-299.

[65] Santos RD. Tratamento das dislipidemias. In: Lopes AC, Martinez TL, organizadores. *Dislipidemias da teoria à* prática. São Paulo: Atheneu; 2004. p. 395-403.
[66] Santos RD. III Diretrizes brasileiras sobre dislipidemias e diretriz de prevenção da aterosclerose do departamento de aterosclerose da sociedade brasileira de cardiologia. *Arq. Bras. Cardiol.* 2001;77 (Supl III):1-48.
[67] Kohen D. Diabetes mellitus and schizophrenia: historical perspective. *Brit. J. Psychiatry Suppl.* 2004;47:s64-6.
[68] Haddad P. Antipsychotics and diabetes: review of non-prospective data. *Brit J Psychiatry Suppl.* 2004;47:s80-6.
[69] Meltzer HY. Illuminating the molecular basis for some antipsychotic drug-induced metabolic burden. *Proc. Natl. Acad. Sci. U S A.* 2007;104(9):3019-20.
[70] Basile VS, Masellis M, McIntyre RS, Meltzer HY, Lieberman JA, Kennedy JL. Genetic dissection of atypical antipsychotic-induced weight gain: novel preliminary data on the pharmacogenetic puzzle. *J. Clin. Psychiatry.* 2001;62(Suppl 23):45-66.

In: The International Psychiatry and Behavioral ...
Editor: Nash Boutros ISBN: 978-1-62257-566-4

Chapter 5

Severe Catatonic Schizophrenia in a 17-Year-Old Adolescent Female*

Barbara Sixt#, Claas van Aaken, Klaus Hennighausen, Christian Fleischhaker and Eberhard Schulz
University Hospital of Freiburg, Department of Child and Adolescent Psychiatry, Freiburg, Germany

Abstract

Objectives: Catatonic symptoms in children and adolescents have not been well investigated and there are hardly any evaluated recommendations for treatment. The present report deals with the course of disease and the therapy of a severe case of catatonic schizophrenia. *Methods:* Reported is the case of a 17-year-old adolescent female suffering from severe, life-threatening catatonic schizophrenia. *Results:* Following unsuccessful pre-treatment, medication with Clozapine markedly improved the pathology. *Conclusions:* Further investigations and case reports about the course of disease and the therapy of the uncommon clinical picture of severe catatonic schizophrenia in children and adolescents are necessary.

Keywords: Catatonic schizophrenia, electroconvulsive therapy, Clozapine, case report

Introduction

Catatonia describes a life threatening, stuporous condition that might occur in various neurological, psychiatric or general medical conditions. The catatonic syndrome is not specific to a certain type of diagnosis.

---

* Original Publication: Sixt B, van Aaken C, Hennighausen K, Fleischhaker C, Schulz E. Severe catatonic schizophrenia in a 17-year-old adolescent. *Z Kinder Jugendpsychiatr Psychother.* 2009 May;37(3):209-14.

Corresponding Author: Barbara Sixt. Department for Child and Adolescent Psychiatry and Psychotherapy - University Clinic Freiburg.

In the psychiatric context, catatonic syndromes occur in schizophrenia (catatonic schizophrenia, ICD-10: F20.2), in organic brain syndromes (organic catatonic disorder, F06.1), in severe depressive episodes with psychotic symptoms (stupor) (F32.3) or in mania (F30.2) as well as in dissociative stupor (F44.2).

Catatonic schizophrenia (F20.2) as a differential diagnosis constitutes a subcategory of schizophrenia according to ICD-10. Primary and essential characteristics are psychomotor disturbances that may alternate between extremes such as agitation and stupor, or between automatic obedience and negativism. Besides the general criteria for the diagnosis of schizophrenia, at least one of the following catatonic symptoms must be present for a minimum of two weeks:

1. Stupor (i. e. significant decrease in responsiveness to the environment and in spontaneous movements and activity) or mutism.
2. Agitation (i. e. apparently futile motor activity, which is not influenced by external stimuli).
3. Posturing (i. e. inappropriate or bizarre postures which are taken and maintained voluntarily).
4. Negativism (i. e. apparently unmotivated resistance against all instructions or attempts to be moved.
5. Rigidity (i. e. maintaining rigid postures resisting efforts to be moved).
6. Waxy flexibility (i. e. maintaining of limbs or body in externally imposed postures).
7. Automatic obedience (i. e. following instructions automatically).

As the most extreme form of catatonia, malignant catatonia (pernicious catatonia) may lead to potential failure of internal organs and is therefore a life-threatening condition. Symptoms are extreme psychomotor disturbance (hypokinetic in most cases), a lack of affective responsiveness, and high fever (without evidence of infection and without inflammation markers in routine laboratory testing). Also a sympathetic, vegetative dysregulation along with tachycardia, electrolyte imbalance and elevated CK levels (as consequences of extreme muscular tension), and possibly also respiratory insufficiency (reduced tidal volume as well as elevated respiration rate). At this time, the underlying biologic dysfunction has not yet been identified.

As a rare side effect of neuroleptic medication, the malignant neuroleptic syndrome (MNS) constitutes a life-threatening, psychiatric emergency in the same manner as malignant catatonia. Its symptoms are similar to those of malignant catatonia while the etiology diverges. The only way to differentiate between MNS and malignant catatonia is by examining the patient's medication history. MNS generally develops within two weeks after commencing a neuroleptic therapy. However, it might occur after months of constant-dose neuroleptic treatment as well. The incidence of MNS is estimated at 0.07 - 0.5 %. In their review, Silva et al. (1999) have found the duration of this illness to be 1 - 119 days. Nine percent of patients had died while 20 % suffered from severe secondary damage. Patients that had been treated with low-dose neuroleptics showed a poorer treatment result. Treatment with Dantrolene had not been reported to have beneficial effects.

All in all, there has been little research on catatonic symptoms in childhood and adolescence up to now. Established therapy recommendations hardly exist.

Case Presentation

Reason for Presentation at Clinic

At the end of July 2005 - five weeks prior to admission to ward at our clinic - Claudia showed acute psychiatric symptoms including ideas of relationships, ideas of persecution, feelings of derealisation, illusionary misjudgement as well as olfactory and gustatory hallucinations according to her parents.

Claudia felt watched. She reported that she could no longer use the telephone, as both the phone and the computer were tapped. Furthermore, she claimed that she was being watched when using the bathroom. On August 3rd, 2005 Claudia completely stopped eating as this would be "disgusting". Moreover, paging through a newspaper on that very day, Claudia looked at a picture showing Franziska van Almsick (a German swimmer) and believed that the photograph would not show the right person and the newspaper "Sport-Bild" was selling lies. Her familiar surroundings seemed "unreal" to her.

Due to an exsiccosis, Claudia was admitted to an internal medicine clinic on August 5th, 2005. Once there, Claudia merely answered questions sporadically in a "yes / no" fashion. According to the ward physician, she was already in a motorically limited and partially agitated condition. She did, however, eat on her own and handle personal hygiene by herself. After one day in the clinic, she withdrew into a corner and appeared to be tense and agitated. She showed merely sporadic responses like "I did not want that" or "I have killed my grandfather".

Claudia positively confirmed that she heard voices. However, she did not answer to the question whether these were familiar voices. Drug screening had been negative for cannabis, amphetamines and heroin. Other laboratory values had been without pathological findings as well.

Eventually, Claudia was admitted to the clinic for child and adolescent psychiatry where she had been treated previously. Upon admission to the clinic, it was decided that it was not possible to meaningfully communicate with her. Claudia suffered from an increasingly severe, muscular hypertension, combined with waxy flexibility, cogwheel phenomenon as well as cataplexy. To some extent, Claudia tracked the examiner with the eyes while rarely showing any spontaneous physical movements (e.g., thumbing through newspapers without reading). Suspecting the diagnosis of catatonic schizophrenia, the initial medication consisted of Zuclopenthixole 50 mg intramuscular and Diazepame 10 mg, 2 times daily followed by a change of medication to Lorazepame 1 mg, 3 times daily up to 2.5 mg, 5 times daily.

This medication regime did not lead to any change of her condition. After three days, a treatment with Olanzapine 15 mg per day was tried. This lead to an initial improvement followed by a change for the worse. After nine days, it was decided that treatment with haloperidole 10 mg i. v., 2 times daily as well as Akineton retard, 4 mg daily be tried. Under this medication, Claudia's withdrawal and muscular catatonia kept progressing, remaining unresponsive and in need of complete nursing care. Intermittently, there had been incidences of elevated body temperature up to 38.5° C without any indication of infection. Other markers for early identification of pernicious catatonia such as myocloniae, pyramidal signs, leukocytosis, increases of creatin kinasis or transaminase, or an elevation of the ESR (erythrocyte sedimentation rate) could not be found. Three weeks after admission to ward,

Claudia was transferred to us for further treatment. At this time, medication had been consisting of haloperidole 10 mg, Atkineton 4 mg and diazepam10 mg, 3 times daily orally.

Patient's Medical History

The patient's medical history completely lacks any pathological findings. In summer 2005, Claudia successfully graduated from school (General Certificate of Secondary Education) with good grades and an average of 2.6. She had planned a gap year in order to do voluntary social work at a kindergarten.

Family Medical History

According to the parents, there had not been any psychiatric disorders in the family. However, in conversations with the patient's mother, she (i.e., the mother) was observed to show a flat affect and barely displays the ability to express changes in emotion.

Psychopathologic Findings at Admission

Patient was a 17-year-old, bed-ridden teenage girl, with physical development appropriate for her age. She was awake but not responsive at most times. However, she sometimes tracks the examiner's finger with her eyes, if asked to. Orientation, attention and memory skills were not verifiable at the time. Content-based train of thought were also not verifiable and hallucinations could not be established.

At times, the patient's mood seemed to be depressed while the ability to express changes in emotion was lacking. She exhibited completely inhibited drive along with inhibited psychomotor activity. Her physical condition, with muscular catatonia, catalepsy and rigor, necessitated full nursing care. Finally, she also exhibited occasional intense vegetative agitation along with recurring subfebrile temperatures up to approximately 38 °C as well as tachycardia up to 120 beats per minute.

Physical / Neurological Findings As Well As Laboratory Values and Somatic Diagnostic Investigation

During the physical examination upon admission to the children's hospital, Claudia presented as a 17-year-old, age-appropriate female adolescent. No other pathological findings except for tachycardia, cataplexia, waxy flexibility and a condition of stuporous vigilance along with dry mucosal membranes in a sense of severe dehydration were found. All analysed laboratory parameters remained in the normal range except for a mild form of iron deficiency anaemia. Lumbar puncture, MRI of skull, EEG, ECG, chest x-ray as well as abdominal sonography showed no pathological findings.

Therapy and Course of Disease

Being in a completely mute condition of severe catatonia, Claudia was transferred to us from the clinic for child and adolescent psychiatry where she had been treated previously. Claudia's distinctive psychopathological abnormalities along with a lack of contact with the external world as well as her severe muscular catatonia, the intermittent fever and tachycardia, required further diagnostic examination. Therefore, we transferred Claudia to our University Clinic Children's Hospital on the very same day of admission.

In our consultative function, we discontinued Haloperidole while keeping Akineton owing to the half-life period of haloperidole. The next day, we changed the medication to lorazepame 7.5 mg i. v. per day, which did not lead to any significant improvement.

Having eliminated any somatic cause and having additionally consulted the psychiatric department for adult patients, we changed the medication to Risperidone 6 mg and Akineton 8 mg maximum. Owing to the severity of symptoms and the resulting high mortality risk, we simultaneously initiated preparations for an electroconvulsive treatment (ECT), as further treatment with neuroleptic medications alone did not seem promising.

With regards to carrying out the ECT without Claudia's consent, we consulted the family court. We were advised, that this can be carried out without any judicial concerns as long as both parents (respectively the persons having the custody and care of a child) give their consent following precise information.

Following Claudia's re-transferral to our clinic and her parents' informed consent, the senior physician in charge of the adjacent adult psychiatry department carried out the first, unitemporal ECT treatment with Claudia's condition remaining psychopathologically unchanged.

During a second, bitemporal ECT treatment two days later, a ventricular tachycardia with subsequent ventricular fibrillation necessitated defibrillation. This made another transfer to the intensive care unit of the University Clinic Children's Hospital necessary. As another questionable cardiac incident happened during the course of Claudia's stay at the Children's Hospital, we kept close contact with the cardiologists, which did not see any indications against a continuation of the ECT's as long as stand-by resuscitation was provided.

While Claudia's psychopatholgogic condition and the catatonic-stuporous rigor remained unchanged, we started treatment with Clozapine in preparation of the next ECT. The parents had been repeatedly informed and had given their consent for the ECT. Under medication with Clozapine, it took a few days until Claudia could re-establish contact with the external world and start communicating by using single words as well as moving with less support from outside.

We rapidly raised the medication dosage to 350 mg/day, which was tolerated well by the patient, who did not suffer from any significant side effects. We cancelled the already planned next ECT.

Eight weeks after admission to the Children's Hospital, Claudia was re-transferred to our clinic on October 04th, 2005. At this time, Claudia had already been able to carry out personal hygiene by herself, eat on her own, move her body and to communicate. At this time, strong fears accompanied by paranoid ideas, fear of intoxication, self-perturbance along with thought diffusion and acoustic hallucinations arose.

As she suffered from negative symptomatology accompanied by increased sleep requirement, a decrease of drive and missing emotional reactivity, Claudia and her parents agreed on gradually increasing the Clozapine dosage up to 425 mg / day. This measure particularly improved social interaction. As a side effect, we observed a gain of weight from 50 to 74 kg at a height of 1.67 m over the period of 11 months (BMI = 27 kg/m²). Furthermore, Claudia suffered from tachycardia, severe constipation and micturition difficulties, which we treated with metoprolol succinate, movicole and pyridostigmine bromide. The negative symptomatology, which had been our main focus during the weeks of treatment that followed, decreased but very slowly and incompletely.

Cognitive performance diagnostics carried out in May 2006, suggested that Claudia's cognitive performance level being slightly below the normal range. There was a slight discrepancy between verbal and performance scales along with a remarkable strength in the retentive auditive memory. Claudia showed weaknesses in both her visual skills with regards to the perception of important visual details and in her spatio-constructive abilities. She also showed slight weaknesses in mathematical thinking, an impairment of concentration and great distractibility.

These findings were considerably worse than one could have possibly expected from a female adolescent with good school grades such as our patient. We therefore took the continuing reduction of cognitive abilities as illness-related.

A retrograde amnesia has existed for the time between start of August and mid-September 2005. Up to her discharge from hospital in July 2006, Claudia had been in need of a structured daily routine and showed distinct negative symptomatology, as well as an increased sleep requirement, lack of drive and significantly reduced emotional reactivity. Follow-up therapy was done in a rehabilitation facility.

DISCUSSION

When 17-year-old Claudia was transferred to us from the Clinic for Child and Adolescent Psychiatry, where she had been treated previously, she had been in a completely mute condition of severe catatonia. The physical examination showed no pathological findings.

No clear treatment recommendations specific to this distinctive symptomatology among female adolescents are provided in the literature.

Solely single case reports regarding treatment by ECT as well as atypical neuroleptics (i. e. Risperidone, Olanzapine, Clozapine) were described in the literature.

Neither pre-treatment with Olanzapine, Haloperidole, Risperidone nor Lorazepame led to any improvement of symptoms. While treatment with ECT had no positive impact on the psychopathological condition, it caused cardiac complications which required resuscitation during the second ECT treatment. Treatment with quickly rising dosages of Clozapine up to 350 mg improved the catatonic symptomatology abruptly. Up to the present day, more than two years after onset, Claudia has stayed free of any relapse under continuous Clozapine treatment.

Regarding the neuroleptic treatment of our patient, we referred to already published single case reports. Kopala and Caudle (1998) have described successfully treating an adolescent suffering from catatonic schizophrenia by treatment with Risperdal (4 mg / day).

The Clinic for Child and Adolescent Psychiatry's attempt (the clinic where Claudia had been treated previously) of a treatment with Olanzapine seems reasonable, given the positive results of treating catatonia with Olanzapine as described in the literature. For instance, Del Bello et al. (2000) have reported on having successfully treated a 16-year-old male adolescent with Olanzapine (20 mg / day) in combination with Valproate (1000 mg / day) and Lorazepame (6 mg / day).

Regarding the ECT in adolescents, which was performed at our premises, life-threatening pernicious catatonia can be considered as the sole legitimate indication, according to the guidelines of the German Society for Child and Adolescent Psychiatry and Psychotherapy (Deutsche Gesellschaft für Kinder- und Jugendpsychiatrie und -pychotherapie). However, there has been no sufficient evidence on treating adolescents with ECT.

Cohen et al. (1999) have found in their review that - even in adolescent patients - both malignant illness course and failure of pharmacotherapy are indicators for the application of ECT. Forty-two adolescents showing catatonic symptoms along with varying principle diagnoses such as bipolar disorder, depressive episodes and schizophrenia have been surveyed in this meta-analysis. ECT was described to be an efficient treatment method for 22 of them.

In their review on catatonia in children and adolescents, Takaoka and Takata (2003) have come to the conclusion that ECT was an efficient method for the treatment of catatonic adolescents, although there have not been any systematic studies yet.

In their review, Moise and Petrides (1996) have described 13 adolescents with varying psychiatric diseases, which have been treated with ECT (1 - 20 treatments) in accordance with the so-called "adult house-standard" at the University Clinic of Stony Brook between 1983 and 1993. Out of these patients, ten have been described as responders while three have been described as non-responders. ECT has proved to be most effective for patients suffering from affective disorders, unspecific psychosis and catatonia.

Etain et al. (2001) have also considered the ECT to be a sensible form of treatment for adolescent patients, especially when it comes to severe psychiatric disorders such as catatonia and the neuroleptic malignant syndrome.

Concerning the legal aspects of treatments with ECT, Zaw et al. (1999) have given recommendations concerning the indication for ECT's as follows: regarding patients < 12 years of age, the indication for an ECT should be assessed by two external experts, while regarding patients > 12 years of age, the ECT should be indicated by at least one external expert.

According to the AACAP's Practice Parameters for the Use of Electroconvulsive Therapy with Adolescents (2004), procedure, risks and benefit of the ECT have to be explained to both patients and their parents. A written consent of at least one of the parents is mandatory. Additionally, the patient should be asked to give either his consent or denial, whereas the patient's ability to give any consent at all is dependent on his mental maturity and the severity of the psychiatric symptoms.

Concerning adult patients with urgent indication for ECT treatment, who are not able to give any consent, the Bundesärztekammer (German Medical Association) postulates the appointment of legal guardians according to the Betreuungsgesetz (law on guardianship). In line with that, the family court in charge informed us that carrying out the ECT treatment without Claudia's consent required detailed information and a written informed consent of both parents (the persons having the custody and the care of the child, respectively).

With regards to ECT treatment in adolescents, the following predominant side effects have been described in various studies according to Remschmidt et al. (2001): headache (42 -

80 %), nausea /vomiting (2 - 64 %) and disturbances of memory (9 - 52 %), cf. Cohen et al. (1997), Ghazziudin et al. (1996), Kutcher and Robertson (1995) and Walter and Rey (1997).

Regarding ECT treatments, Zaw (2006) has described the potential risks of disturbances of the cardio-vascular system, of status epilepticus, of laryngospasms and of peripheral nerve paralysis.

Overall, there is no evidence from available literature that ECT treatments in adolescents are of higher risk compared to adults. Hence, our patient's ventricular tachycardia with subsequent ventricular fibrillation has to be considered as a rare side effect. The consulting pediatricians and cardiologists did not see any contraindications against continuing the ECT treatments. They merely recommended that special attention be paid in order to prepare for a possible resuscitation.

However, having talked to the parents, we decided to start a probationary treatment with Clozapine before the next planned ECT session.

Clozapine as a receptor antagonist ranks among the most potent neuroleptics and shows high affinity for D_4-H_1- and Ach-M_1-receptors, a middle affinity for D_1-, D_3-, Alpha$_1$- and $_5$-HT_2-receptors and a low affinity for D_2-receptors. Numerous studies have described its clear superiority to other typical and atypical neuroleptics - especially when it comes to therapy-resistent schizophrenia (Naber, 2000).

Moreover, the positive outcome of treatment in our case corresponds with the results of the case report of Dursun et al. (2005).

Other new treatment methods could also gain importance in treating catatonic disorders in adolescents. Saba et al. (2002) described the successful treatment of an 18-year-old catatonic female adolescent by transcranial magnet stimulation (TMS) (10 sessions, 1600 stimuli / day, 10 Hz). According to the guidelines of the Deutsche Gesellschaft für Psychatrie, Psychotherapie und Nervenheilkunde (DGPPN), (i. e. German Society for Psychiatry, Psychotherapy and Neurology), however, TMS cannot yet be recommended for the treatment of schizophrenia except for study purposes due to insufficient evidence on its effectivity.

All in all, few case reports and studies on the treatment of children and adolescents suffering from catatonia can be found in the literature. In order to establish sufficient therapy guidelines to help affected patients, further studies and case reports are absolutely necessary.

REFERENCES

Cohen, D., Paillere-Martinot, M. L. and Basquin, M. (1997). Use of electroconvulsive therapy in adolescents. *Convulsive Therapy, 13,* 25-31.

Cohen D., Flament M., Dubos P. F. and Basquin M. (1999). Case series: Catatonic Syndrome in Young People. *Journal of the American Academy of Child and Adolescent Psychiatry, 38,* 1040-1046.

DelBello M., Foster K. D. and Strakowski S. M. (2000). Case report: Treatment of Catatonia in an Adolescent Male. *Journal of Adolescent Health, 27,* 69-71.

Dursun S. M., Hallak J. E. C., Haddad P., Leahy A., Byrne A., Strickland P. L., Anderson I. M., Zuardi A. W. and Deakin J. F. W. (2005). Clozapine monotherapy for catatonic schizophrenia: Should clozapine be the treatment of choice, with catatonia rather than psychosis as the main therapeutic index? *Journal of Psychopharmacology, 19,* 432-433.

Etain B., Le Heuzey M. F. and Mouren-Simeoni M. C. (2001). Electroconvulsivethérapie chez l´adolescent: considérations cliniques á propos d´une série d´observations. *Canadian journal of Psychiatry, 46,* 976-981.

Saba G., Rocamora J. F., Kalalou K., Benadhira R., Plaze M., Aubriot-Delmas B. and Januel D. (2002). Catatonia and Transcranial Magnetic Stimulation. *American Journal of Psychiatry, 159,* 1794.

Ghaziuddin, N., King, C. A., Naylor, M. W., Ghaziuddin, M., Chaudary, C. Giordani, B., DeQuardo, J. R., Tandon, R. and Greden, J.F. (1996) Electroconvulsive treatment in adolescents with pharmacotherapy refractory depression. *Journal of Child and Adolescent Psychopharmacology, 6,* 259-71.

Hung Y., Yang P. and Huang T. (2006). Clozapine in schizophrenia patients with recurrent catatonia: Report of two cases. *Psychiatry and Clinical Neurosciences, 60,* 256-258.

Kopala L. C. and Caudle C. (1998). Acute and longer-term effects of risperidone in a case first-episode catatonic schizophrenia. *Journal of Psychopharmacology, 12,* 314-317.

Kutcher, S. and Robertson, H. A. (1995). Electroconvulsive therapy in treatment resistant bipolar youth. *Journal of Child and Adolescent Psychopharmacology, 5,* 167-75.

Moise F. and Petrides G. (1996). Case study: Electroconvulsive Therapy in Adolescents. *Journal of the American Academy of Child and Adolescent Psychiatry, 35,* 312-318.

Naber, D. (2000) *Atypische Neuroleptika in der Behandlung schizophrener Patienten.* Bremen: UNI-MED. 103-104.

Silva, R. S., Munoz, D. M., Alpert, M., Perlmutter, I. R. and Diaz, J. (1999). *Journal of the American Academy of Child and Adolescent Psychiatry, 38,* 187-193.

Remschmidt H., Martin, M., Hennighausen, K., Schulz, E. (2001) Treatment and rehabilitation in Remschmidt H., *Schizophrenia in children and adolescents, Cambridge University Press*, 192-267.

Takaoka K. and Takata T. (2003). Catatonia in childhood and adolescence. *Psychiatry and Clinical Neurosciences, 57,* 129-137.

Walter, G. and Rey, J. M. (1997). An epidemiological study of the use of ECT in adolescents. *Journal of the American Academy of Child and Adolescent Psychiatry, 36,* 809-15.

Zaw F.K.M., Bates G.D., Murali V. and Bentham P. (1999). Catatonia, autism and ECT. *Developmental Medicine and Child Neurology, 41,* 843-845.

Zaw F.K.M. (2006). ECT and the youth: Catatonia in Context. *International Review of Neurobiology, 72,* 207-231.

In: The International Psychiatry and Behavioral ...
Editor: Nash Boutros
ISBN: 978-1-62257-566-4

Chapter 6

THE EFFECTS OF PHARMACOTHERAPY IN PSYCHIATRY: IMPACT, PERCEPTION AND INTERPRETATION

Slawomir Murawiec *
Mental Health Centre, The Institute of Psychiatry and Neurology,
Warszawa, Poland

ABSTRACT

Biological activity of psychopharmacological agents extends from intracellular level to its impact on highly integrated mental functions. On this last mentioned level, pharmacological agents modulate salience (antipsychotics) and emotional processing, processing of social cues, emotional memory, attentional vigilance, and threat processing (antidepressants and anxiolitics). This level of the effect of medication is situated at the border of person's abilities to perceive it and then verbalize it. The effect of medication is then subjectively perceived in the context of individual insight and personality (on the basis of emotional, cognitive, behavioural or social context). The perceptions of the effects of medication are then interpreted by patient, physician and all other persons directly or indirectly involved in psychopharmacological process. The ultimate description and evaluation of pharmacology is based on this last process of interpretation.

Keywords: pharmacotherapy, psychiatry, perception, interpretation, psychosis, anxiety, depression

INTRODUCTION

It is the aim of this paper to present the observations made in the course of clinical work, against the background of recent scientific publications on the impact of medication in the

* Contact details: Sławomir Murawiec, Centrum Zdrowia Psychicznego, Instytut Psychiatrii i Neurologii, Al. Sobieskiego 9, 02-957 Warszawa, e-mail: smurawiec@gmail.com, Tel : +48 22 45 82 751

pharmacotherapy of mental diseases and disorders. Based on these two sources (clinical observation and analysis of the literature) an attempt has been made here to form certain generalizations, and draw conclusions from a range of basic phenomena taking place in the course of pharmacological treatment in psychiatry.

The effects of medication are perceptible on many levels; starting with sub-cellular levels, the effects that drugs have on the activity of receptors and neurotransmitters, following to more complex neurological brain systems, and finally to the modification of the perception of essential stimuli and representations, including the ways information is processed in the brain. None of these stages are available to direct subjective perception; no one is directly aware of them and they cannot be verbalised. In fact, the effects of medication are verbalized after a subjective perception of their impact. The perception of the activity of medication takes place on a level different to where it actually happens, yet it is accessible to consciousness. For example, let us assume that antidepressants have an impact on processing emotional information. Our subjective perceptions will not be about this level of their activity, instead, they will focus on the indirect effects of medication, which might be verbalized as "I cry less" or "I go out more". Individually observed effects of medication are a far-transformed and based on individual factors way of transcribing the real impact of medication into subjectively perceived changes, and ways of verbalising them, whereas the subjectively perceived impact of medication and the related change in patient's behaviour provide a basis for interpreting the impact of medication and the effects of treatment. These interpretations are made by everyone involved in the treatment process directly or indirectly. They are of individual character and are a combination of individual contexts of all these people, and therefore might be, and often are, mutually contradictory. It is, however, only the interpretation level that gives a final shape to the effects of treatment and makes its evaluation possible.

Perceptions of the clinical effects of medication in a medical context i.e. as "improved mood", "disappearance of psychotic symptoms" are processes very far from the real activity of medication, based on the complex cognitive concepts (e.g. depression, psychosis) that are encoded through education in a doctor's mind, but they are nevertheless useful.

And so the processes that take place between the time medication is administered, taken and the effects of its activity are observed, are rarely noticed as they happen on many levels. The aim of this paper is therefore to propose three separate stages, each of them with a very complex inner structure and practically unlimited number of variations. These stages are:

- basic biological activity of medication on many levels of brain/mind functions
- perceptions of this biological activity
- interpretation of the biological impact by many people involved in therapy and in a variety of contexts.

Each of the stages proposed here, involves a great deal of phenomena, taking place on many levels and in many contexts. It is enough to realize how much information we actually have on the biological activity of medication, starting with sub-cellular and cellular level, all the way to its impact on information processing, and the level of its activity affecting psychopathological symptoms in the course of pharmacologically treated illnesses.

The presentation of such knowledge would require a multifaceted approach, in which the principal concept of this paper would be lost. This is why it is important to be aware of the fact that each of the stages of pharmacotherapy sketched here has practically infinite number of variations and is influenced by multiple factors, yet listing them all is not a subject of this work. The main reason for leaving out excessive detail is opting out for clear presentation the main concept. So going back to the example quoted before, the possible number of genetic, metabolic, individual pharmacokinetic, possible interactions, and other variables that have an impact on the pharmacological workings of medication is difficult to evaluate and practically almost impossible to describe. So for the clarity of argument, I suggest accepting the premise that medication causes biological activity, although in other contexts it is important to realize that this is not the case in all circumstances and that the impact we are talking about here might be extremely individually varied. Similarly, it is impossible within one paper do discuss all the factors that influence the stage of perceiving the activity of medication. This is because the number of factors influencing the interpretation of the activity of medication, the number of contexts in which interpretations are made and their changeability throughout time leave us with two options: choosing casuistic descriptions and making high level generalizations that summarise the discussed phenomena or grouping them into very spacious categories.

Biological Activity of Medication

Biological activity of drugs takes place on many levels, beginning with sub-cellular structures, through the level of synapses and receptors, activities of neuronal systems (dopaminergic, serotoninergic etc.), neuroplasticity, lipid peroxidation and finally more complex brain systems and probably in many other dimensions. The activity of medication within the biological systems mentioned here is not accessible to direct subjective observation.

It is expressed on the level of more integrated brain/mind functions, which lie beyond the boundary open to direct perception and verbalization based on subjective experience. For example antipsychotic drugs dampen excessive salience of external stimuli and internal representations [1, 2, 3]. In this case the mesolimbic dopamine system that is overactive in psychosis is calmed down, which stops the psychotic process of attributing aberrant salience to otherwise neutral external stimuli. In effect, a persons treated with antipsychotic drugs experiences lower intensity of signals and representations identified as "meaningful", and clinically they no longer refer all external signals originating in their environment to themselves. Similar processes can be detected in the treatment of depression. As many recent research results indicate [4, 5, 6, 7, 8, 9], the impact of antidepressants may change the ways in which emotionally relevant information or social stimuli are being processed. It also dulls the sensitivity to information in interactions with other people and affects emotional memory. Depressive persons display certain characteristic bias in processing emotionally charged information and interactions, and the research quoted above also implies that the effects of antidepressants can modify the distorted reception of signals and information analysis. Also new studies are being published that discuss the way in which anxiolytics (diazepam) modify perception centres, processing information of a social character or stimuli that cause anxiety. [10] Yet still these changes are still impossible to be perceived and named directly.

A helpful analogy may be found in the impact of antibiotics on bacteria that respond to it – the process is also outside of the reach of subjective perception. What can be perceived, however, at the beginning of the treatment is general impressions, such as "I feel somehow better", and then specific manifestations of clinical improvement, such as "lowering body temperature, or intensity of other symptoms, such as cough, muscle pains etc."

Psychoactive drugs can be discussed in the analogical context. Their impact on both sub-cellular and receptor level, and the level of integrated neuronal systems is not subjectively perceived. The way this medication works at the higher levels of the organisation of neurological systems can not be perceived subjectively (patients never mention the "improvement in processing emotional information" as the description of what is happening to them or "the reduction in attributing excessive salience to external stimuli").

Future research will certainly provide new data about the way medication used in psychiatry essentially works, especially with respect of more integrated brain/mind functions. They will certainly focus on the complex impact of medication on processing information in the brain, its influence on the analysis of information perceived from the outside, attention, memory and other functions. However, it seems that the principle described in this paper may still be treated as universal. The biological activity of medication on many levels remains impossible to perceive subjectively. On more complex levels, however, such as for example information processing, it lies on the boundary between unclear subjective perception originating at a biological level and the possibility to perceive things consciously. It is clear though that the clinical effects of medication must be perceived and noticed in the context of an individual person, and it is only as a result of this subjective perception that the information that "the drug works" emerges in the awareness of the treated person.

PERCEPTION OF THE IMPACT OF MEDICATION

The effect of the activity of medication must be subjectively perceived by a patient, doctor or other people, such as the patient's family, other patients, nurses, ward managers etc. This perception does not take place, however, on the level that the drug „actually" works at i.e. on the level described above. It is rather focused on the subjective perception of change in perceiving things, thinking, emotional responses, behaviour, relations with other people etc.

This perception can vary in character, for example it can be:

- sensory ("I have begun to notice colours")
- somatic ("I'm not in so much pain now")
- cognitive ("My thoughts are clearer")
- emotional ("I can feel my emotions again")
- observation of behaviour ("I cry less and smile more")
- mood changes ("My mood has improved")
- physical fitness ("I can walk faster")
- increased level of activity ("I began going out again")
- social relations ("I'm in touch with people again")

And so a patient who is treated with an antipsychotic drug can, for example, notice that she is no longer stared at in the street. A patient with depression can notice that she cries less or that she can see colours more vividly. She will not notice how the drug actually affects her subjective experience but the perception will be indirect in character; a patient will simply notice certain subjective displays of the impact of medication.

In the first stages of the activity of medication, the process itself takes place on the border between a biological and subjective level, which means that the effects of its activity, such as changes in the way one feels might be subjectively felt on a psychosomatic level (feelings, impressions, sensations of unspecific general change), but they can not be fully verbalized on the conscious level. In schizophrenia, this is reflected in the research on the early subjective response to neuroleptics. [11]. The response, tested 24 and 48 hours after the first dosage of medication is taken, is based on subjectively felt biological changes caused by medication. What's important and interesting is that it allows for forecasting the efficiency of treatment over a period of a few weeks (early positive response correlates with positive clinical response to administered medication.) In this and the next stages of the activity of medication, a process takes place which has an additional effect on the dimensions described above – the process referred to as a "placebo effect". Kapsambelis has noted that "... the notion of placebo effect is somehow inaccurately used when it comes to psychoactive drugs." [12]

It is because the problem that appears in psychiatry is that the impact area of psychoactive drugs is identical to the area where the effect of the influence of one mind on another takes place, one psyche on another." [12, p.123]. In biological dimensions the "placebo" and "nocebo" effects are accompanied by a corresponding increase or decrease of endogenous dopamine transmission and excretion of opioids. [13]

And so both of these effects have simultaneously a psychological (expectations of the impact of medication) and biological (through the activity of appropriate neuronal systems linked to controlling the way one feels) components. The impact of medication in this context can be identified as the combined biological activity of the medication and the psychological/biological impact of the placebo or nocebo effect.

In some cases a patient might not notice the effect of the medication even if the effect is clearly perceived by other people. Sometimes a doctor or patient's family notice the changes in patient's behaviour brought about by the treatment, whereas the patient neither notices it or talks about it. This might happen for various reasons, such as the patient's intellectual deficits, lack of insights into their own emotional states, the activity of medication being different to the patient's expectations or the unconscious rejection of noticing the impact of medication due to intrapsychic conflicts.

Interpretation of the Activity of Medication

The stage described above involves noticing certain specific manifestations of how the medication is actually working for a patient. In the next stage, these very manifestations are being interpreted by:

- the person under the treatment
- the doctor

- other professionals in the treatment context (nurses, psychologists, other doctors)
- persons close to the patient (family)
- other people in the patient's social network (acquaintances, colleagues)
- bosses, directors, insurers and other institutions involved in the process of controlling the treatment etc.

The main problem with describing this phase of treatment is linked to the fact that there might be as many of these individual interpretations as there are individual treatment processes. The interpretations can take place in very different contexts (occurring simultaneously in the same person). The interpretations of the changes observed in the patients are made by the patient, the doctor in charge, and the patient's family. Each of these people might notice different changes and interpret them differently. The contexts of these interpretations are fully individual.

For example, increased activity of a schizophrenic patient might be interpreted by the patient as a sign that the previously administered medication was harmful, and therefore it is best to stop treatment; a doctor in charge may think in terms of reduced intensity of negative symptoms, and the patient's family might feel endangered and fear that the patient's aggressive behaviour that occurred in the past might return on this occasion. Each one of the people involved in this treatment process interprets, and therefore evaluates the change that they observe differently, and this is why their treatment-related behaviour might be entirely different. These interpretations will also change throughout time. For example if a patient's increased level of activity results in his or her increased involvement in housework or employment, the family might be willing to change their interpretation of the same treatment-related processes. Because of the complexity of this stage of treatment, it is often described on two levels: first on the casuistic level and second on grouping certain phenomena related to the individual interpretations of treatment. Casuistic descriptions provide examples of very individual situations which may take place during pharmacological treatment, whereas other illustrative work provides summaries of what is going on, taking into the account various groups of phenomena that influence the interpretation of the treatment process, linked with, for example, psychopathological symptoms, levels of insight, characteristics of medication, adverse reactions to treatment etc.

Interpretation of the Effects of Medication in the Context of Diagnosing Illnesses and Dysfunctions

It is worth noting here that a doctor in charge of treatment interprets and evaluates these processes on the basis of a certain system of reference points.

- first of all, the doctors extract from the patient's account the information that they consider important in the overall context of treatment, most frequently in the context of psychopathological symptoms (for example they will consider it relevant if the patient says what she or he is in a better mood, but not if the patient has a stronger sense of smell)

- secondly the doctor makes use of very complex conceptual notions, such as depressive disorder, positive symptoms, negative symptoms, psychosis.

Therefore, it appears there is a very complex correlation in many intermediate stages between the "real" activity of medication and the doctor noticing it on a clinical level, in relation how the psychopathological symptoms are disappearing or to the treatment of a specific illness. This "real" activity of medication may include, for example, its impact on distorted processing of information, whereas the clinical evaluation is formulated on the level of the overall improvement in a certain group of symptoms distinguished "apriori" or based on the fact that "the episode of the illness is disappearing". Between these effects of medication and their interpretations on a clinical level there is a large space for the phenomena that are actually taking place and the concepts used for describing them, whose existence usually goes unnoticed.

Relevance of Doctor Patient Relationship

The doctor –patient relationship has an important impact on the phenomena presented here, at each of the stages I have attempted to identify so far. Even before a pharmacological treatment is actually undertaken, the person that comes for treatment has certain expectations and ideas about the doctor and the medication that they will be exposed to. These preconceptions are then reflected in the workings of the placebo and nocebo effect. In reference to the pharmacological impact of medication, the impact of the patient-doctor relationship on the effects of medication used in psychiatry has been described on more than one occasion. Various factors linked with this relationship such as emotional aspects, conscious and unconscious elements of the dyad (transference and countertransference) may seriously modify and sometimes even block the effects of the biological activity of medication. [14, 15, 16] Psychiatrists are often the key persons at the stage of making observations about how medication works. Based on the patient's account, they often select the one change, that is actually the result of medication and communicate this to the patient. The doctors also communicate what is a desirable (good) effect of the medication and what is "bad" or undesirable. In this way, they essentially or sometimes even exclusively influence the subjective perceptions of the effects of the activity of medication. A similar role is played by the patient-doctor relationship at the stage of interpreting the changes in the way a patient feels and behaves. Psychiatrists provide their own interpretations and communicate them to the patient directly or indirectly by their behaviour or emotional responses to the patient), thus essentially influencing the patient's evaluation of the observed effects of medication, their behaviour and compliance.

Conclusion

This paper makes an attempt to justify the thesis that there are many levels at which the biological activity of medication used in psychiatry cannot be perceived subjectively. Their impact on the integrated mental functions (for example processing of social and emotional information, memory and attention) take place in the border areas of the possibilities of subjective perceptions, whereas the effect of the activity of medication remains observed by the patients in the context of their individual capacity for insight, mood changes in the context of personality changes. Later on, this effect is subjectively interpreted in many contexts, which gives a final shape to the evaluation of the impact of the medication used.

REFERENCES

[1] Kapur S. Psychosis as a state of aberrant salience: a framework linking biology, phenomenology, and pharmacology in schizophrenia. *Am. J. Psychiatry.* 2003 Jan;160(1):13-23.

[2] Kapur S.: How antipsychotic become anti-psychotic – from dopamine to salience to psychosis. *Trends Pharmacol. Sc,* 2004; 25: 402-406.

[3] Kapur S., Mizrahi R., Li M.: From dopamine to salience to psychosis –linking biology, pharmacology and phenomenology of psychosis. *Schizophr. Res.*, 2005; 79: 59-68. 16.

[4] Harmer C.J., Bhagwagar Z., Perrett D.I., Völlm B.A., Cowen P.J., Goodwin G.M.: Acute SSRI administration affects the processing of social cues in healthy volunteers. *Neuropsychopharmacol.*, 2003; 28: 148-152.

[5] Bowins B.: How psychiatric treatments can enhance psychological defense mechanisms. *Am. J. Psychoanalysis*, 2006;66,2, DOI: 10.1007/s11231-006-9014-6.

[6] Harmer C.J.: Serotonin and emotional processing: does it help explain antidepressant drug action? *Neuropharmacology,* 2008; 55:1023-1028.

[7] Harmer CJ, O'Sullivan U, Favaron E, Massey-Chase R, Ayres R, Reinecke A, Goodwin GM, Cowen PJ.: Effect of acute antidepressant administration on negative affective bias in depressed patients. *Am. J. Psychiatry.* 2009 Oct;166(10):1178-84.

[8] Arnone D., Horder J., Cowen P.J., Harmer C.J.: Early effects of mirtazapine on emotional processing. *Psychopharmacol.*, 2009; 203: 685-691.

[9] Tang TZ, DeRubeis RJ, Hollon SD, Amsterdam J, Shelton R, Schalet B.: Personality change during depression treatment: a placebo-controlled trial. *Arch. Gen. Psychiatry.* 2009 Dec;66(12):1322-30.

[10] Murphy S.E., Downham C., Cowen P.J., Harmer C.J.: Direct effect of diazepam on emotional processing in healthy volunteers. *Psychopharmacol.,* 2008; 199: 503-513.

[11] Awad A.G.: Subjective response to neuroleptics in schizophrenia. Schizophr. Bull. 1993;19: 609-617.

[12] Kapsambelis V.: Pacjent, przepisujący receptę i psychosomatyczne doświadczenie leku. podejście psychoanalityczne. W: Murawiec S., Żechowski C. (red.): Od neurobiologii do psychoterapii. *Instytut Psychiatrii i Neurologii*, Warszawa 2009. s.122-139.

[13] Scott D., Stohler C.S., Egnatuk C.M., wang H., Koeppe R.A., Zubieta J.K.: Placebo and nocebo effects are defined by opposite opioid and dopaminergic responses. *Arch. Gen. Psychiatry* 2008; 65(2): 220-231.

[14] Murawiec S.: Psychodynamiczna interpretacja działania leków psychotropowych. W: Murawiec S., Żechowski C. (red.): Od neurobiologii do psychoterapii. *Instytut Psychiatrii i Neurologii,* Warszawa 2009. s.140-219.

[15] Mintz D.: Meaning and medication in the care of treatment-resistant patients. *Am. J. Psychotherapy* 2002;56: 322-335.

[16] Mintz D., Belnap B.: A view from Riggs. Treatment resistance and patient authority – III. What is psychodynamic psychopharmacology? An approach to pharmacologic treatment resistance. *J. Am. Acad. Psychoanal. Dyn. Psychiatr.* 2006; 34: 581- 600.

In: The International Psychiatry and Behavioral ...
Editor: Nash Boutros
ISBN: 978-1-62257-566-4

Chapter 7

THE SCHIZOPHRENIA COGNITION RATING SCALE JAPANESE VERSION (SCORS-J)*

***Yasuhiro Kaneda**[*1], **Yoshinori Ueoka**[2], **Tomiki Sumiyoshi**[3], **Norio Yasui-Furukori**[4], **Toru Ito**[3], **Yuko Higuchi**[3], **Ichiro Kawamura**[5] **and Michio Suzuki**[3], **Tetsuro Ohmori**[2]*

[1]Department of Psychiatry, Iwaki Clinic, Anan, Japan
[2]Department of Psychiatry, Tokushima University Hospital, Tokushima, Japan
[3]Department of Neuropsychiatry, University of Toyama Graduate School of Medicine and Pharmaceutical Sciences, Toyama, Japan
[4]Department of Neuropsychiatry, Graduate School of Medicine, Hirosaki University, Hirosaki Japan
[5]Department of Psychiatry, Fujii Hospital, Anan, Japan

ABSTRACT

The assessment of cognitive function is important for patients with schizophrenia because cognitive impairment is a core feature of the disease, and is a major determinant of functional outcome. So far, an extensive neuropsychological test battery, consisting of several tests of key domains of cognition, has been employed to evaluate cognitive deficits of schizophrenia. To implement a practical assessment tool, we previously developed the Japanese-language version of the Brief Assessment of Cognition in Schizophrenia (BACS-J) that objectively measures cognitive domains relevant to outcome. The Schizophrenia Cognition Rating Scale (SCoRS) has been developed as a new interview-based measure of cognition. It consists of 20 questions to measure attention, memory, reasoning and problem solving, working memory, language production, and motor skills, which are related to day-to-day functioning. For its clinical application, we developed the Japanese-language version of the SCoRS (SCoRS-J) through back-translation into English, which was checked by the author of the scale. In

* Corresponding author: Yasuhiro KANEDA, M.D., Ph.D. Department of Psychiatry, Iwaki Clinic, 11-1 Kamimizuta, Gakubara, Anan, Tokushima 774-0014, Japan, Telephone number: +81-884-23-5600, Facsimile number: +81-884-22-1780, E-mail: kaneday-tsh@umin.ac.jp

this paper, psychometric properties of the SCoRS-J are presented with data from patients with schizophrenia.

Keywords: Cognitive function, Japanese version, Neuropsychology, Psychometrics, Schizophrenia, Schizophrenia Cognition Rating Scale (SCoRS)

1. Introduction

The assessment of cognitive function is an important step in evaluating patients with schizophrenia because of the extensive evidence that cognitive impairment is a core feature of schizophrenia, as well as a key determinant of functional outcome [4, 5]. Cognitive domains specifically impaired in schizophrenia include attention (vigilance) /information processing, executive function, learning memory, working memory, and verbal fluency. For assessing cognitive function in schizophrenia, an extensive neuropsychological test battery (NTB), usually consisting of 8-12 tests tapping each of several tests for the putative neurocognitive domains, has been employed. These NTBs are, generally, time consuming, technically difficult, and costly. Thus, a quick and efficient tool for measuring cognition would be useful for clinicians in considering psychosocial rehabilitation, as well as for researchers implementing clinical trials to assess cognitive improvement.

In this regard, we introduced the Brief Assessment of Cognition in Schizophrenia (BACS), and prepared the Japanese-language version (BACS-J) [7, 8]. Meanwhile, the National Institute of Mental Health Measurement and Treatment Research to Improve Cognition in Schizophrenia (NIMH-MATRICS) Initiative was created to stimulate the development of cognition-enhancing drugs for schizophrenia, and developed a consensus cognitive battery for clinical trials of cognition-enhancing treatments for schizophrenia through a broadly based scientific evaluation: the MATRICS Consensus Cognitive Battery. However, the U.S. Food and Drug Administration (FDA) indicated at the MATRICS meetings that significant improvement on a consensus cognitive performance endpoint would be necessary, but not sufficient, for drug approval. In addition to changes in cognitive performance, the FDA required improvements on a functionally meaningful co-primary measure that would have more face validity for consumers and clinicians than cognitive performance measures. Panel members from an FDA-NIMH-MATRICS Workshop on Clinical Trial Designs for Neurocognitive Drugs for Schizophrenia suggested two potential types of assessment techniques for consideration as co-primary measures [11]: functional capacity (Maryland Assessment of Social Competence; MASC [2] and University of California at San Diego Performance-Based Skills Assessment; UPSA [13]) and interview-based assessment of cognition (Schizophrenia Cognition Rating Scale; SCoRS [9] and Clinical Global Impression of Cognition in Schizophrenia ; CGI-CogS [14]). Psychometric properties of all of the measures were considered acceptable [6].

Previous studies of interview-based assessments of cognitive function have reported either nonsignificant or small correlations with cognitive performance [9]. In addition, these studies have relied merely upon a self-report or clinicians' impression, and observation from a caregiver is required to obtain a more accurate view of functioning levels of patients. Accordingly, the SCoRS was developed as an interview-based measure which meets the validity criteria defined by the FDA-NIMH-MATRICS panel [9]. The SCoRS includes informant reports about cognitive performance relevant to real-world functioning [9], and has high test-retest reliability [6]. The aim of this study was to test the validity and usefulness of the Japanese-language version of the SCoRS (SCoRS -J).

2. METHODS

2.1. Translation of the SCoRS

Table 1 shows the SCoRS–J items. In order to have an approved translation of the SCoRS, the following translation methodology was used: two independent forward translations, reconciliation, two independent back translations, and pilot testing on five people with schizophrenia. The author of the scale checked the back-translation.

Table 1. The Schizophrenia Cognition Rating Scale Japanese version (SCoRS-J)

1．知人あるいは面識のある人の名前を覚える
2．場所への行き方を覚える
3．テレビ番組の筋を追う
4．物を置いた場所を覚える
5．用事や責務を覚える
6．道具や機器の使用法を学び，使う
7．与えられたばかりの情報および，あるいはまた教示を覚える
8．言おうとしていたことを覚えておく
9．お金を管理する
10．混乱せずに話す
11．集中して新聞あるいは本を読む
12．慣れた作業を行う
13．集中を持続させる
14．新しい事を学習する
15．考えを言葉にして，思ったとおり迅速に話す
16．物事を迅速に行う
17．日課の変更に対応する
18．話かけられていることの意味を理解する
19．他人が物事をどう感じているか理解する
20．集団の中で会話についてゆく

2.2. Subjects

Subjects for the present study were in/outpatients with chronic schizophrenia seen mainly at the University Hospital of Tokushima, Toyama, and Hirosaki. Sixty-four patients were recruited. The diagnosis was based on Diagnostic and Statistical Manual of the American

Psychiatric Association (DSM)-IV criteria for schizophrenia [1], a detailed clinical interview, and review of the prior records. In the subjects, hepatic and renal functions were normal, and subjects were excluded if they presented with any organic central nervous system disorder, significant substance abuse, or mental retardation. The study was performed in accordance with the Declaration of Helsinki II. The patients who gave informed consent to the research participated in this study. Table 2 shows the demographic characteristics of the subjects.

Table 2. Demographic characteristics of the sample

	Total (n=64)	Tokushima (n=15)	Toyama (n=29)	Hirosaki (n=20)
Age	36.7 (13.8)	52.0 (14.1)	29.1(8.3)	36.3(9.5)
Duration of the illness (years)	13.2 (12.5)	25.6(14.6)	5.1(4.8)	15.4(9.5)
Education (years)	13.1 (2.4)	12.0 (3.3)	14.1(2.2)	12.3(1.0)
BPRS-J (total)	38.0 (9.6)	34.8 (10.3)	39.5(9.4)	38.9(9.1)
SCoRS-J (interviewer global rating)	4.0 (1.8)	2.7 (1.1)	3.8(1.7)	5.2 (1.7)

Data are given as mean (SD).
BPRS-J=Brief Psychiatric Rating Scale Japanese version.

2.3. Assessment Procedures

The SCoRS is a 20-item interview-based assessment of cognitive deficits and the degree to which they affect day-to-day functioning. A global rating is also generated. The items were developed to assess the cognitive domains of attention, learning and memory, reasoning and problem solving, working memory, language production, processing/motor skills, and social cognition.

These areas were chosen due to the severity of impairment of these domains in many patients with schizophrenia, and the demonstrated relationship of these areas of cognitive deficit to impairments in aspects of functional outcome [4, 5]. Two examples of items from the SCoRS are: "Do you have difficulty with remembering names of people you know?" and "Do you have difficulty following a TV show?" Each item is rated on a 4-point rating scale. Higher ratings reflect a greater degree of impairment. It is possible to make a rating of "N/A" for "not applicable" (e.g., if the patient is illiterate, items related to reading are rated as "N/A").

Each item has anchor points for all levels of the 4-point scale. The anchor points for each item focus on the degree of impairment and the degree to which the deficit impairs day-to-day functioning. Interviewers considered cognitive deficits only and did their best to rule-out non-cognitive sources of the deficits. For example, a patient may have had severe difficulty managing money because he/she never learned how to count money, which would suggest that the limitation was related to level of education and not cognitive impairment.

Complete administration of the SCoRS included two separate sources of information that generated three different ratings: an interview with the patient, an interview with a caregiver of the patient (family member, friend, social worker, etc.) and a rating by the interviewer who administered the scale to the patient and caregiver. The caregiver based his or her responses on interaction with and knowledge of the patient; we aimed to identify as the caregiver the person who had the most regular contact with the patient in everyday situations. The interviewer's rating reflected a combination of the two interviews incorporating the interviewer's observations of the patient.

The caregiver ratings were completed within 7 days of the administration of the patient scale. A global scale was rated by the patient, caregiver, and interviewer after the 20 items were rated. For the patient and caregiver interviews, the global rating reflects the informant's (patient or caregiver) overall impression of the patient's level of cognitive difficulty in the 20 areas of cognition assessed, and is rated 1 – 10. In order to examine the validity of the SCoRS-J, the relationship of the SCoRS-J to BACS-J was determined. The BACS-J takes approximately 30 minutes, and is devised for easy administration and scoring by non-psychologists.

It is specifically designed to measure treatment-related improvements, and includes alternate forms. The BACS-J has high test-retest reliability, and is as sensitive to cognitive dysfunction in schizophrenia as standard 2 ½ hour batteries. The BACS-J includes brief assessments of verbal memory, working memory, motor speed, verbal fluency, attention and processing speed, and executive function, and its composite scores are calculated by averaging all z-scores of the six primary measures from the BACS-J, using means and standard deviations. The 18-item Brief Psychiatric Rating Scale (BPRS [12], 1-7 score) was completed by a trained psychiatrist along with the SCoRS-J and BACS-J.

2.4. Data Analyses

Data analyses were conducted using JMP-8.0.1.J for Mac software. Descriptive statistics were used to report socio-demographic and clinical data. Cronbach's alpha [3] was used to determine the internal consistency of the SCoRS-J. The relationship between the measures was determined by calculating Pearson correlations among the scores. The level of significance was set at $p<0.05$.

3. Results

3.1. Reliability Assessments

Internal consistency using Cronbach's coefficient alpha was found to be 0.95. Examination of the contribution of the individual items to the total scale scores indicated that there were no items whose deletion would have improved the overall internal consistency of the scale more than 0.01. The interviewer global ratings were highly correlated with a mean of the 20 items (r=0.85, $p<0.0001$; Table 3).

The interviewer global ratings were also highly correlated with the global ratings based upon the interview with the caregiver (r=0.87, $p<0.00001$) and those with the patient (r=0.82, $p<0.0001$).

Table 3. The relationship between SCoRS-J interviewer global ratings and items

Item	r
1	0.28*
2	0.52****
3	0.56****
4	0.45***
5	0.45***
6	0.41***
7	0.65****
8	0.55****
9	0.60****
10	0.75****
11	0.57****
12	0.55****
13	0.68****
14	0.63****
15	0.67****
16	0.67****
17	0.73****
18	0.73****
19	0.65****
20	0.68****
Mean of 20 items	0.85****

*p<0.05, **p<0.01, ***p<0.001, and ****p<0.0001.

3.2. Validity Assessments

The SCoRS-J interviewer global ratings significantly correlated with the BACS-J composite scores (r=-0.33, $p<0.01$). In addition, the mean of the 20 items in the SCoRS-J interviewer form significantly correlated with the BACS-J composite scores (r=-0.51, $p<0.0001$).

Table 4. The relationship between SCoRS-J interviewer ratings and BACS-J composite scores

		SCoRS-J interviewer global rating	Mean of 20 items in the SCoRS-J interviewer form
BACS-J composite score	Total	-0.33**	-0.49**
	Tokushima	-0.53*	-0.47
	Toyama	-0.48**	-0.48**
	Hirosaki	-0.38	-0.42

*$p<0.05$ and **$p<0.01$.

BACS-J= Brief Assessment of Cognition in Schizophrenia Japanese version.

Table 4 also shows the relationship between SCoRS-J interviewer global ratings and BACS-J composite scores for each site: site=Tokushima, r=-0.53, n=15, $p < 0.05$; Toyama, -0.48, n=29, $p < 0.01$, Hirosaki, -0.38, 20, N.S. The relationship between the mean of 20 items in the SCoRS-J interviewer form and BACS-J composite scores for each site was as follows: site=Tokushima, r=-0.47, n=15, N.S.; Toyama, -0.48, 29, $p < 0.01$, Hirosaki, -0.42, 20, N.S.

DISCUSSION

The original SCoRS met two of the criteria established by the FDA-NIMH-MATRICS Panel for co-primary outcome measures for cognitive enhancement trials in schizophrenia: the SCoRS global ratings were strongly correlated with cognitive performance and real-world functioning [10]. In this study, SCoRS-J global ratings showed a weak but significant correlation with composite scores of cognitive performance generated from the BACS-J.

In a previous study, Keefe et al. [10] reported that when the patient's and caregiver's ratings were discrepant, an interviewer was more likely to use the caregiver's ratings when determining the global ratings. However, in this study, patients and caregivers provided good accordance in terms of both the ratings for each item and those for the global ratings. Although this may be due to a small sample size of the current study, the authors cannot exclude the possibility that information from patients, in addition to that from caregivers is necessary in the analysis of an interview-based assessment of cognition. The SCoRS-J interviewer global ratings were correlated with cognitive performance as evaluated by the BACS-J. This finding fulfills the validity criterion, which is clearly the most important in determining whether the SCoRS-J assesses behaviors that are related to cognition. Basically, cognitive assessments by an interview with the SCoRS-J and those by performance on the BACS-J are different modalities. In spite of this, there was considerable shared variance in these two outcome measures, suggesting that a common substrate mediating cognition are measured by the two scales. Meanwhile, the correlation coefficient between the mean of 20 items in the SCoRS-J interviewer form and BACS-J composite scores was larger than that between SCoRS-J interviewer global ratings and BACS-J composite scores.

This may be explained by the fact that there were no clear anchor points for SCoRS-J interviewer global ratings. Therefore, for any research, particularly multicenter study, it is quite important to establish a good level of interrater reliability, or the mean of the 20 items in the SCoRS-J interviewer form maybe a good alternative to the SCoRS-J interviewer global rating. One of the limitations of this study was that test-retest reliability and inter-rater reliability were not assessed due to the cross-sectional nature, which should be addressed in future studies with a larger sample. Also, associations between the SCoRS-J and real-world functioning should deserve further study.

CONCLUSION

This preliminary study indicates that the SCoRS-J, a new interview-based assessment of cognition designed to measure cognitive deficits based on information from patients, caregivers and interviewers, provides a reliable and valid measure of cognitive function. The

SCoRS-J may thus prompt clinicians to consider neurocognitive deficits as one of the important targets in treating patients with schizophrenia.

ACKNOWLEDGMENTS

This study was presented in part at the 27th annual meeting of the Japanese Society for Psychiatric Diagnosis, Tokushima, Japan, 2007, the 7th and 8th annual meeting of the Mental Illness and Cognitive Function, Tokyo, Japan, 2007 and 2008, and the 105th annual meeting of the Japanese Society of Psychiatry and Neurology, Kobe, Japan, 2009. Part of this work was supported by Health and Labour Sciences Research Grants and grants from Japan Society for Promotion of Sciences.

REFERENCES

[1] American Psychiatric Association: Diagnostic and Statistical Manual of Mental Disorders, Fourth Edition (DSM-IV), *American Psychiatric Association*, Washington, D.C., 1994.

[2] Bellack AS, Sayers M, Mueser KT, et al: Evaluation of social problem solving in schizophrenia. J. Abnorm. Psychol. 103(2): 371-378, 1994.

[3] Cronbach LJ: Coefficient alpha and the internal structure of tests. *Psychometrika* 16: 297-334, 1951.

[4] Green MF: What are the functional consequences of neurocognitive deficits in schizophrenia? *Am. J. Psychiatry* 153(3): 321-330, 1996.

[5] Green MF, Kern RS, Braff DL, et al: Neurocognitive deficits and functional outcome in schizophrenia: are we measuring the "right stuff"? *Schizophr. Bull* 26(1): 119-136, 2000.

[6] Green MF, Nuechterlein KH, Kern RS, et al: Functional co-primary measures for clinical trials in schizophrenia: results from the MATRICS Psychometric and Standardization Study. *Am. J. Psychiatry* 165(2): 221-228, 2008.

[7] Kaneda Y, Sumiyoshi T, Keefe R, et al: Brief assessment of cognition in schizophrenia: validation of the Japanese version. *Psychiatry Clin. Neurosci.* 61(6): 602-609, 2007.

[8] Kaneda Y, Sumiyoshi T, Nakagome K, Numata S, Tanaka T, Ueoka Y, Ohmori T, Keefe R: The Brief Assessment of Cognition in Schizophrenia Japanese version (BACS-J), Seishin Igaku (Clinical Psychiatry), 50(9), 913-917, 2008.

[9] Keefe RS, Poe M, Walker TM, et al: The Schizophrenia Cognition Rating Scale: an interview-based assessment and its relationship to cognition, real-world functioning, and functional capacity. *Am. J. Psychiatry* 163(3): 426-432, 2006.

[10] Keefe RS, Poe M, Walker TM, Kang JW, Harvey PD: The Schizophrenia Cognition Rating Scale: an interview-based assessment and its relationship to cognition, real-world functioning, and functional capacity. *Am. J. Psychiatry* 163(3):426-32.

[11] Marder SR, Fenton W: Measurement and Treatment Research to Improve Cognition in Schizophrenia: NIMH MATRICS initiative to support the development of agents for improving cognition in schizophrenia. *Schizophr. Res.* 72(1): 5-9, 2004.

[12] Overall JE, Gorham DR: The brief psychiatric rating scale. Psychol Rep 10: 799-812, 1962.

[13] Patterson TL, Goldman S, McKibbin CL, et al: UCSD Performance-Based Skills Assessment: development of a new measure of everyday functioning for severely mentally ill adults. *Schizophr. Bull* 27(2): 235-245, 2001.

[14] Ventura J, Cienfuegos A, Boxer O, et al: Clinical global impression of cognition in schizophrenia (CGI-CogS): reliability and validity of a co-primary measure of cognition. *Schizophr. Res.* 106(1): 59-69, 2008.

Mood Disorders

In: The International Psychiatry and Behavioral ... ISBN: 978-1-62257-566-4
Editor: Nash Boutros

Chapter 8

FORMALIZED CONSENSUS GUIDELINES (FCG) SCREENING AND MANAGEMENT OF BIPOLAR DISORDER*

***Pierre-Michel Llorca*[#1], *Philippe Courtet*[2], *Patrick Martin*[3], *Mocrane Abbar*[4], *Christian Gay*[5], *Jean-Albert Meynard*[6], *Franck Baylé*[7], *Michel Hamon*[7], *Christophe Lançon*[8], *Florence Thibaut*[9], *Sylvie Lancrenon*[10], *Sébastien Guillaume*[2] and *Ludovic Samalin*[1]**

L'Association Française de Psychiatrie
Biologique et Neuropsychopharmacologie (AFPBN)
[1]CHU de Clermont-Ferrand, France
[2]CHU de Montpellier, France
[3]CHU St Antoine Paris, France
[4]CHU de Nimes, France
[5] Clinique de Garches, France
[6]CH La Rochelle, France
[7]UMR894 INSERM-CPN UPMC France
[8]CHU St Marguerite Marseille, France
[9]CHU de Rouen, France
[10]SYLIA-STAT, France

INSTRUCTIONS FOR USE

The aim of these guidelines is to help practitioners to offer appropriate patient care in a broad range of clinical situations.

---

* Original Publication: Screening and management of bipolar disorders: methodology

Corresponding author: E-mail : pmllorca@chu-clermontferrand.fr

The guidelines come under five headings:

- Screening and diagnosis
- Acute phase treatment
- Long-term treatments
- Non-pharmacological treatments
- Allowance for somatic and psychiatric comorbidities and the specific features of certain populations.

The sections for the two domains concerning drug treatments start with a list of drugs considered by the experts as efficacious for acute phase treatment or prophylaxis. They are presented by drug class and in alphabetical order.

The various recommendations will then refer back to the drug class.

For example:
For an acute manic episode
The anticonvulsant (AC) drugs recommended are:

- First-line: valproate, valpromide
- Second line: carbamazepine and oxcarbazepine

When the experts recommend an AC in a patient presenting an acute manic phase you can choose from among these four drugs.

The recommendations for the care management of a thymic episode (mania or bipolar depression) are set out as follows:

- A first series of therapeutic strategies (taking into account any prior treatment),
- Approaches to take if the first-line treatment proves inefficacious or leads only a partial response,
- Expert proposals for patient care after resolution of the acute episode.

For example:
Patient care management for a first manic episode with psychotic symptoms.

The first recommended therapeutic strategy is either to initiate monotherapy with a second generation antipsychotic (SGA) or to combine an SGA with lithium (Li) or an anticonvulsant (AC).

If you decide to use an SGA monotherapy, then:

- A 3-week period before re-assessment is recommended,
- If the treatment is not efficacious, you are advised to check patient compliance, optimize dosage and combine a second MS.

Prophylactic treatment corresponds to therapeutic strategies following remission of an acute episode. As for acute phase patient care, the recommendations are set out as follows:

- At outset, indications for initiating patient care,
- The first therapeutic strategies (taking into account any prior treatment),
- Duration of prophylactic treatment.

Abbreviations (in Order of Appearance)

MDE:	Major Depressive Episode
MDQ:	Mood Disorder Questionnaire
BD:	Bipolar Disorder
AC:	Anticonvulsant
FGA:	First Generation Antipsychotic
SGA:	Second Generation Antipsychotic
ECT:	ElectroConvulsive Therapy
MS:	Mood Stabilizer
Li:	Lithium
AD:	Antidepressant
SRI:	Serotonin Re-uptake Inhibitor
SNRI:	Serotonin-Norepinephrin Re-uptake Inhibitor
CBT:	Cognitive-Behavioural Therapy
PCM:	Patient Care Management
ADHD:	Attention Deficit Hyperactivity Disorder

1. Screening and Diagnosis

Population at Risk

Screening for bipolar disorder must be done systematically among subpopulations at risk, such as:

- Patients presenting a major depressive episode (MDE)
- Patients at risk for suicide
- Patients with an addiction

In these risk groups, the use of screening questionnaires such as the Mood Disorder Questionnaire (MDQ) is recommended.

Diagnosis of Disorder

The diagnosis of mood disorder is clinical. **It is based on the occurrence of manic, hypomanic or mixed episodes in the patient's history**.

Although isolated occurrence of such episodes does not permit a diagnosis, certain features should alert the clinician to the possible presence of a bipolar disorder.

- A bipolar disorder may be suspected in any patient with:
  - A family history of bipolar disorder
  - A past history of multiple depressive episodes
  - Post-partum psychosis
  - A family history of suicide

- A bipolar disorder may be suspected in a patient with depression:
  - Starting at an early age
  - Showing features of melancholia
  - Combined with agitation
  - With a past history of severe suicidal behaviour
  - With a post-partum MDE

To help diagnosis, a structured interview is recommended, such as the MINI, together with a mood diary.

A diagnosis of bipolar disorder must be confirmed by a psychiatrist

The diagnosis of bipolar disorder needs:

- Confirmation by family questioning
- A somatic clinical examination

Unless the clinical examination calls for them, biological or imaging examinations do not help to make a diagnosis.

2. Acute Phase Therapy

Choice of a drug during the acute phase

The choice will depend on:

- The clinical features of the current episode
- The type of bipolar disorder: I or II

- The patient's thymic history throughout his or her life (predominance of manic, hypomanic, or mixed episodes, or depressive episodes)
- Whether or not rapid cycles occur (patients who have also had at least four thymic episodes per year according to DSM IV-TR criteria)

Modalities of prescription during the acute phase

The modalities will depend on:

- Initially: whether or not a prophylactic treatment is being administered
- When the therapeutic efficacy is being assessed: the treatment duration and the drug used
- After resolution of the episode: whether or not therapies are combined

Criteria for hospital admission during the acute phase

Hospitalization **must** be considered in the following situations:

- Manic or mixed episode
- Severe depressive episode
- Depressive episode with psychotic features
- High level of suicidality
- Recent increase in addictive behaviour
- Somatic state giving cause for concern

Hospitalization **may** also be proposed if the treatment is inefficacious or meets resistance.

2.1. Treatment of Manic, Hypomanic and Mixed Episodes

Drugs or Therapies Recommended for the Treatment of Mania or Hypomania

The drugs are presented in alphabetical order in each drug class

- Lithium (Li)
- Anticonvulsants (AC): carbamazepine, oxcarbazepine, valproate, valpromide
- Second generation antipsychotics (SGAs): amisulpride, aripiprazole, clozapine, olanzapine, risperidone
- First generation antipsychotics (FGAs): haloperidol
- Electroconvulsive therapy (ECT)

Drugs or therapies recommended for the treatment of mania or hypomania according to the type of bipolar disorder and the occurrence of rapid cycles

	Without rapid cycle		With rapid cycle	
	BD I	BD I	BD I	BD II
First line	Li AC: valproate, valpromide SGA: aripiprazole, olanzapine, risperidone FGA: haloperidol ECT	Li AC: valproate, valpromide SGA: aripiprazole, olanzapine, risperidone	Li AC: carbamazepine, oxcarbazepine, valproate, valpromide SGA: olanzapine, risperidone ECT	Li AC: carbamazepine, oxcarbazepine, valproate, valpromide SGA: olanzapine, risperidone
Second line	AC: carbamazepine, oxcarbazepine SGA: amisulpride clozapine	AC: carbamazepine, oxcarbazepine SGA: amisulpride	SGA: amisulpride, aripiprazole, clozapine	SGA: amisulpride, aripiprazole, clozapine

The experts recommend haloperidol for first-line treatment of mania without a rapid cycle. International recommendations consider its benefit-risk ratio to be unfavourable for second- or third-line treatments [1-4].

2.1.1. First episode or patients not treated with mood stabilizers (MSs)

Subtypes of mania and therapeutic strategies

Dysphoric mania: consider monotherapy with Li, AC or SGA or direct bitherapy with two MSs (Li+SGA, AC+SGA, Li+AC)

Mania with psychotic symptoms: consider SGA monotherapy or direct bitherapy with another antimanic MS (SGA+AC or SGA+Li)

Irritable mania (definition in annex 1): consider monotherapy with AC or SGA, or direct bitherapy with two antimanic MSs including one SGA (SGA+AC or SGA+Li)

Mixed state (definition in annex 2): consider monotherapy with AC or SGA, or direct bitherapy with AC+SGA

Hypomania: consider monotherapy with AC or SGA

For mania with psychotic symptoms, SGAs are always recommended in monotherapy or combination. Monotherapy with Li is not recommended for hypomania and only in second line for irritable mania and mixed state.

Dealing with incomplete response before re-assessment

If the treatment is inefficacious or leads only to partial response, the therapeutic strategy should be modified after a duration of treatment that will be defined according to the MS used:

- 4 weeks for Li,
- 3 weeks for AC, SGAs and ECT,
- 2 weeks for FGAs.

If an MS is combined, in case of partial response before re-assessment treatment duration will be adjusted according to the last MS administered.

Incomplete response to treatment for acute mania or hypomania

When the treatment is inefficacious or leads only to partial response, the sequence below should be followed:

- Check patient adherence to treatment
- Optimize the MS dosage
- Add a second MS
- Maintain an SGA in the combination of 2 MSs when psychotic symptoms are observed

2.1.2. Manic, hypomanic or mixed relapse during long-term treatment

Therapeutic sequences

When faced with a type I or II bipolar disorder with or without a rapid cycle, the sequence below should be followed:

- Stop any current antidepressant (AD) treatment
- Check patient adherence to treatment
- Optimize the current MS dosage
- Add an antimanic MS with the current MS
- Switch from one of the two MSs to another antimanic MS (if the long-term treatment was two MSs).
- Maintain an SGA in the combination of two MSs when there are psychotic symptoms

IMPORTANT
If there are manic symptoms, all AD treatment must be stopped.
Treatment with an MS that has an antidepressant effect may be continued.
Combinations of antipsychotics (FGA+FGA and FGA+SGA) should be avoided

Dealing with incomplete response before re-assessment

If the treatment is inefficacious or leads only to partial response, the therapeutic strategy should be modified after a duration of treatment that will be defined according to the MS used:

- 4 weeks for Li,
- 3 weeks for AC, SGAs and ECT,
- 2 weeks for FGAs (incisive or sedative).

If an MS is combined, in case of partial response before re-assessment treatment duration will be adjusted according to the last MS administered.

If the patient is resistant to the treatment, a combination of three MSs can be considered. Clozapine and ECT must be considered in the most resistant cases.

2.1.3. Cases of Aggressiveness or Agitation

Recommendations are to:

– Prefer the oral formulation to the injectable formulation
– Add an SGA, a sedative FGA or a benzodiazepine with the current anti-manic treatment.

2.1.4. After Resolution of the Manic Episode

If an MS is combined you should:
– in first-line treatment, discontinue antipsychotics (FGA or SGA)
– if possible, maintain monotherapy for 3 months after resolution of the manic episode.

2.2. Treatment of BIPOLAR DEPRESSION

Drugs or therapies with antidepressant effects during the acute phase

The drugs are presented in alphabetical order in each drug class.

✓ ECT
✓ Li
✓ AC: lamotrigine, valproate, valpromide
✓ SGA: aripiprazole, olanzapine *
✓ AD associated with an antimanic MS

* Quetiapine was not available in France when the recommendations were elaborated.

The experts consider that the *combination antimanic MS + AD* has an antidepressant effect in the acute phase:

Antimanic MS: Li, AC or SGA

AD: first line: serotonin re-uptake inhibitor (SRI), serotonin-norepinephrine re-uptake inhibitor (SNRI);

second line: mirtazapine, mianserine, tianeptine

Drugs or therapies with antidepressant effects during the acute phase according to their grades of recommendation

First line	AC: lamotrigine ECT
Second line	Li AC: valproate, valpromide SGA: aripiprazole, olanzapine

Expert recommendations concerning drugs or therapies are the same for BD I and BD II, and do not depend on whether or not rapid cycles occur.

IMPORTANT
FGAs should be avoided.

2.2.1. Non-Treated Patients

Subtype of bipolar depression and therapeutic strategies

Mild to moderate depressive episode: consider monotherapy with Li or AC

Severe MDE with no psychotic symptom:

- no rapid cycle: consider bitherapy AD + MS (Li, AC or SGA) for first-line treatment
- with rapid cycle: consider monotherapy with Li or AC

MDE with psychotic symptoms:

- no rapid cycle: consider bitherapy; SGA + AD for first-line treatment, and AD + (Li or AC) and SGA + Li for second-line treatment
- with rapid cycle: consider bitherapy SGA + AC or SGA + Li

Mixed depressive episode (definition in annex 3)

- no rapid cycle: consider monotherapy with AC or bitherapy with AC + SGA for first-line treatment, and monotherapy with Li or bitherapy with Li + SGA for second-line treatment
- with rapid cycle: consider bitherapy with AC + SGA for first-line treatment and Li + SGA for second-line treatment

Experts consider that a mixed episode and (or) a rapid cycle are factors favouring weaker response to Li. MDE in a patient who has an history of treatment-induced mania: no consensus found. There is no consensus either in the scientific literature or among the experts concerning the therapeutic approach recommended in this clinical situation.

First-line ECT

ECT is recommended in first-line treatment when the clinical condition is life-threatening

Dealing with incomplete response before re-assessment

If the treatment is inefficacious or leads only to partial response, the therapeutic strategy should be modified after a treatment time that will depend on the MS used:

- At least 4 weeks for Li,
- At least 3 weeks for AC, SGAs, and ECT,
- 2 weeks for FGAs.

If an MS is combined, in case of partial response before re-assessment treatment duration will be adjusted according to the last MS administered

Partial response to treatment for acute bipolar depression

When a treatment is inefficacious or leads only to partial response, the sequence below should be followed:

- Check patient compliance
- Optimize dosage of MS and (or) AD
- Add a second MS
- Consider ECT
- Consider adding an AD in a BD with no rapid cycle
- For a mixed depressive episode, combine an MS that has an antidepressant effect with an antimanic MS
- Maintain an SGA in the combination of two MSs when there are psychotic symptoms

2.2.2. Depressive Relapse During Long-Term Treatment

Therapeutic sequences

For a type I or II bipolar disorder the sequence below should be followed:

- Check patient compliance
- Optimize the current MS dosage
- Add to the current MS:
- No rapid cycle: consider adding an AD
- With rapid cycle: consider adding an MS with an antidepressor effect
- Consider ECT
- Maintain an SGA in the combination of two MSs when there are psychotic symptoms

Strategies taking into account the predominant polarity

These strategies apply when there is no rapid cycle. They concern the choice between AD and an MS with an antidepressant effect.

If the patient displays depressive polarity and is already being treated with an antimanic MS + AD, then an MS with an antidepressant effect should be considered.

If the patient displays manic polarity and is already being treated with an antimanic MS + AD, then the AD therapeutic strategy should be reconsidered.

2.2.3. After Resolution of the Depressive Episode

If an MS is combined with an AD, the AD should be discontinued on average 6 months after resolution of the episode.

3. Long-Term Therapy

Choice of prophylactic strategy

The choice will depend on:

- The predominant polarity
- Whether suicidal or risk-seeking behaviour are reported
- The efficacy of acute phase treatment
- The severity of the episodes
- Whether rapid cycles occur
- Whether there is a treatment-induced mania
- Any comorbidities
- The tolerance profile of the drug chosen
- The patient's preference
- The patient's compliance

Indication for prophylactic treatment

Prophylactic treatment should be considered: – Systematically at the first manic episode – As soon as BDII is diagnosed – After two hypomanic episodes As early as the first hypomanic episode if the following factors are recorded: • Early age of onset, • First degree family history of bipolar disorder, • Presence of psychotic features at index episode • Presence of residual symptoms • Past history of suicidal behaviour, observed at index episode • Occurrence of psychiatric comorbidities

Drugs or therapies with preventive effect on manic or depressive relapses in BD

The drugs are presented in alphabetical order in each drug class

Preventive effect on manic relapses	Li AC: carbamazepine, oxcarbazepine, valproate, valpromide SGA: amisulpride, aripiprazole, clozapine, olanzapine, risperidone Maintenance ECT
Preventive effect on depressive relapses	Li AC: carbamazepine, lamotrigine, oxcarbazepine, valproate, valpromide SGA: olanzapine Maintenance ECT

Drugs with preventive effects on manic or depressive relapses in bipolar disorders I and II with and without rapid cycles

<table>
<tr><th colspan="2" rowspan="2"></th><th colspan="2">BDI</th><th colspan="2">BDII</th></tr>
<tr><th>Without CR</th><th>With CR</th><th>Without CR</th><th>With CR</th></tr>
<tr><td rowspan="3">Preventive effect on manic relapses</td><td rowspan="2">First line</td><td colspan="4">Li
AC: carbamazepine, oxcarbazepine, valproate, valpromide
SGA: aripiprazole, olanzapine</td></tr>
<tr><td>clozapine
risperidone,</td><td>clozapine</td><td>risperidone</td><td></td></tr>
<tr><td>Second line</td><td>amisulpride
ECT</td><td>amisulpride
risperidone
ECT</td><td>amisulpride</td><td>amisulpride
risperidone</td></tr>
</table>

		BDI		BDII	
		Without CR	With CR	Without CR	With CR
Preventive effect on depressive relapses	First line	Li AC: lamotrigine SGA: olanzapine	AC: lamotrigine, valproate, valpromide SGA: olanzapine	Li AC: lamotrigine	Li AC: lamotrigine, valproate, valpromide
	Second line	AC: carbamazepine, oxcarbazepine, valproate, valpromide SGA: amisulpride aripiprazole, clozapine ECT	Li AC: carbamazepine, oxcarbazepine SGA: aripiprazole, clozapine ECT	AC: carbamazepine, oxcarbazepine, valproate, valpromide SGA: amisulpride aripiprazole, clozapine, olanzapine	AC: carbamazepine, oxcarbazepine SGA: amisulpride aripiprazole, clozapine, olanzapine

Classes of AD recommended in combination with an MS in the prophylactic treatment of a BD patient

- First line: SRI
- Second line: SNRI, mirtazapine, mianserine

IMPORTANT
FGAs should be avoided

After an acute episode

It is advised:

- either to continue the acute phase treatment when this was efficacious (if the current drugs have a preventive effect),
- or propose a drug therapy with a specific preventive effect on the predominant polarity of the bipolar disorder

Relapse during prophylactic treatment

In the event of a relapse during prophylactic treatment, you should do the following:

- Optimize the dosage of the prophylactic treatment
- Consider bitherapy after trying out two MSs in monotherapy
- Consider direct bitherapy according to the following:

- First degree family history of BD
- Severity of the episode
- Suicidal behaviour at index episode
- Any psychiatric comorbidities

The experts did not mention early age of onset, family history of psychiatric disorders, presence of psychotic symptoms, or social isolation

- Prefer combinations of MSs in different drug classes
- Avoid AD in patients with rapid cycles

Duration of prophylactic treatment

The prophylactic treatment should be continued as long as possible in both BD I and BD II. Regular re-assessment is needed.

Lifelong continuous treatment should be considered, according to the following factors:

- First-degree family history of bipolar disorder
- Severity of episode
- Suicidal behaviour at index episode
- Psychiatric comorbidities
- Persistent residual symptoms
- Number of thymic episodes
- Early age of onset
- Short time intervals between episodes

4. Non-Pharmacological Treatments

4.1. Psychotherapies

Aims of psychotherapies

- To inform the patient about the illness and its care management
- To allow regular assessment of mood to screen for early signs of relapse
- To enhance the therapeutic alliance and drug compliance
- To enable the patient to grow more adaptable, in particular when faced with stress-inducing factors.

The objective is to improve the overall prognosis of the disorder and the patient's psychosocial health and quality of life.

Implementation and choice of psychotherapy

- During hospitalization or during a manic, mixed or major depressive episode of severe intensity, informing the patient and family and the support therapy form the first-line non-drug care.
- During a depressive episode of mild to moderate intensity or in a remission phase, the following are systematically recommended:

- Information for patient and family
- Support therapy
- Keeping a diary of mood and sleep patterns
- Reading advice
- Orientation towards self-help support groups or patient associations
- Communication of emergency numbers
- Participation in psychoeducation groups

The experts recommend:

- Cognitive-behavioural therapy (CBT)
- Interpersonal and social rhythm therapy

Improving patient compliance

The following are recommended:

- Raising the issue regularly during consultations
- Systematic checking for and consideration of side effects
- Promote awareness and involvement of family and friends
- Directing poorly compliant patients to psychoeducation groups.

4.2. Part-Time Care

Day hospitalization **must be systematically** considered when faced with:

- Occurrence of rapid cycles
- Marked addictive comorbidities
- Social isolation and significant interactional impairment

Day hospitalization **may be** offered in the event of:

- Poor compliance
- Residual symptoms.

5. Somatic and Psychiatric Comorbidities

5.1. Somatic comorbidities

Initial pretherapeutic examination

Examination necessary irrespective of MS
Blood cell count
Blood electrolytes
Fasting blood sugar
Urea and creatinine, proteinuria
TSHus
Lipids
Liver function
β HCG
ECG

Treatment tolerance monitoring schedule

	Every 2 months	Every 3 months	Every 4 months	Every 6 months	Every year
BMI	SGA	Li	AC		
Umbilical waist circumference		SGA, Li		AC	
Blood pressure		SGA, Li	AC		
Full blood count				SGA, AC	Li
Blood glucose			SGA		AC, Li
Lipid profile			SGA	AC	Li
Liver function				AC, SGA	Li
Thyroid function				Li, AC	SGA
Renal function				Li	AC, SGA

Preexisting diabetes

Preexisting diabetes is to be taken into account if SGAs are prescribed, for both acute phase and long-term treatment. Another MS is best prescribed.

Preexisting thyroid dysfunction

Preexisting thyroid dysfunction is to be taken into account if lithium is prescribed, for both acute phase and long-term treatment. Another MS is best prescribed.

Management of side effects

Cessation of MS treatment

In a patient taking a mood stabilizer, cessation of treatment should be considered if any of the following side effects occur:

- Metabolic syndrome
- Arterial hypertension
- Diabetes
- Clinically significant drug interaction

Occurrence of thyroid dysfunction

If thyroid dysfunction occurs under MS, then:

(A) If it is not clinically significant:

- The treatment must not be stopped
- Clinical monitoring must be set up with re-assessment of thyroid function after 1 month
- If it persists, expert advice must be taken and in the event of hypothyroidism, thyroid hormone supplementation must be considered

(B) If it is clinically significant:

- Expert advice must be sought
- The benefit-risk ratio must be discussed (discontinuing the treatment is generally not recommended)
- Systematic thyroid hormone supplementation must be offered.

Occurrence of weight gain

If an MS induces weight gain, the following recommendations are:

- Give simple dietary advice (set mealtimes, quantity and type of food to be preferred, etc.)
- Motivate the patient for physical activity
- Offer specialized dietary care if the weight gain is appreciable (>7%)
- Discuss stopping treatment if the weight gain is appreciable (>7%)
- Do not stop the treatment if the weight gain is moderate (<7%)

There is no consensus among the experts concerning the addition of topiramate.

5.2. Psychiatric Comorbidities

5.2.1. Bipolar Disorder and Addiction

The presence of an addictive comorbidity calls for specific care management

Care management strategies

Care management for bipolar disorder and addictive disorder must be concomitant.

- The only exception to this rule is the combination of mild to moderate depression with alcohol addiction, when the thymic state will be assessed after withdrawal.
- In the case of dependence, care **must** involve professionals of addiction, a psychotherapy centred on prevention of addictive relapse, and include psychoeducation groups.
- In the case of abuse, care **may** involve professionals of addiction and specific psychotherapeutic care.

Drug treatment

SGAs and AC in monotherapy should be the first-line treatment for both an episode of mania and prophylaxis.

In depression, the existence of an addiction does not warrant any specific drug treatment.

Cases of agitation not linked to withdrawal

If addition of a sedative treatment is necessary, sedative FGAs must be used in preference to benzodiazepines owing to the risk of inducing dependence.

Opiate substitution treatment

The presence of a manic or depressive episode must not lead to an interruption of opiate substitution treatment

5.2.2. Bipolar Disorder and Personality Disorder

Borderline or antisocial personality type

The existence of a borderline or antisocial type personality disorder:

- Modifies prescription strategy during manic episodes and in prophylaxis with the preferential use of an SGA in monotherapy or in combined therapy
- Needs systematic specific psychotherapeutic care

The experts were unable to reach a consensus on whether a specific drug treatment was useful during a major depressive episode occurring in a patient with a BD and a borderline or antisocial personality.

Other personality disorders

The existence of another type of personality disorder does not modify the care management of bipolar disorder

5.2.3. Bipolar Disorder And Suicidal Behaviour

The risk of suicidal behaviour is high in patients suffering from bipolar disorder.

Regular, precise assessment of suicide risk must be made systematically in the following situations:

- At the beginning of any evolution of the disorder
- During a depressive episode
- In case of a mixed episode
- During hospitalization
- During a manic episode
- During negative life events
- At the start or end of a treatment
- If therapy is interrupted

Suicide risk factors to be identified

Highly specific risk factors	Specific risk factors
• Suicidal ideation • Current depression (and more particularly agitated or anxious depression) • Psychotic symptoms • Impulsive aggressive personality traits • Previously attested suicidal behaviour	• Access to lethal means • Nefarious social environment • Current mixed episode • Presence of rapid cycles • Family history of suicide • Addictive comorbidities • History of self-mutilation • Negative life events • Type II bipolar disorder

The co-occurrence of these factors increases suicide risk correspondingly.

Specific strategy

In patients presenting a long-term suicide risk, MS treatment with lithium is to be preferred, and more intensive psychotherapeutic care should be offered.

Bipolar disorder and anxiety disorder

> In the presence of anxiety disorder associated with the bipolar disorder, the first-line treatment of the anxiety disorder must be CBT.

SUMMARY OF COMORBIDITIES MODIFYING DRUG-BASED CARE MANAGEMENT

Clinical situation	Manic episode	Depressive episode	Prophylactic phase
Associated diabetes	Li, AC or Li+AC	Li, AC, AD+Li, AD+AC	Li, AC
Associated thyroid dysfunction	AC, SGA or AC+SGA	AC, AD+AC, AD+SGA	AC, SGA
Addictive comorbidity	First line: AC or SGA Second line: AC+SGA; AC+Li; SGA+Li	No modification of patient care management (PCM)	Monotherapy with SGA or AC
Cluster B personality comorbidity	First line: SGA or SGA+AC or SGA+Li*	No consensus	First line: SGA or SGA+AC or SGA+Li* Second line: AC Systematic association of specific psychotherapeutic care
Cluster A or C personality comorbidity	No change in PCM	No change in PCM	No change in PCM

* If there is a past history of severe suicidal behaviour or family history of response to lithium.

6. SPECIAL POPULATIONS

6.1. Bipolar Disorder in Adolescents

Diagnosis of bipolar disorder

> Before diagnosing bipolar disorder in an adolescent it is necessary **systematically** to:
>
> - Carry out a family interview

- Look for an attention deficit hyperactivity disorder (ADHD)
- Seek paediatric advice to rule out an organic disorder

In most cases the following is recommended:

- Make a detailed assessment of growth and development (prenatal history, psychomotor development, etc.)
- Contact the patient's teachers

Drug prescription

The drug prescription must obey to certain rules:

- It must be made only by a specialist
- The dosage must be adjusted to the patient's weight
- Initiation must be more gradual than in adults
- Medical follow-up must be more closely spaced than in adults
- In young girls who can become pregnant, an efficacious method of contraception must be considered

If there is a manic episode

The treatment must be:

- First line: monotherapy with AC or SGA, or the two combined
- Second line: lithium monotherapy, or combined with AC or SGA

If there is a depressive episode

The treatment must be:

- Not limited to psychotherapeutic care alone
- First line: AC monotherapy.
- Second line: monotherapy with Li or SGA or combined AD + MS (Li, AC or SGA)

Prophylactic treatment

The treatment must be:

- Not limited to psychotherapeutic care alone
- First line: AC monotherapy or continuation of treatment found efficacious during the acute phase.
- Second line: monotherapy with Li or SGA

6.2. Bipolar Disorder in the Elderly

Diagnosis

In the late-onset forms, before making a diagnosis it is necessary **systematically** to :

- Take expert advice on the possible presence of a somatic pathology
- Eliminate dementia
- Make a detailed assessment of drug treatments and any drug interactions
- Conduct a family interview
- Make a neuropsychological assessment

Drug strategy

The drug prescription must obey to certain rules:

- Prescription only by a specialist
- Gradual titration
- Dosage adjusted to renal and hepatic function
- Medical follow-up and regular monitoring of tolerance
- Precise assessment of any drug interactions

If there is a manic episode

- The first-line treatment must be AC or lithium
- Second-line may be SGA alone or combined with an AC
- Prescription of the SGA must follow benefit-risk ratio assessment
- For third-line treatment, ECT may be discussed

If there is a depressive episode

- First-line care must be AC monotherapy or combined AC + AD or ECT
- Second-line treatment may be Li monotherapy or combined Li + AD
- Third-line treatment may be SGA alone or combined with an AD

Prophylactic treatment

The drug treatment must be monotherapy with Li or AC or continuation of treatment found efficacious in the acute phase

6.3. Bipolar Disorder during Pregnancy

Actual or planned pregnancy modifies the care management of bipolar disorder.

If a pregnancy is planned:

- If the patient is under treatment with AC or lithium:
  - Gradual cessation before pregnancy
  - According to the clinical situation, SGA treatment may be prescribed, or care may be limited to monitoring, followed by resumption of treatment during the second trimester for lithium or after birth for AC.
- If the patient is under treatment with SGA:
  - For type I bipolar disorder, the treatment must be maintained
  - For type II bipolar disorder, the SGA may be either maintained or discontinued in the light of a benefit-risk assessment.

If pregnancy is discovered fortuitously:

- AC treatment must be discontinued
- Lithium can be maintained after the patient has been told about the benefit-risk ratio and provided specialized, closely-spaced monitoring (echography, in particular) is available
- Prescription of SGA may be maintained.

Manic episode during pregnancy

- The first-line treatment must be an SGA
- The second-line treatment may be a FGA
- The third-line treatment may be ECT

Depressive episode during pregnancy

In the event of a mild to moderate depressive episode, the treatment must be psychotherapeutic.

In the event of a severe episode:

- Combined SGA and AD (avoiding paroxetine), or ECT may be offered.
- The type of bipolar disorder (type I or II) has no bearing on the patient care management

Summary of Specific Situations Modifying Drug-Based Care Management

Clinical situation	Manic episode	Depressive episode	Prophylactic phase
Adolescent	First line: AC or SGA or AC+SGA Second line: Li or combination Li+ (SGA or AC)	First line: AC Second line: Li or SGA Combination AD + MS (Li, AC SGA)	First line: AC or continuation of treatment found efficacious in the acute phase. Second line: Li or SGA
Elderly patient	First line: Li or AC Second line: SGA or AC + SGA Third line: ECT	First line: AC or AC + AD or ECT Second line: Li or Li+AD Third line: SGA or SGA+AD	First line: Li or AC or continuation of treatment found efficacious in the acute phase.
Pregnancy	SGA Second line: FGA Third line: ECT	If depression is mild: psychotherapy If depression is severe: ECT or SGA +AD	If patient is under SGA: maintain SGA If patient is under AC: stop AC and SGA or monitoring (especially in BD2) If patient is under Li and pregnancy is planned: stop Li and resume in second trimester or at birth (especially in BD2) or SGA If patient is under Li and pregnancy discovered: Maintenance and specialized monitoring

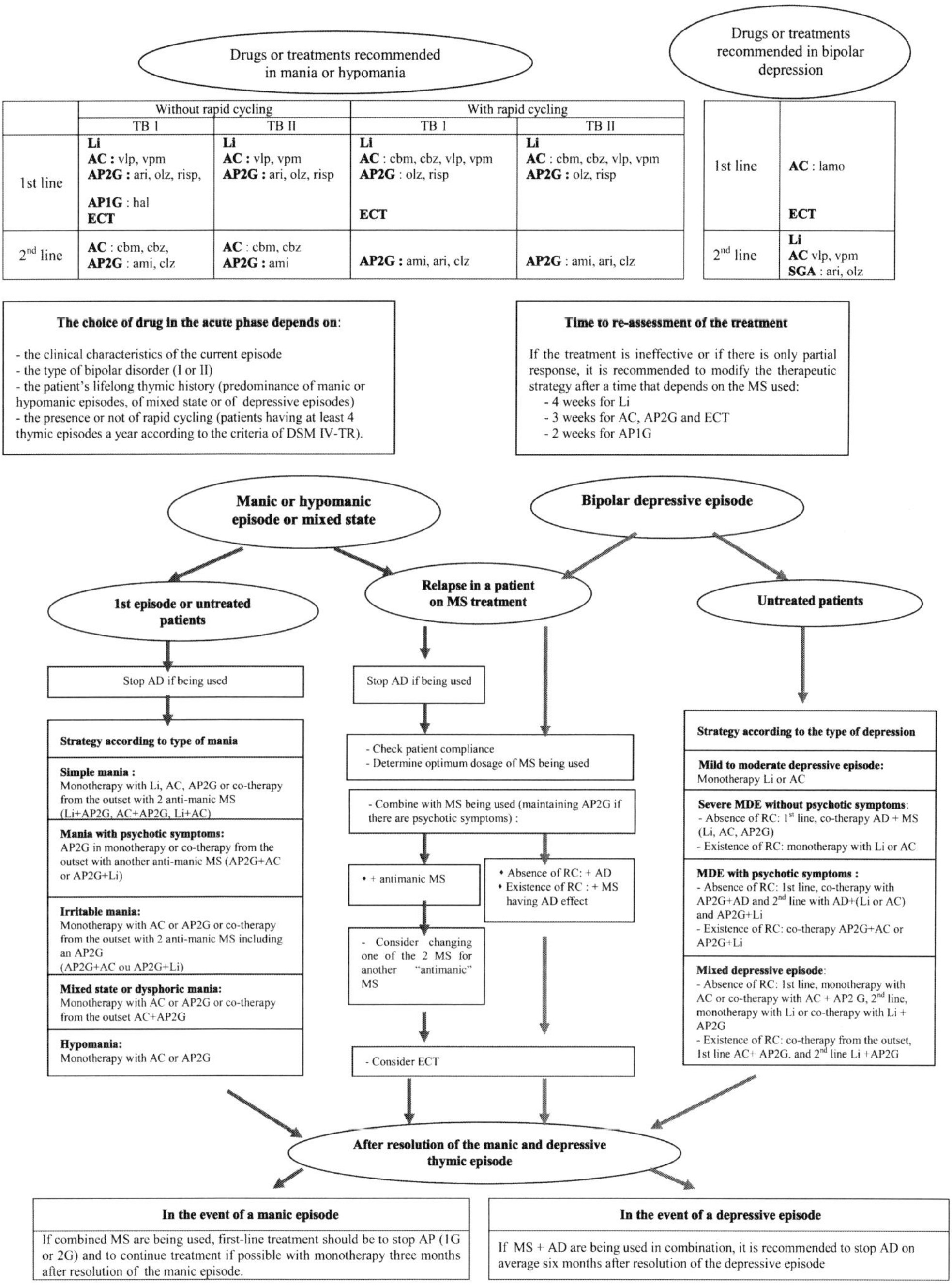

Abbreviations: BD bipolar disorder, RC rapid cycling, MS mood stabiliser, AD antidepressant, AC anticonvulsant, cbm carbamazepine, cbz oxcarbazepine, Vlp valproate, vpm valpromide, lamo lamotrigine, AP1G/AP2G antipsychotic of 1st/2nd generation, hal haloperidol, ami amisulpride, ari aripiprazole, clz clozapine, risp risperidone, olz olanzapine , ECT electroconvulsive therapy, Li lithium.

Figure 1. Treatment in the acute phase of bipolar disorder (Llorca et al, 2010).

The choice of maintenance strategy depends on the:
- predominant polarity of the disorder
- presence of risk or suicidal behaviours
- efficacy of the treatment in the acute phase
- severity of the episodes
- presence of rapid cycling
- possibility of inducing a mood switch
- existence of co-morbidities
- tolerance profile of the drug chosen
- patient's preference and ability to comply

Drugs or treatments recommended for long-term therapy

		BIPOLAR DISORDER I		BIPOLAR DISORDER II	
		WITHOUT RC	WITH RC	WITHOUT RC	WITH RC
Preventive effect on mania relapse	1st line	**Li** **AC** : carbamazepine, oxcarbazepine, valproate, valpromide **AP2G** : aripiprazole, olanzapine			
		clozapine risperidone	clozapine	risperidone	
	2nd line	amisulpride **ECT**	amisulpride risperidone **ECT**	amisulpride	amisulpride risperidone
Preventive effect on depression relapse	1st line	**Li** **AC :** lamotrigine **AP2G** : olanzapine	**AC :** lamotrigine valproate,valpromide **AP2G** : olanzapine	**Li** **AC :** lamotrigine	**Li** **AC :** lamotrigine valproate, valpromide
	2nd ligne	**AC** : carbamazepine, oxcarbazepine, valproate, valpromide **AP2G** : amisulpride aripiprazole, clozapine **ECT**	**Li** **AC :** carbamazepine, oxcarbazepine **AP2G** : aripiprazole, clozapine **ECT**	**AC** : carbamazepine, oxcarbazepine, valproate, valpromide **AP2G** : amisulpride aripiprazole, clozapine olanzapine	**AC :** carbamazepine, oxcarbazepine **AP2G** : amisulpride aripiprazole, clozapine, olanzapine

Initiation of maintenance therapy
- 1st manic episode
- Diagnosis of BP II
- 2nd hypomanic episode

- Continue treatment for the acute phase if it has been effective (if the drugs used have a proven preventive effect).
- Drug treatment with one preventive effect specific to the predominant polarity of the disorder (see. table).

Relapse on maintenance therapy

- Check patient compliance
- Determine the optimum dosage of the maintenance treatment
- Consider a co-therapy after trying 2 MS in monotherapy or consider co-therapy from the outset (depending on the presence of family history of BD in first-degree relatives, on the severity of the episode, on suicidal behaviour during the index episode and on psychiatric co-morbidity)
- Give priority to a combination of MS from different drug classes and prescribe AD for patients with RC.

Duration of course of treatment

- Continue maintenance therapy as long as possible whatever the type of bipolar disorder (I or II)
- Continue treatment for life in the event of poor prognostic factors:
(family history of BD in first-degree relatives, severity of the episode, suicidal behaviour during the index episode, psychiatric co-morbidity, persistence of residual symptoms, high number of thymic episodes, early-age onset, short interval between episodes).

Figure 2. Maintenance therapy (Llorca et al, 2010).

Annexes

Annex 1. Irritable Mania

Mania in which the patient's prevailing mood is characterized by irritability.

Annex 2. Dysphoric Mania

Dysphoric mania, described by Bauer et al. [5], is a form of manic state combining depressive symptoms and dysphoric mood. Dysphoric mania is more prevalent in women and in persons with depressive tendencies. It is said to be characterized by a poor response to lithium, a more favourable response to anticonvulsants and possible induction by antidepressants. For S. McElroy, it is defined by the simultaneous presence of a manic state, according to the criteria of DSM III-R and at least three depressive symptoms from among the major depressive episode criteria according to DSM III-R [6].

Annex 3. Mixed Depressive State

Mixed depressive states, which are not a category of DSM-IV, are characterized according to a certain number of authors by the presence of manic symptoms during a major bipolar depressive episode. The patient does not, of course, meet the criteria of a mixed state.

For these same authors, antidepressants may trigger or worsen these states. An example of a clinical picture would be: irritability, need to talk against a background of slowed responsiveness, extreme tiredness, ruminations of guilt feelings, diffuse anxiety, panic attacks, refractory insomnia, increased libido, histrionic appearance but with an expression of depressive suffering and suicidal impulses.

References

[1] Goodwin, G.M., Evidence-based guidelines for treating bipolar disorder: revised second edition--recommendations from the British Association for Psychopharmacology. *J. Psychopharmacol*, 2009. 23(4): p. 346-88.

[2] Grunze, H., et al., The World Federation of Societies of Biological Psychiatry (WFSBP) guidelines for the biological treatment of bipolar disorders: update 2009 on the treatment of acute mania. *World J. Biol. Psychiatry,* 2009. 10(2): p. 85-116.

[3] Malhi, G.S., et al., Clinical practice recommendations for bipolar disorder. *Acta Psychiatr. Scand. Suppl*, 2009(439): p. 27-46.

[4] Yatham, L.N., et al., Canadian Network for Mood and Anxiety Treatments (CANMAT) and International Society for Bipolar Disorders (ISBD) collaborative update of CANMAT guidelines for the management of patients with bipolar disorder: update 2009. *Bipolar Disord*, 2009. 11(3): p. 225-55.

[5] Bauer, M.S., et al., Testing definitions of dysphoric mania and hypomania: prevalence, clinical characteristics and inter-episode stability. *J. Affect. Disord,* 1994. 32(3): p. 201-11.

[6] McElroy, S.L., et al., Clinical and research implications of the diagnosis of dysphoric or mixed mania or hypomania. *Am. J. Psychiatry*, 1992. 149(12): p. 1633-44.

In: The International Psychiatry and Behavioral ... ISBN: 978-1-62257-566-4
Editor: Nash Boutros

Chapter 9

THE STUDY OF EFFECTS OF 20-HZ REPETITIVE TRANSCRANIAL MAGNETIC STIMULATION (rTMS) IN PATIENTS WITH MEDICATION RESISTANT MAJOR DEPRESSIVE DISORDER

Sanaz Khomami*, Reza Rostami, Reza Kazemi and Abbas Rahiminezhad

Department of Psychology,
Faculty of Psychology and Educational Sciences, Tehran University, Tehran, Iran

ABSTRACT

Introduction: The aim of this study was to examine the efficacy of the repetitive transcranial magnetic stimulation (rTMS) in medication-resistant patients with major depressive disorder.

Materials and Methods: In a quasi-experimental one group time-series study in summer and autumn 2008, 12 patients with major depressive disorder were assessed with available sampling and treated with rTMS (20 Hz) over left dorsolateral prefrontal cortex for 30 sessions. All the patients were appraised with the Beck Depression Inventory before first session of treatment, immediately after the 30th session and 1.5 months after treatment course.

Results: rTMS could decrease the symptoms of depression significantly ($P<0.001$) in patients with major depressive disorder and these effects lasted 1.5 months after rTMS sessions were finished.

Conclusion: rTMS has therapeutic effects in patients with medication resistant major depressive disorder and these effects lasted 1.5 month after treatment.

Keywords: Major depression disorder, Resistant, Transcranial magnetic stimulation

---

* Corresponding Author: Tel: +982184012128, skhomami@ut.ac.ir

INTRODUCTION

Depression is one of the most common neuropsychiatric disorders with a lifetime possibility of 17% [1, 2] and about 10% of people worldwide need significant treatment.

Depression can be treated with different methods like medications, psychotherapy and electroconvulsive therapy (ECT). But in some patients the symptoms still remain and over 20 percent show minimal response to treatment, while others don't have response to any treatment [3-6]. Antidepressants are considered as the first line treatment of mood disorders and ECT mostly can be used for patients who don't respond to any drug or perhaps medical treatments aren't tolerable for them [7]. Despite the effective use of ECT in treatment of mood disorders like depression, gradually the mind of psychiatrists shifted to other modes of therapies that can provide therapeutic effects in treatment of depression with focal stimulation without inducing a generalized seizure [6].

First in 1985, Barker stimulated some areas of cortex with transcranial magnetic stimulation (TMS) and then several studies were carried out on the effectiveness of this method on depression, Parkinson disease and pain [8]. TMS is a safe and non invasive technique which through the sending of magnetic fields and changing the glucose levels and neurotransmitters activity can affect the target area [9-12].

In this method, a strong electric current through the coil which is placed on the head, induces a magnetic field and then leads to milder electrical fields in the cortex and thus induces action potential in stimulated nerve tissues [13].

The strength of generated magnetic fields by TMS is equivalent with MR scanners and bones and stimulated tissues don't show resistance to them [5]. The magnetic stimulator devices can produce pulses with 1 to 100 Hz frequency that, based on the frequency, can create excitation or inhibition effects. Low frequency (less than or equal 1 Hz) has inhibition effects while high frequency (more than 1 Hz) induces excitatory effects in neurons. Although these mechanisms are not fully elucidated, the evidence suggests that therapeutic effects caused by TMS are due to changes in neurotransmitters and neurons neuroplasticity.

One of the cortical brain regions which is available to TMS coil is dorsolateral prefrontal cortex (DLPFC). According to functional neuroimaging studies this area of the brain includes the middle frontal gyrus and because of its connectivity to limbic system, has an important role in mood regulations and treatment of major depressive disorder (MDD) [14].

Based on the evidence obtained via cerebral imagings in depression, this region has a low activity in left hemisphere and we can stimulate this area with repetitive TMS (rTMS). Over the past decades, the numbers of studies that have examined the effects of this therapy on depression have increased [8, 15, 16]. The majority of these researches indicate that TMS can be equal or close to ECT in treatment of drug- resistant depression [17- 22].

Based on metaanalysis results, stimulation with high frequency in left DLPFC decreases the symptoms of depression significantly [18, 23, 19]. Also there are other studies which indicate that this improvement is sustained after stimulation is ended [24].

Regarding the effectiveness of this method in the majority of studies, there are still reports that show this new technique to be ineffective or is equal to placebo [8]. Therefore, experimental studies for the study of effectiveness of this method and achievement of optimal parameters of rTMS in treatment of depression remain necessary.

Given the importance of this treatment method for depressive disorder, there hasn't been any local investigations in this area and as was mentioned the efficacy depends on various factors like intensity, duration of sessions and trains. Since the efficacy of rTMS with 20 Hz frequency during long sessions (30 sessions) with 3000 pulses per day (9000 pulses totally) hasn't been studied, we decided to conduct the current study. So the main question of this study is whether 30 sessions rTMS (thirty consecutive days) with high frequency and delivering 3000 pulses every session influences medication resistant depression or not and if it can change it, whether these changes will last or the effects are temporary?

METHOD

This quasi- experimental study was a single time series design and approved in Tehran university research committee. The subjects of study completed the consent form and were between 20 to 50 year old. Exclusion criteria were the history of head trauma or seizure in patients or their relatives, dependency to drug, pregnancy, having any metals or shunt in cranium and having peacemaker. 12 subjects who were referred to ATIEH clinic (Comprehensive Nerve and Psyche center) in summer to autumn 2010 were entered to the study after the diagnosis of a psychiatrist based on having MDD according to DSM-IV-TR.

By definition, being resistant to medications is that the patient did not show a therapeutic response to two different antidepressants agents [25]. The Beck Depression Inventory (BDI) was used to measure depression. This test has 21 items and each item is associated with a depressive symptoms. The validity and reliability has been reported high [26, 27].

The subjects were assessed with BDI two weeks and one week before the rTMS, and then were treated with rTMS in 30 daily sessions (except holidays). During the studies the subjects continued their medications without any changes. In follow up periods the medications were stable as well. The parameters were considered in left DLPFC (9 and 46 Brodman area), 60 trains with 20 Hz frequency, 2.5 seconds was the length of train and the intertrain pulse was 10 seconds. The figure-of-eight coil was selected and the intensity of stimulation was 100% of motor threshold. For each subject 3000 pulses were delivered in every session.

In each session patients sat on a chair for 20 minutes and put an earplug in their ears and had minimum communication with therapist. The BDI was completed immediately after the 30th session and 6 week later. For data analyzing, we applied the repeated measure ANOVA.

RESULTS

Totally 15 patients were considered for participating in the study, but subjects were excluded because of some reasons like having no cooperation, using of psychotherapy during rTMS or headache. The demographic characteristics of the 12 completers are provided in Table 1. The descriptive findings have been indicated in Table 2 and figure 1 in four steps (the first pre test, the second pre test, post test (i.e., after rTMS) and follow up).

For studying that whether the intervention was able to make changes in means of BDI in post test and follow up or not, we applied the repeated measure analysis of variance (rANOVA). It is worth noting that homogeneity of covariance assumptions by Mauchly's test of sphericity was mentioned and their results are in Table 3.

Table 1. Demographic characteristics of patients with MDD

Patient	Gender	age	medications
1	Female	44	Desipramine, Alprazolam
2	Female	20	Citalopram
3	Female	25	Clomipramine, lamotrigine
4	Male	45	Imipramine , Diazepam
5	Female	24	Depakin, trimipramine, Respridone
6	Female	50	Flouxtine, Xanax
7	Female	48	Serteraline
8	Male	37	Flouxtine, Desipramine
9	Female	50	-
10	Female	31	Desipramine, Lamotrigine, Clonazepam
11	Female	37	Desipramine, chloro diazopoxide
12	Female	39	Amitriptiline

Table 2. Results summary of Beck questionnaire

Step	Means of BDI	Standard deviations of BDI
First pre test (two weeks before rTMS)	23/33	7/53
Second pre test (one week before rTMS)	24/92	7/41
After rTMS	9/83	2/85
Follow up	10/42	2/87

Table 3. The Mauchly's Test of Sphericity

Scale	Mauchly W	K squares estimation	df	Sig
Depression	0/58	39.20	5	0.01

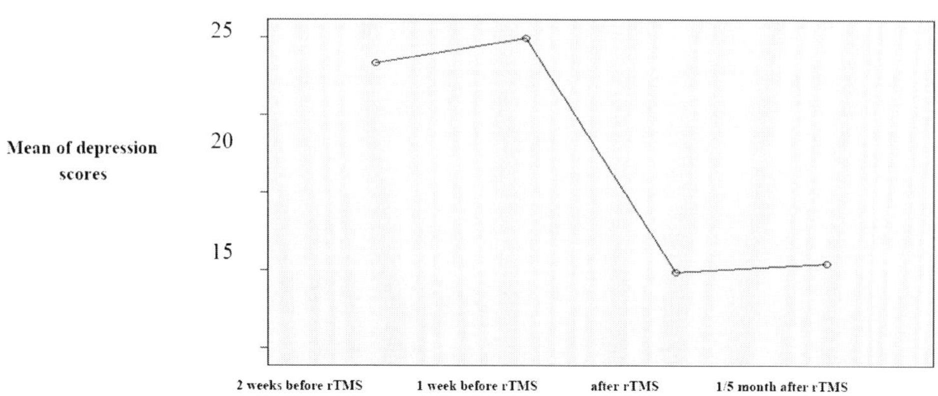

Figure 1. The changing of depression scores from the first to 1.5 month after rTMS.

This table results show that the homogenous covariance condition was established in this variable and analysis of variance with repeated measures in the data is permitted. Table 4 shows that the treatment could significantly improve the BDI scores ($p \leq 0.001$). For indicating that these changes are between what steps, we studied the mean of comparisons.

Table 4. The summary of within subjects effects

ecruoS	df	Sum squares	Mean squares	F	sig
Treatment	1/16	2369/08	2041/36	32/70	0/01
Error	12/77	796/92	62/43		

Table 5. The summary of changes in depression scores from the first pre test to follow up step

		Mean differences	Standard Error
First pre test	Second pre test	-1.58	0.65
	After rTMS	13.50	2.52
	Follow up	12.92	2.40
Second pre test	After rTMS	15.08	2.48
	Follow up	14.50	2.23
Post test	Follow up	-0.58	0.72

The results indicate that there were a mean difference between the first and second pre test and post test and follow up, while there weren't any differences between the first and second pre test (Table 5).

CONCLUSION

The aim of this research was to study of effectiveness of repetitive transcranial magnetic stimulation in medication resistant depression. Results show that rTMS with high frequency (20 Hz) is effective in patients with major depression. This finding is consistent with other findings [24, 17, 29, 34]. Long term changes in cortical excitability may explain the beneficial results which have obtained from patients. These changes are dependent on several factors like frequency, intensity, site and duration of stimulation. Some of these factors like site of stimulation in left prefrontal cortex are mostly the same in majority of studies, while other factors such as frequency, stimulation's time and sessions are inconclusive and optimizing and integration of them is essential [19].

As was stated, the duration of stimulation can be an important factor in effectiveness of this method. Results of meta analysis on depression and rTMS show that the stimulation with high frequency on DLPFC isn't associated with improvement of depression after two weeks treatment [35]. Most studies consider at least 4 consecutive weeks of treatment to achieve a significant therapeutic effects on depression [36]. One reasons for conflicting results is the limitation in duration of experiment. Most studies that have applied rTMS in 10 sessions or less have failed to obtain the meaningful results in treatment of depression. Therefore in this study, delivering 30 sessions can be raised as one of the reasons which is associated with efficacy of rTMS and this issue can be related to possible changes in long term potentiation (LTP) in neurons [37]. The frequency is another important factor. High frequency (more than 1 or equal) in rTMS and ECT has a similar effect in brain monoamine [38], beta adrenergic receptors [39], adenosine mono phosphate cycle [40], gene expression in nerve cells of mice [38- 41].

rTMS with high frequency in comparison to sham rTMS has been associated with the significant increase of 1A serotonin and NMDA receptors [42]. In Muller study, the results indicate that rTMS with high frequency like antidepressants and ECT is related to increasing of BDNF, mRNA and CCK in brain of mice [16]. Also in brain imagings like PET, dopamine has an important role in depression.

According to findings high frequency of rTMS in left dorsolateral prefrontal cortex increases the dopamine in ipsilateral nucleus accumbance [43]. rTMS with high frequency can induce mania and normalizes dexamethazone suppression test in depressed patient as well [44, 45]. Given the above, we conclude that high frequency rTMS can result in a significant antidepressant effect. Other effective factors in rTMS are the intensity of stimulation that has been reported as an important factor for inducing of LTP in most studies [46]. Due to the important role of rTMS in cortical excitability, like other studies the intensity was determined at 100% of motor threshold. However, a review of preview studies indicate that using high intensity, can however increase the risk of seizures.

Secondary objective of this study was the determination of the duration of treatment effects. Results show that the positive therapeutic effects lasted 6 weeks after the acute treatment. This finding is equivalent with other studies in terms of long lasting therapeutic effects. Bortolomasi with using 20 Hz rTMS during 20 sessions and totally with 800 pulses every session showed that the therapeutic effects have lasted about one month [47].

The duration of the therapeutic effect is one of the most important issues in this area and according to review that has been done by Gershon, the integration of some factors either in treatment or in long lasting effects can provide better results [11]. Due to the lack of time, there wasn't possible to follow up more than 6 weeks. For determining of long lasting effects, longer follow up with larger samples studies is essential.

One of the limitations of current study is the lack of control group with sham rTMS. Placebo can cause clinical response and its diagnosis is difficult without a control group. Therefore, the subjects were observed in a time series design and were as their control group, but the treatment environment could affect the results. Hence, nowadays the TMS companies with designing sham coils have provided that the patients experience a real sense of actual treatment without receiving the magnetic pulses [8].

Also due to individual differences in the form and cerebral anatomy, one of the limitation of this research is using of traditional method for determining the site of stimulation. In this study, the site stimulation was selected by international 10-20 system which is commonly used for electroencephalographic electrode placement and despite of the ease of use, there is a possibility of error in positioning of site stimulation correctly.

Nevertheless, further studies are necessary to determine optimal factors like intensity, frequency, duration of stimulation and the number of sessions in treatment of depression.

Also, it's necessary to have a comparison between this method an ECT and investigation of rTMS as a maintenance therapy after ECT. More studies in this fields cause to more knowledge about neuroanatomic structures in patients with resistant major depression.

ACKNOWLEDGMENTS

This study was approved and financially supported by research committee of faculty of psychology of Tehran University. The authors had no conflict of interest with the results.

ORIGINAL REFERENCE

Khomami S, Rostami R, Kazemi R, Rahiminezhad A. The study of effects of 20-Hz repetitive transcranial magnetic stimulation (rTMS) in medication resistant patients with major depression disorder. Journal of Fundamentals of Mental Health 2010; 12(3): 552-61.

REFERENCES

[1] Kessler RC, Berglund P, Demler O, Jin R, Merikangas KR, Walters EE. Life time prevalence and age-of-onset distributions of DSM-IV disorders in the National Comorbidity Survey Replication. *Arch. Gen. Psychiatry* 2005; 62: 593-602.

[2] World Health Organization. Fact Sheet N 130. Mental Health 1996 August. Geneva, Switzerland: *World Health Organization*; 2000: 120.

[3] Fava M. Diagnosis and definition of treatment-resistant depression. *Biol. Psychiatry* 2003; 53: 649-59.

[4] Keller MB, Lavori PW, Mueller TI, Endicott J, Coryell W, Hirschfeld RM, et al. Time to recovery, chronicity and levels of psychopathology in major depression. A 5-year prospective follow-up of 431 subjects. *Arch. Gen. Psychiatry* 1992; 49: 809-16.

[5] Fink M. Convulsive therapy: A review of the first 55 years. *J. Affect Disord.* 2001; 63: 1-15.

[6] Sackeim HA. The definition and meaning of treatment-resistant depression. *J. Clin. Psychiatry* 2001; 62: 10-7.

[7] Janicak PG, Davis JM, Gibbons RD, Ericksen S, Chang S, Gallagher P. Efficacy of ECT: A metaanalysis. *Am. J. Psychiatry* 1985; 142: 297-302.

[8] Mantovani A, Lisanby S. Transcranial magnetic stimulation in major depression. In: George MS, Belmaker R. (editors). Transcranial magnetic stimulation in clinical psychiatry. Washington. DC: *American Psychiatric Association*; 2007: 113-51.

[9] George MS, Nahas Z, Molloy M, Speer AM, Oliver NC, Li XB, et al. A controlled trial of daily left prefrontal cortex TMS for treating depression. *Biol. Psychiatry* 2000; 48: 962-70.

[10] Pascual-Leone A, Rubio B, Pallardo F, Catala M. Rapid-rate transcranial magnetic stimulation of left dorsolateral prefrontal cortex in drug resistant depression. *Lancet* 1996; 348: 233-7.

[11] Gershon AA, Dannon PN, Grunhaus L. Transcranial magnetic stimulation in the treatment of depression. *Am. J. Psychiatry* 2003; 160: 835-45.

[12] Loo C, Mitchel P, Sachdev P, McDarmont B, Parker G, Gandevia S. Double-blind controlled investigation of transcranial magnetic stimulation for the treatment of resistant major depression. *Am. J. Psychiatry* 1999; 156: 946-8.

[13] Keck ME. Repetitive transcranial magnetic stimulation effects in vitro and in animal models. In: Marcolin MA, Padberg F. (editors). Transcranial brain stimulation for treatment of psychiatric disorders. Switzerland: Karger publishing; 2007: 18-34.

[14] Soares JC, Mann JJ. The functional neuroanatomy of mood disorders. *J. Psychiatr. Res.* 1997; 31: 393-432.

[15] Hoflich G, Kasper S, Hufnagel S, Ruhrmann S, Moeller H. Application of transcranial magnetic stimulation in treatment of drug-resistant major depression: A report of two cases. *Hum. Psychopharmacol.* 1993; 8: 361-5.

[16] Muller M, Toschi N, Kresse A, Post A, Keck M. Long-term repetitive transcranial magnetic stimulation increases the expression of brain-derived neurotrophic factor and cholecystokinin mRNA, but not neuropeptide tyrosine mRNA in specific areas of rat brain. *Neuropsychopharmacol.* 2000; 23: 205-15.

[17] Berman RM, Narasimhan M, Sanacora G, Miano AP, Hoffman RE, Hu XS, et al. A randomized clinical trial of repetitive transcranial magnetic stimulation in the treatment of major depression. *Biol. Psychiatry* 2000; 47: 332-7.

[18] Burt T, Lisanby SH, Sackeim HA. Neuropsychiatric application of transcranial magnetic stimulation: A meta analysis. *Int J. Neuropsychopharmacol.* 2002; 5: 73-103.

[19] Martin JL, Barbanoj MJ, Schlaepfer TE, Thompson E, Kulisevsky J. Repetitive transcranial magnetic stimulation for the treatment of depression. Systematic review and and meta-analysis. *Br. J. Psychiatry* 2003; 182: 480-91.

[20] Schlaepfer TE, Kosel M, Nemeroff CB. Efficacy of repetitive transcranial magnetic stimulation (rTMS) in the treatment of affective disorders. *Neuropsychopharmacol.* 2003; 28: 201-5.

[21] Rowny S, Lisanby S. Other brain stimulation methods. In: Sadock B, Sadock V,Ruiz P. (editors). Comprehensive textbook of psychiatry. 9th ed. Philadelphia: Lippincott Williams and Wilkins; 2009: 3301-13.

[22] Herrmann LL, Ebmeier KP. Factors modifying the efficacy of transcranial magnetic stimulation in the treatment of depression a review. *J. Clin. Psychiatry* 2006; 67: 1870-6.

[23] Holtzheimer PE, Russo J, Avery DH. A meta-analysis of repetitive transcranial magnetic stimulation in the treatment of depression. *Psycho Pharmacol. Bull* 2001; 35: 149-69.

[24] Triggs WJ, McCoy KJ, Greer R, Rossi F, Bowers D, Kortenkamp S, et al. Effects of left frontal transcranial magnetic stimulation on depressed mood, cognition, and corticomotor threshold. *Biol. Psychiatry* 1999; 45: 1440-6.

[25] Rossini D, Magri L, Lucca A. Does rTMS hasten the response to escitalopram, sertraline, or venlafaxine in patients with major depressive disorder? A double-blind, randomized, sham-controlled trial. *J. Clin. Psychiatry* 2005; 66: 1569-75.

[26] Sarduee Gh. [The introduction on Beck revised questioner normalization]. MA. Dissertation. Tehran: Allame Tabatabaee University, College of psychology, 1995: 122-5. (Persian)

[27] Azadi F. [The appraisal of Beck depression inventory in Farabi Hospital (in one hundred and thirty depresses patients)]. MD. Dissertation. Kermanshah University of Medical Sciences, 1996. (Persian)

[28] Wassermann EM. Risk and safety of repetitive transcranial magnetic stimulation: Report and suggested guidelines from the International Workshop on the Safety of

Repetitive Transcranial Magnetic Stimulation, June 5-7, 1996. *Electroencephalogr. Clin. Neurophysiol.* 1998; 108: 1-16.

[29] George MS, Wassermann EM, Williams WA, Callahan A, Ketter TA, Basser P, et al. Daily repetitive transcranial magnetic stimulation (rTMS) improves mood in depression. *Neuroreport* 1995; : 1853-6.

[30] Manes F, Jorge R, Morcuende M, Yamada T, Paradiso S, Robinson RG. A controlled study of repetitive transcranial magnetic stimulation as a treatment of depression in the elderly. *Int. Psychogeriatr.* 2001; 13: 225-31.

[31] Garcia-Toro M, Pascual-Leone A, Romera M, Gonzalez A, Mico J, Ibarra O, et al. Prefrontal repetitive transcranial magnetic stimulation as add on treatment in depression. *J. Neurol. Neurosurg. Psychiatry* 2001; 71: 546-8.

[32] Hoppner J, Schulz M, Irmisch G, Mau R, Schlafke D, Richter J. Antidepressant efficacy of two different rTMS procedures. High frequency over left versus low frequency over right prefrontal cortex compared with sham stimulation. *Eur. Arch. Psychiatry Clin. Neurosci.* 2003; 253: 103-9.

[33] Mosimann UP, Schmitt W, Greenberg BD, Kose M, Muri R, Berkhoff M, et al. Repetitive transcranial magnetic stimulation: A putative add-on treatment for major depression in elderly patients. *Psychiatry Res.* 2004; 126: 123-33.

[34] Koerselman F, Laman DM, van Duijn H, van Duijin M, Willems M. A 3-month, follow-up, randomized, placebo-controlled study of repetitive transcranial magnetic stimulation in depression. *J. Clin. Psychiatry* 2004; 65: 1323-8.

[35] Couturier JL. Efficacy of rapid-rate repetitive transcranial magnetic stimulation in the treatment of depression: A systematic review and meta-analysis. *J. Psychiatry Neurosci.* 2005; 30: 83-90.

[36] Rumi DO, Gattaz WF, Rigonatti SP, Rosa M, Fregni F, Rosa M, et al. Transcranial magnetic stimulation accelerates the antidepressant effect of amitriptyline in severe depression: A double-blind placebo-controlled study. *Biol. Psychiatry* 2005; 57: 162-6.

[37] Wassermann EM, Lisanby SH. Therapeutic application of repetitive transcranial magnetic stimulation: A review. *Clin. Neurophysiol.* 2001; 112: 1367-77.

[38] Ben-Shachar D, Belmaker R, Grisaru N, Klein E. Transcranial magnetic stimulation induces alterations monoamines in brain. *J. Neural. Transmis.* 1997; 104: 191-7.

[39] Ben-Shachar D, Gazawi H, Riboyand-Levin J, Klein E. Chronic repetitive transcranial magnetic stimulation alters beta-adrenergic and 5-HT2 receptor characteristics in rat brain. *Brain Res.* 1999; 816: 78-83.

[40] Fujiki M, Steward O. High frequency TMS mimics the effects of ECS up regulating astroglial gene expression in the murine CNS. *Molecul. Brain Res.* 1997; 44: 301-8.

[41] Ji R, Schlaepfer T, Aizenman C, Epstein CM, Qiu D, Huang J, et al. Repetitive transcranial magnetic stimulation activates specific regions in rat brain. Proceedings National Academy Science USA 1998; 95: 15635-40.

[42] Kole M, Fuchs E, Ziemann U, Paulus W, Ebert U. Changes in 5-HT1A and NMDA binding sites by a single rapid transcranial magnetic stimulation procedure in rats. *Brain Res.* 1999; 826: 309-12.

[43] Strafella A, Paus T, Barrett J, Dagher A. Repetitive transcranial magnetic stimulation of the human prefrontal cortex induces dopamine release in the caudate nucleus. *J. Neurosci.* 2001; 21: 1-4.

[44] Dolberg O, Schreiber S, Grunhaus L. Transcranial magnetic stimulation-induced switch into mania: a report of two cases. *Biol. Psychiatry* 2001; 49: 468-70.

[45] Pridmore S. Rapid Transcranial magnetic stimulation (rTMS) and normalization of the dexamethasone suppression test (DST). *Psychiatr. Clin. Neurosci.* 1999; 53: 33-7.

[46] Kozel A, Nahas Z, deBrux C, Molloy M, Lorberbaum J, Bohning D, et al. How coil-cortex distance relates to age, motor threshold, and antidepressant response to transcranial magnetic stimulation. *J. Neuropsychiatr. Clin. Neurosci.* 2000; 12: 376-84.

[47] Bortlomasi M, Minelli A, Fuggetta G, Perini M, Comencini S, Fiaschi A, et al. Long-lasting effects of high frequency repetitive transcranial magnetic stimulation in major depressed patients. *J. Clin. Psychiatry* 2007; 150: 181-6.

NEUROPSYCHIATRY

In: The International Psychiatry and Behavioral ... ISBN: 978-1-62257-566-4
Editor: Nash Boutros

Chapter 10

ADVOCACY OF ELDERLY PERSONS WITH DEMENTIA AND EVALUATION OF THEIR MENTAL CAPACITY: CONSISTENCY BETWEEN RESULTS OF INTELLIGENT AND COGNITIVE TESTS AND CAPACITY TO PERFORM FINANCIAL AND EVERYDAY ACTIVITIES

***Osamu Matsuda**[*1] and Masahiko Saito*[2]

[1]Tokyo Gakugei University, Japan
[2]Tokyo Metroporitan Matsuzawa Hospital, Tokyo, Japan

ABSTRACT

This study examined the relationship between results of psychological tests (WAIS-R, MMSE, and COGNISTAT) of 96 patients with dementia and their capacity to perform everyday activities, including the capacity to manage their finances. The financial capacity did not correspond with their IQ scores when they were above average (89/90). It also did not correspond with the MMSE score when they were above the cutoff point (23/24). Approximately 80% of the patients whose IQ was above average did not have enough capacity to manage their finances. However, in these patients, the likelihood that they could not manage their finances was high when their scaled-score on the orientation subtest of the COGNISTAT was at the impaired level. This study suggests a possibility that patients with dementia do not have enough capacity to manage their finances even if their IQ and MMSE scores are above average or normal. We must note this point in cases of psychiatric evidence for adult guardianship.

Keywords: Dementia, advocacy, capacity assessment, adult guardianship, psychiatric evidence

---

* Corresponding Author: Osamu Matsuda, PhD Associate Professor of Tokyo Gakugei University, Nukuikita 4-1-1, Koganei-shi, Tokyo 184-8501, Japan ; Phone and Fax: +81-42-329-7373; E-mail: matsuda@u-gakugei.ac.jp
Reprinted with permission from The Japanese Journal of Geriatric Psychiatry. Original Publication: The Japanese Journal of Geriatric Psychiatry Vol 22 (6): 723–733, 2011.

Background and Purpose

The age structure of the world population in 2005 (United Nations, 2008) indicated that elderly people accounted for an estimated 7.3% of the world's population. For Japan, the figure was 20.1%, which is the highest in the world, and is expected to rise further, reaching 48.0% in 2025. The unprecedented aging of the Japanese population has markedly increased the number of persons at risk for dementia, particularly Alzheimer's disease (AD). In such circumstances, guardianship for elderly persons with dementia has become increasingly important.

Various capacities are needed for elderly persons to live safety and independently in their communities. These include not only the capacities to perform everyday activities, such as shopping and going to the doctor, but also other capacities such as for managing finances. The financial capacity is a fundamental ability to continue independent living. Presently, elderly persons with dementia are often victims of financial crimes and unfair contracts in Japan because they continue to manage their financial affairs despite being unable to do so appropriately. The Japanese new adult guardianship system is expected to protect the rights of such Japanese persons.

Judging about whether an individual has the mental capacity to manage the financial affairs is a curial procedure in adult guardianship proceedings. In Japan, traditionally, while making a civil statement, a psychiatrist has to evaluate the symptoms related to psychosis, organic mental disorders like dementia and any other disorders that affect conscious cognition, and other psychological functions (Saito, 2001). When no psychotic symptoms are observed, the level of intelligence (IQ) is often the only judgment criterion. However, this conventional method is unsuitable for judging the mental capacity of elderly patients with dementia, particularly AD. In the procedure of judging the mental capacity or financial capacity, psychological assessment is used as an important tool to assess the mental capacity of elderly persons. Structured psychological tests such as the Wechsler Adult Intelligence Scale (WAIS-R) and dementia screening tests such as the Mini-Mental State Examination (MMSE) have often been used for obtaining information about mental capacity. In Japan, the results of the IQ or MMSE scores have been regarded as one of the most important indicators of the financial capacity of elderly persons. In general, if the subjects' psychological test results shown them to be at an impaired level, they are regarded as not having enough financial capacity (Igarashi, 2006). On the other hand, if their test scores are within the normal range (e.g., IQ $\geq$ 90 or MMSE score $\geq$ cut-off point), they are likely to be regarded as having enough capacity and judged to have little need of protective intervention (Saito, 1997; Saito, 2001). However, this conventional strategy is not always adequate to judge the financial capacity of elderly persons with dementia because of two considerations regarding the interpretation of test results. The first consideration is the interpretation of IQ. Saito (2001) pointed out that many patients with dementia of the Alzheimer type, even with an IQ of 100 or higher, are unable to perform simple actions such as withdrawing cash from their bank account. Major intellectual tests such as WAIS-R include no items to evaluate episodic memory and orientation, which are commonly impaired in patients with dementia. Some patients with high premorbid IQ exhibit a relatively higher IQ after the onset of dementia, in particular, during the stage of mild dementia. As a result, some patients who have impairments in the episodic memory and orientation still exhibit normal IQ levels (e.g., IQ $\geq$

90). However, these impairments are often associated with many everyday activities, including managing finances (Matsuda and Saito, 2005). Therefore, some patients whose IQ is above average do not have enough capacity to manage their finances. The second consideration is the interpretation of the scores of dementia screening tests. Needless to say, these tests were developed as a screening test for dementia and not to judge financial capacity. The cut-off point of these tests is the criterion for separating persons with dementia from those without, but not for separating persons who have enough financial capacity from those who do not. As a result, some dementia patients do not always have enough financial capacity even though their MMSE score is less than the cut-off point. We hypothesized that even when the results of psychological tests are within the normal range, they do not always correspond with having enough financial capacity (e.g., IQ or MMSE score). Furthermore, in patients with dementia, even though these results are normal, the patients may be unable to perform activities that are linked to specific cognitive abilities such as episodic memory and orientation. However, data-based studies addressing these points are scarce, particularly in Japan. In this study, we examined the relationship between the results of neuropsychological tests (e.g., WAIS-R, MMSE, and Neurobehavioral Cognitive Status Examination (COGNISTAT)) of 96 patients with dementia and their capacity to perform everyday activities, including financial capacity.

METHODS

1. Subjects

The subjects of this study were 96 community-dwelling patients with dementia who were treated in a psychiatric clinic from April 2001 until March 2005 (Male = 30, Female = 66). All subjects fulfilled the diagnostic criteria for dementia of Japanese translation of DSM-IV-TR (Takahashi, 2003). Eighty-seven subjects were diagnosed as having dementia of the Alzheimer's type, six were diagnosed as having vascular dementia, and three were diagnosed as having front temporal dementia. The mean age of the subjects was 74.9 years (SD = 8.4), ranging from 50 to 89. The mean years of education was 12.9 (SD = 2.6), ranging from 6 to 18. According to the Japanese translation of the Clinical Dementia Rating (Honma, 1991), the subjects of this study included 21 (21.9%) of CDR0.5, 48 (50.0%) of CDR1, 26 (27.1%) of CDR2, and 1 (1.0%) of CDR3. About 70% of the subjects were classified as patients with mild dementia.

2. MEASUREMENTS

2.1. Neuropsychological Assessment

We used three psychological tests, including the Japanese version of the WAIS-R (Shinagawa et al., 1990), the Japanese translation of the MMSE (Kitamura, 1991), and the Japanese version of the COGNISTAT (Matsuda and Nakatani, 2004). IQ was calculated using the Japanese version of the WAIS-R (Shinagawa, et al., 1990). According to the manual of the WAIS-R, one's IQ is regarded as average if it is 90 or higher. Based on this criterion, we classified subjects into two groups according to their IQ (IQ-high group and IQ-low group). The IQ-high group consisted of subjects whose IQ was 90 or higher, and the IQ-low group consisted of those whose IQ was less than 90. For the MMSE score, we classified subjects into two groups (MMSE-high group and MMSE-low group) based on the cut-off point (23/34). The COGNISTAT includes ten subtests of cognition: orientation, attention, comprehension, repetition, naming, construct ability, memory, calculation, similarities, and judgment. According to the manual of the COGNISTAT, the cut-off point for each subtest was set between 8 and 9. Based on this cut-off point, we classified the subjects into two groups for each subtest (impaired-level (IMP) group and within normal limits (WNL) group).

Table 1 shows the number of subjects in each group. All assessments were conducted by the first author who is a licensed, certified clinical psychologist.

2.2. Functional Assessment

The capacities to perform financial and everyday activities were evaluated by a 35-item questionnaire that covered basic and instrumental ADLs. As shown in Table 2, the questionnaire covered items about managing finances, using public transportation, taking precautions, self-care, housekeeping, communication, and taking medicine.

The degree of the patients' ability to perform each activity was rated on a 4-point scale (1 = cannot do at all to 4 = can do well) by relatives familiar with the patients' everyday activities. If a subject was rated 1 or 2 for an activity, we judged that the subject was unable to perform that activity. The subjects rated 1 or 2 were classified as the "unable group," and the others were classified as the "able group." The subjects who had not undertaken a particular activity until that time were not included in the analysis for that activity.

3. Data Analysis

In this study, we examined the consistency between the results of neuropsychological assessments and those of functional assessment. To examine consistency, we calculated a kappa coefficient between each pair of the results of neuropsychological assessment (IQ-high group vs. IQ-low group, MMSE-high group vs. MMSE-low group, and IMP group vs. WNL group) and the performance of 35 activities (unable group vs. able group). According to Landis and Koch (1977), a Kappa coefficient is regarded fair if ranging 0.21–0.40, moderate if ranging 0.41–0.60, substantial if ranging 0.61–0.80, and almost perfect if ranging 0.81–1.00. In this study, we judged the kappa coefficients of more than 0.40 as acceptable.

4. Ethical Considerations

The research protocol of this study was approved by the ethical committee of Tokyo Gakugei University.

Table 1. Frequency of each group based on the results of the neuropsychological tests

	Groups					
	Low or IMP		High or WNL		Sum	
Neuropsychological tests	n	%	n	%	n	%
IQ group (IQ-low group vs. IQ-high group)	59	61.5	37	38.5	96	100
MMSE group (MMSE-low group vs. MMSE-high group)	71	81.6	16	18.4	87[a]	100
COGNISTAT orientation (IMP group vs. WNL group)	79	82.3	17	17.7	96	100
COGNISTAT attention (IMP group vs. WNL group)	35	36.5	61	63.5	96	100
COGNISTAT comprehension (IMP group vs. WNL group)	45	46.9	51	53.1	96	100
COGNISTAT repetition (IMP group vs. WNL group)	31	32.3	65	67.7	96	100
COGNISTAT naming (IMP group vs. WNL group)	39	40.6	57	59.4	96	100
COGNISTAT construct ability (IMP group vs. WNL group)	79	82.3	17	17.7	96	100
COGNISTAT memory (IMP group vs. WNL group)	90	93.8	6	6.3	96	100
COGNISTAT calculation (IMP group vs. WNL group)	35	36.5	61	63.5	96	100
COGNISTAT similarities (IMP group vs. WNL group)	50	52.1	46	47.9	96	100
COGNISTAT judgment (IMP group vs. WNL group)	27	28.1	69	71.9	96	100

Note: IMP = Impaired level. WNL = Within normal limits. [a] Missing value for MMSE (n= 9).

Table 2. Consistency between IQ and functional activities

Functional Activities		IQ-low group (IQ≦89)		IQ-high group (IQ≧90)		Kappa		Odds[a]	
No.	Items	n/N	%	n/N	%				
1	Managing immovable items or property	27/40	67.5	17/26	65.4	0.02		1.10	
2	Paying money correctly	26/50	52.0	9/31	29.0	0.21	*	2.64	
3	Managing a bank account	30/53	56.6	12/30	40.0	0.15		1.96	
4	Use of a credit card	14/27	51.9	9/18	50.0	0.02		1.08	
5	Contract for a loan, rental, and sale	23/28	82.1	14/18	77.8	0.05		1.31	
6	Buying expensive things	24/33	72.7	13/17	76.5	-0.04		0.82	
7	Buying things of daily necessity	18/56	32.1	4/35	11.4	0.18	*	3.67	*
8	Taking medicine properly	36/59	61.0	13/36	36.1	0.24	*	2.77	*
9	Going to hospital	37/57	64.9	17/37	45.9	0.19		2.18	
10	Applying for a social welfare service	38/39	97.4	15/19	78.9	0.23	*	10.13	
11	Driving a car	17/19	89.5	10/13	79.9	0.14		2.55	
12	Taking a train or subway	35/56	62.5	16/37	43.2	0.19		2.19	
13	Taking a bus	34/55	61.8	13/37	35.1	0.26	*	2.99	*
14	Taking a taxi	27/50	54.0	13/35	37.1	0.16		1.99	
15	Gifting	32/48	66.7	13/23	56.5	0.10		1.54	
16	Writing letters	31/55	56.4	12/36	33.3	0.22	*	2.58	
17	Using a telephone	13/57	22.8	3/34	8.8	0.11		3.05	
18	Using e-mail	13/14	92.9	4/6	66.7			6.50	
19	Preparing a menu	32/44	72.7	7/20	35.0	0.35	**	4.95	*
20	Cooking	30/47	63.8	9/19	47.4	0.15		1.96	

Functional Activities		IQ-low group (IQ≦89)		IQ-high group (IQ≧90)		Kappa		Odds[a]	
21	Arranging the room	28/58	48.3	8/35	22.9	0.23	*	3.15	*
22	Clearing the room	25/53	47.2	10/30	33.3	0.12		1.79	
23	Operating a washing machine	19/47	40.4	7/22	31.8	0.07		1.45	
24	Managing and handling a gas range	16/54	29.6	3/32	9.4	0.17	*	4.07	
25	Locking doors	14/58	24.1	2/35	5.7	0.15	*	5.25	*
26	Operating televisions or radios	16/57	28.1	3/36	8.3	0.17	*	4.29	*
27	Operating heaters or air conditioners	22/57	38.6	5/34	14.7	0.20	*	3.65	*
28	Preparing for a bath	24/52	46.2	4/32	12.5	0.29	**	6.00	**
29	Taking a bath	10/58	17.2	1/36	2.8	0.12	*	7.29	
30	Toilet	2/58	3.4	0/36	0.0	0.03			
31	Eating	3/58	5.2	1/35	2.9	0.02		1.86	
32	Choosing suitable clothes for the season	16/58	27.6	3/34	8.8	0.15	*	3.94	
33	Dressing	8/58	13.8	1/35	2.9	0.09		5.44	
34	Being careful of one's appearance	11/58	19.0	3/36	8.3	0.09		2.57	
35	Washing one's face and teeth and managing false teeth	7/58	12.1	0/36	0.0	0.10	*		

Note "n" represents the number of the subjects who were judged as unable to perform. It does not include the number of the subjects who had not performed the activities previously. "N" represents the number of the subjects who had not performed the activity previously. The sum of N on the same line represents the number of the subjects who had performed the activity previously. aBlank indicates that the odds ratio could not be calculated because the figure in the cell was zero. * $p < 0.05$, ** $p < 0.01$.

Table 3. Consistency between MMSE and functional activities

Functional Activities		MMSE-low group (MMSE ≤ 23)		MMSE-high group (MMSE ≥ 24)		Kappa		Odds[a]	
No.	Items	n/N	%	n/N	%				
1	Managing immovable items or property	37/49	75.5	5/11	45.5	0.24	*	3.70	
2	Paying money correctly	31/60	51.7	2/15	13.3	0.23	**	6.95	*
3	Managing a bank account	38/60	63.3	2/15	13.3	0.33	**	11.23	**
4	Use of a credit card	21/36	58.3	1/6	16.7	0.21		7.00	
5	Contract for a loan, rental, and sale	30/36	83.3	4/7	57.1	0.24		3.75	
6	Buying expensive things	31/38	81.6	4/8	50.0	0.28		4.43	
7	Buying things of daily necessity	21/66	31.8	1/16	6.3	0.13	*	7.00	
8	Taking medicine properly	42/71	59.2	5/16	31.3	0.18	*	3.19	
9	Going to hospital	47/70	67.1	2/16	12.5	0.36	**	14.30	**
10	Applying for a social welfare service	43/45	95.6	5/8	62.5	0.39	**	12.90	*
11	Driving a car	23/26	88.5	1/3	33.3	0.43	*	15.33	
12	Taking a train or subway	42/69	60.9	4/15	26.7	0.21	*	4.28	*
13	Taking a bus	41/68	60.3	2/15	13.3	0.29	**	9.87	**
14	Taking a taxi	35/63	55.6	3/14	21.4	0.20	*	4.58	*
15	Gifting	39/53	73.6	3/11	27.3	0.33	**	7.43	**
16	Writing letters	36/66	54.5	4/16	25.0	0.18	*	3.60	
17	Using a telephone	14/67			6.7	0.06		3.70	
18	Using e-mail	15/16	93.8	1/3	33.3	0.60	**	30.00	
19	Preparing a menu	35/45	77.8	3/13	23.1	0.46	**	11.67	**
20	Cooking	33/46	71.7	3/14	21.4	0.40	**	9.31	*

Functional Activities		MMSE-low group (MMSE ≤ 23)		MMSE-high group (MMSE ≥ 24)		Kappa		Odds[a]	
21	Arranging the room	31/68	45.6	3/16	18.8	0.15	*	3.63	
22	Clearing the room	29/59	49.2	4/15	26.7	0.14		2.66	
23	Operating a washing machine	22/50	44.0	2/14	14.3	0.18	*	4.71	
24	Managing and handling a gas range	18/64	28.1	1/15	6.7	0.10		5.48	
25	Locking doors	15/69	21.7	0/16	0.0	0.10	*		
26	Operating televisions or radios	18/68	26.5	0/16	0.0	0.12	*		
27	Operating heaters or air conditioners	24/67	35.8	1/16	6.3	0.15	*	8.37	*
28	Preparing for a bath	24/61	39.3	3/16	18.8	0.12		2.81	
29	Taking a bath	9/69	13.0	1/16	6.3	0.03		2.25	
30	Toilet	2/69	2.9	0/16	0.0	0.01			
31	Eating	3/68	4.4	0/16	0.0	0.02			
32	Choosing suitable clothes for the season	18/68	26.5	1/16	6.3	0.09		5.40	
33	Dressing	8/68	11.8	0/16	0.0	0.05			
34	Being careful of one's appearance	12/69	17.4	1/16	6.3	0.05		3.16	
35	Washing one's face and teeth and managing false teeth	6/69	8.7	1/16	6.3	0.01		1.43	

Note: "n" represents the number of the subjects who were judged as unable to perform. It does not include the number of the subjects who had not performed the activities previously. "N" represents the number of the subjects who had not performed the activity previously. The sum of N on the same line represents the number of the subjects who had performed the activity previously. aBlank indicates that the odds ratio could not be calculated because the figure in the cell was zero. * $p < 0.05$, ** $p < 0.01$.

Table 4. Consistency between COGNISTAT and functional activities

COGNISTAT	Functional Activities		Groups				Kappa		Odds[a]	
			IMP group		WNL group					
	No.	Items	n/N	%	n/N	%				
Orientation	1	Managing immovable items or property	40/51	78.4	4/15	26.7	0.44	**	10.00	**
	2	Paying money correctly	32/65	49.2	3/16	18.8	0.18	*	4.20	
	3	Managing a bank account	39/68	57.4	3/15	20.0	0.22	**	5.38	*
	5	Contract for a loan, rental, and sale	30/34	88.2	7/12	58.3	0.33	*	5.36	
	6	Buying expensive things	34/41	82.9	3/9	33.3	0.42	**	9.71	**
	9	Going to hospital	48/77	62.3	6/17	35.3	0.18	*	3.03	
	11	Driving a car	23/25	92.0	4/7	57.1	0.39	**	8.63	
	13	Taking a bus	44/76	57.9	3/16	18.8	0.23	**	5.96	*
	15	Gifting	40/57	70.2	5/14	35.7	0.26	*	4.24	*
	16	Writing letters	40/74	54.1	3/17	17.6	0.21	**	5.49	*
	32	Choosing suitable clothes for the season	19/75	25.3	0/17	0.0	0.11	*		
Comprehension	7	Buying things of daily necessity	14/41	34.1	8/50	16.0	0.19	*	2.72	
	9	Going to hospital	32/45	71.1	22/49	44.9	0.26	*	3.02	*
	13	Taking a bus	27/41	65.9	20/51	39.2	0.26	*	2.99	*
	14	Taking a taxi	23/38	60.5	17/47	36.2	0.24	*	2.71	*
	15	Gifting	28/36	77.8	17/35	48.6			3.71	*
	16	Writing letters	25/42	59.5	18/49	36.7			2.53	
	17	Using a telephone	13/43	30.2	3/48	6.3	0.25	**	6.50	**
	24	Managing and handling a gas range	13/39	33.3	6/47	12.8	0.22	*	3.42	*

COGNISTAT	Functional Activities		Groups					Kappa		Odds[a]	
			IMP group			WNL group					
			n/N	%		n/N	%				
	25	Locking doors	13/44	29.5		3/49	6.1	0.24	**	6.43	**
	26	Operating televisions or radios	13/43	30.2		6/50	12.0	0.19	*	3.18	
	28	Preparing for a bath	17/38	44.7		11/46	23.9	0.21	*	2.58	
	32	Choosing suitable clothes for the season	14/43	32.6		5/49	10.2	0.23	**	4.25	*
Repetition	7	Buying things of daily necessity	11/29	37.9		11/62	17.7	0.22	*	2.83	
	17	Using a telephone	10/30	33.3		6/61	9.8	0.27	**	4.58	*
	19	Preparing for a menu	17/21	81.0		22/43	51.2	0.24	*	4.06	*
	27	Operating heaters or air conditioners	13/28	46.4		14/63	22.2	0.24	*	3.03	*
	28	Preparing for a bath	15/29	51.7		13/55	23.6	0.28	**	3.46	*
	32	Choosing suitable clothes for the season	10/29	34.5		9/63	14.3	0.22	*	3.16	
	33	Dressing	7/30	23.3		2/63	3.2	0.25	**	9.28	**
	35	Washing one's face and teeth and managing false teeth	5/30	16.7		2/64	3.1	0.17	*	6.20	
Naming	2	Paying money correctly	21/33	63.6		14/48	29.2	0.34	**	4.25	**
	3	Managing a bank account	23/34	67.6		19/49	38.8	0.28	*	3.30	*
	5	Contract for a loan, rental, and sale	20/21	95.2		17/25	68.0	0.26	*	9.41	
	7	Buying things of daily necessity	13/36	36.1		9/55	16.4	0.21	*	2.89	
	8	Taking medicine properly	26/38	68.4		23/57	40.4	0.27	**	3.20	*
	9	Going to hospital	29/39	74.4		25/55	45.5	0.27	**	3.48	*
	12	Taking a train or subway	28/38	73.7		23/55	41.8	0.30	**	3.90	**
	13	Taking a bus	27/37	73.0		20/55	36.4	0.35	**	4.73	**

Table 4. (Continued)

COGNISTAT	Functional Activities		Groups					Kappa		Odds[a]	
			IMP group			WNL group					
			n/N	%		n/N	%				
	14	Taking a taxi	24/34	70.6		16/51	31.4	0.38	**	5.25	**
	15	Gifting	25/30	83.3		20/41	48.8	0.32	**	5.25	**
	16	Writing letters	22/35	62.9		21/56	37.5	0.24	*	2.82	*
	17	Using a telephone	11/36	30.6		5/55	9.1	0.24	**	4.40	*
	19	Preparing a menu	21/27	77.8		18/37	48.6	0.28	*	3.69	*
	20	Cooking	20/27	74.1		19/39	48.7	0.24	*	3.01	
	22	Clearing the room	19/33	57.6		16/50	32.0	0.25	*	2.88	*
	24	Managing and handling a gas range	11/33	33.3		8/53	15.1	0.20	*	2.81	
	25	Locking doors	10/37	27.0		6/56	10.7	0.18	*	3.09	
	28	Preparing for a bath	17/32	53.1		11/52	21.2	0.33	**	4.22	**
	32	Choosing suitable clothes for the season	12/36	33.3		7/56	12.5	0.23	*	3.50	*
	33	Dressing	7/37	18.9		2/56	3.6	0.18	*	6.30	*
	35	Washing one's face and teeth and managing false teeth	6/37	16.2		1/57	1.8	0.17	**	10.84	*
Construct ability	7	Buying things of daily necessity	22/74	29.7		0/17	0.0	0.14	*		
	9	Going to hospital	48/77	62.3		6/17	35.3	0.18	*	3.03	
	21	Arranging the room	34/76	44.7		2/17	11.8	0.17	*	6.07	*
	24	Managing and handling a gas range	19/71	26.8		0/15	0.0	0.11	*		
	25	Locking doors	16/76	21.1		0/17	0.0	0.09	*		
	32	Choosing suitable clothes for the season	19/75	25.3		0/17	0.0	0.11	*		

COGNISTAT	Functional Activities		Groups					Kappa		Odds[a]	
			IMP group			WNL group					
			n/N	%		n/N	%				
Memory	2	Paying money correctly	35/75	46.7		0/6	0.0	0.12	*		
	5	Contract for a loan, rental, and sale	37/44	84.1		0/2	0.0	0.32	**		
	6	Buying expensive things	37/47	78.7		0/3	0.0	0.31	**		
	11	Driving a car	26/28	92.9		1/4	25.0	0.61	**	39.00	**
Calculation	2	Paying money correctly	18/29	62.1		17/52	32.7	0.28	*	3.37	*
	7	Buying things of daily necessity	12/33	36.4		10/58	17.2	0.21	*	2.74	
	8	Taking medicine properly	23/35	65.7		26/60	43.3	0.21	*	2.51	
	16	Writing letters	21/33	63.6		22/58	37.9	0.24	*	2.86	*
	17	Using a telephone	11/34	32.4		5/57	8.8	0.26	**	4.97	*
	19	Preparing a menu	22/25	88.0		17/39	43.6	0.40	**	9.49	**
	22	Clearing the room	20/33	60.6		15/50	30.0	0.30	**	3.59	*
	26	Operating televisions or radios	11/35	31.4		8/58	13.8	0.19	*	2.87	
	28	Preparing for a bath	17/33	51.5		11/51	21.6	0.31	**	3.86	**
	32	Choosing suitable clothes for the season	11/34	32.4		8/58	13.8	0.20	*	2.99	
	33	Dressing	7/34	20.6		2/59	3.4	0.20	**	7.39	*
	34	Being careful of one's appearance	9/35	25.7		5/59	8.5	0.20	*	3.74	*
	35	Washing one's face and teeth and managing false teeth	7/35	20.0		0/59	0.0	0.24	**		
Similarities	8	Taking medicine properly	31/50	62.0		18/45	40.0	0.22	*	2.45	
	20	Cooking	25/35	71.4		14/31	45.2	0.27	*	3.04	
Judgment	2	Paying money correctly	16/24	66.7		19/57	33.3	0.29	**	4.00	*
	4	Use of a credit card	9/9	100.0		14/36	38.9	0.39	**		

Table 4. (Continued)

COGNISTAT	Functional Activities		Groups				Kappa		Odds[a]	
			IMP group		WNL group					
			n/N	%	n/N	%				
	5	Contract for a loan, rental, and sale	15/15	100.0	22/31	71.0	0.21	*		
	7	Buying things of daily necessity	10/24	41.7	12/67	17.9	0.24	*	3.27	*
	12	Taking a train or subway	20/25	80.0	31/68	45.6	0.26	**	4.77	**
	13	Taking a bus	19/25	76.0	28/67	41.8	0.27	**	4.41	**
	14	Taking a taxi	16/24	66.7	24/61	39.3	0.23	*	3.08	*
	15	Gifting	19/21	90.5	26/50	52.0	0.29	**	8.77	**
	16	Writing letters	19/25	76.0	24/66	36.4	0.32	**	5.54	**
	19	Preparing a menu	14/15	93.3	25/49	51.0	0.27	**	13.44	**
	21	Arranging the room	15/27	55.6	21/66	31.8	0.22	*	2.68	
	23	Operating a washing machine	10/17	58.8	16/52	30.8	0.24	*	3.21	
	24	Managing and handling a gas range	9/23	39.1	10/63	15.9	0.25	*	3.41	*
	28	Preparing for a bath	13/21	61.9	15/63	23.8	0.34	**	5.20	**
	32	Choosing suitable clothes for the season	10/27	37.0	9/65	13.8	0.25	*	3.66	*
	35	Washing one's face and teeth and managing false teeth	5/27	18.5	2/67	3.0	0.20	**	7.39	*

Note: This table shows only those activities whose kappa coefficient was significant. "n" represents the number of the subjects who were judged as unable to perform. It does not include the number of the subjects who had not performed the activities previously. "N" represents the number of the subjects who had not performed the activity previously. The sum of N on the same line represents the number of the subjects who had performed the activity previously. aBlank indicates that the odds ratio could not be calculated because the figure in the cell was zero. * $p < 0.05$, ** $p < 0.01$.

Table 5. Relationship between the results of COGNISTAT and functional activities among the subjects in the IQ-high group and MMSE-high group

Group	Subtests	Functional activities		Groups				Kappa		Odds[a]	
				IMP group		WML group					
		No.	Items	n/N	%	n/N	%				
IQ-high group	Orientation	1	Managing immovable items or property	16/21	76.2	1/5	20.0	0.43	*	12.80	
	Orientation	5	Contract for a loan, rental, and sale	13/14	92.9	1/4	25.0	0.68	**	39.00	*
	Memory	6	Buying expensive things	13/15	86.7	0/2	0.0	0.61	**		
	Orientation	11	Driving a car	10/11	90.9	0/2	0.0	0.76	**		
	Orientation	13	Taking a bus	13/30	43.3	0/7	0.0	0.22	*		
MMSE-high group	Orientation	16	Writing letters	4/7	57.1	0/9	0.0	0.60	**		
	Naming	23	Operating a washing machine	2/3	66.7	0/11	0.0	0.76	**		

Note This table shows only those activities whose kappa coefficient was significant. "n" represents the number of the subjects who were judged as unable to perform. It does not include the number of the subjects who had not performed the activities previously. "N" represents the number of the subjects who had not performed the activity previously. The sum of N on the same line represents the number of the subjects who had performed the activity previously. aBlank indicates that the odds ratio could not be calculated because the figure in the cell was zero. * $p < 0.05$, ** $p < 0.01$.

RESULTS

1. Consistency between IQ and Functional Activities

Table 2 shows the consistency between the scores of the IQ groups and the judgment of functional activities. As shown in the table, there were no kappa coefficients with value of 0.41 or above. More than 75% of the subjects in the IQ-high group were judged as unable to contract a loan, rental, or sale; buy expensive things; apply for social welfare services; or drive a car.

2. Consistency between MMSE and Functional Activities

Table 3 shows the consistency between the scores of the groups of MMSE and the judgment of functional activities. As shown in the table, results for three activities (driving a car, using e-mail, and preparing a menu) were moderately consistent with the MMSE group scores. About half of the MMSE-high group was judged as unable to contract a loan, rental, or sale; buy expensive things; or apply for social welfare services.

3. Consistency between COGNISTAT and Functional Activities

Table 4 shows the consistency between the scores of the groups of each subtest of COGNISTAT and those of functional activities. This table shows only significant kappa coefficients. Within the group of orientation, two activities (managing immovable items or property and buying expensive things) were moderately consistent. Within the group of memory, driving a car was also moderately consistent.

Table 5 shows significantly consistent pairs between the results of the subtest of COGNISTAT and functional activities for the subjects of the IQ-high group and for the MMSE-high group. In the IQ-high group, the results of orientation were substantially consistent with the performance of three activities (managing immovable items or property, buying expensive things, and driving a car). The value of odds ratio between the results of orientation and contract for loan, rental, and sale was significantly high.

DISCUSSION

The financial capacity did not correspond with the IQ score when it was above average (89/90). It also did not agree with the MMSE score when it was above the cutoff point (23/24). More than 75% of the patients with above-average IQ did not have enough capacity to manage their finances. Further, none of the financial activities that were main targets for evaluation of adult guardianship were moderately consistent with the results of the MMSE. This point may be consistent with Saito's opinion that it is impossible to apply the standards of conventional psychiatric judgment emphasizing IQ to the standards of adult guardianship for elderly persons with dementia (Saito, 1997; 2001). Our results also seem consistent with

Mizuno's opinion that the intellectual or cognitive abilities represented by the psychological test scores do not always agree with the diagnostic guidelines for adult guardianship in Japan (Mizuno. 2005).

Unlike the classification of IQ or MMSE, the result of the orientation subtest of the COGNISTAT was moderately consistent with that of financial activities. In addition, for the patients in the IQ-high group, the likelihood that they could not manage their finances was about 40 times higher when their scaled-score of the orientation subtest on the COGNISTAT was at the impaired level. These results suggest that these patients may not have enough capacity to manage their finances even though their IQ and MMSE scores are above average or normal. It may be possible that disorientation makes it difficult to understand the content of the contract (e.g., days or the cooling-off period and due date of payments). This may make it difficult for patients with disorientation to enter into contracts independently. Even if the IQ is relatively high (e.g., IQ $\geq$ 90), financial capacity may possibly be impaired, particularly when patients with dementia have significant impairments in their cognitive ability to manage their finances (e.g., orientation).

The interpretation of the results of this study should be cautiously considered because they contain several limitations. First, the sample size was small. Additionally, because the information about the patients' functional assessment was obtained from relatives, it may be possible that the information was influenced by observer bias. For example, the relatives who experienced high stress may have reported the patients' functional incapacity as being higher than it actually was. Despite these limitations, this study suggests the possibility that elderly patients with dementia do not have enough capacity to manage their finances even if their IQ and MMSE scores are above average or normal. We must note this point in the psychiatric evidence given for determining the need for adult guardianship.

ACKNOWLEDGMENTS

A part of this study was conducted with support by a grant from "Seizon-kagaku-kennkyu-sho." A part of the results of this study was presented at the 2010 World Congress on Adult Guardianship Law (Yokohama, Japan).

REFERENCES

Honma A. Clinical dementia rating (CDR). In: Otsuka T., Homma A. (eds.) Assessment manual of intellectual function for the demented elderly. World Planning 1991: 65–69 (in Japanese) Igarashi Y. Mental capacity and psychiatric evidence. In: Arai M., Akanuma Y., Ohnuki M. (eds.) Adult guardianship law: Theory and practice of the law. Yuhikaku 20063: 63–419.

Kitamura T. Mini-mental state (MMS). In: Otsuka T., Homma A. (eds.) Assessment manual of intellectual function for the demented elderly. World Planning 1991: 35–38 (in Japanese).

Landis J.R., Koch G.G. The measurement of observer agreement for categorical data. *Biometrics* 1977; 33: 159–174.

Matsuda O, Saito M. Functional competency and cognitive ability in mild Alzheimer's disease: relationship between ADL assessed by a relative/carer-rated scale and neuropsychological performance. *International Psychogeriatrics* 2005; 17: 275–288.

Matsuda O., Nakatani, M. Manual for Japanese version of the Neurobehavioral Cognitive Status Examination (COGNISTAT). World Planning 2004 (in Japanese).

Mizuno Y. Adult guardianship system and its application: From the psychiatric view. In: Matsushita M. (ed.) Civil law and Psychiatry. Forensic mental Health Nakayama-shotenn 2005; vol. 4: 107–117.

Saito M. Decision-making in social and medical services for patients with dementia in Japan. In: Aging: Caring for our elders. Weisstub D.N., Thomasma D.C., Gauthier S., Tomossy G.F. (eds.) Kluwer: Netherlands 2001: 191–202.

Saito M. Financial affairs of the elderly people with dementia. *Japanese Journal of Clinical psychiatry* 1997; 26: 1399–1405 (in Japanese).

Shinagawa, F., Kobayashi, S., Fujita, K., Maekawa, H. Japanese Wechsler Adult Intelligence Scale-Revised. Tokyo: *Nihon-bunka-kagaku-sha* 1990 (in Japanese).

Takahashi S., Ohno Y., Someya T. Japanese translation of Diagnostic and Statistical Manual of Mental disorders, Fourth Edition, Text Revision. Tokyo: *Igaku-shiin.* 2003 (in Japanese).

The Committee of Publication of Japanese WAIS-R. Japanese Wechsler Adult Intelligence scale, Third Edition. Tokyo: *Nihon-bunka-kagaku-sha.* 2006 (in Japanese).

United Nations.HYPERLINK "http://www.amazon.co.jp/exec/obidos/search-handle-url?_encoding=UTF8andsearch-type=ssandindex=books-usandfield-author=United%20Nations.Department%20of%20Economic%20and%20Social%20Affairs.%20Population%20Division" *World Population Prospects: The 2006 Revision: Sex and Age Distribution of the World Population (Department of Economic and Social Affairs-Population Studies).* United Nations Pubns, 2007.

In: The International Psychiatry and Behavioral ...
Editor: Nash Boutros
ISBN: 978-1-62257-566-4

Chapter 11

Linguistic Validation of the Japanese Version of the Quality of Life in Epilepsy Inventory (QOLIE-31-P)

Yushi Inoue[1]*, Dai Inayoshi[1], Yoshinobu Kasai[1], Teiichi Onuma[2], Mutsuo Sasagawa[3], Kazuichi Yagi[1] and Joyce A. Cramer[4]

[1]National Epilepsy Center,
Shizuoka Institute of Epilepsy and Neurological Disorders, Shizouka, Japan
[2]Musashino Kokubunji Clinic, Kokubunji, Japan
[3]Nishi-Niigata Chuo National Hospital, Niigata, Japan
[4]Yale University School of Medicine, New Haven, CT, US

Abstract

Although epilepsy is a condition that seriously affects the quality of life (QOL) of patients, few instruments appropriate for measuring the QOL of patients with epilepsy are currently available in Japan. Therefore, QOLIE-31-P, the epilepsy-specific QOL questionnaire for adults that is highly reputed and widely used outside Japan, was translated into Japanese and validated linguistically. During the validation process, ten Japanese patients with epilepsy were asked to fill in the questionnaire and interviewed as to the appropriateness of the expressions used in the translated text. A few expressions had to be amended. Overall, the Japanese version of QOLIE-31-P was found to have content and face validity. The finalized version of QOLIE-31-P is expected to serve as a useful instrument for measuring the QOL in Japanese adults with epilepsy, although its psychometric properties remain to be validated.

Keywords: epilepsy, quality of life (QOL), QOLIE-31-P, questionnaire, linguistic validation

* Corresponding author: Yushi Inoue, Director, National Epilepsy Center, Shizuoka Institute of Epilepsy and Neurological Disorders, Urushiyama 886, Aoi-ku, Shizuoka, 420-8688, Japan, E-mail: yinoue-jes@umin.net

INTRODUCTION

Epilepsy is a condition that seriously affects the quality of life (QOL) of patients and its treatment should target not only on prevention and relief of seizure symptoms but also on improvement of the QOL.

In order to achieve this goal, it is essential to assess the QOL of patients with epilepsy. Not a few epilepsy-specific QOL questionnaires have been developed and used for quantitative assessment of the QOL overseas. There are also many study reports on QOL assessment in patients with epilepsy. In Japan, however, few studies have been conducted on quantitative assessment of the QOL in patients with epilepsy because of few available epilepsy-specific QOL questionnaires. Discussion on treatment targeting on improvement of the patients' QOL is also less active in Japan compared to overseas. We considered it necessary to provide more instruments for appropriate assessment of the QOL in patients with epilepsy in Japan and developed a Japanese version of an epilepsy-specific QOL questionnaire.

METHODS

Selection of an Epilepsy-Specific QOL Questionnaire

Prior to development of a Japanese version of an epilepsy-specific QOL questionnaire, we reviewed QOL questionnaires developed overseas and selected the following four questionnaires as candidates for translation into Japanese: the Epilepsy Foundation of America Concerns Index (EFA Concerns Index), [1] the Epilepsy Surgery Inventory 55 (ESI-55), [2] the Performance, Sociodemographic Aspects, Subjective Evaluation/estimation (PESOS) questionnaire [3] and the Quality of Life in Epilepsy Inventory—31 Problems (QOLIE-31-P).[4]

The content and face validity as well as psychometric properties were compared among these four questionnaires. Their introduction was also validated by reference to an overseas article reviewing epilepsy-specific QOL instruments. [5] As a result, the QOLIE-31-P that is the revised version (Version 2) of the QOLIE-31 was selected for translation and cultural adaptation for use in Japan. The rationale for this selection is as follows: (i) the number of questions in the QOLIE-31-P is adequate; (ii) it includes not only questions on "seizure worry", "emotional well-being" and "medication effects" but also questions on "driving", "employment", "cognitive functioning" and "social problems" that are important factors affecting the QOL of adult patients with epilepsy; [6] (iii) it is sufficiently comprehensive and covers all aspects; (iv) the original QOLIE-31 (Version 1) [7] has been validated for classical psychometric properties (e.g., internal consistency, test-retest reliability, construct validity, criterion-related validity) and reported to have a high level of reliability and validity in every validation study; and (v) the QOLIE-31 has been translated to more than a dozen languages in the world [8] and is one of the most commonly used epilepsy-specific QOL questionnaires all over the world.

As is the case for the QOLIE-31, the QOLIE-31-P consists of questions divided into seven subscales: seizure worry, overall quality of life, emotional well-being, energy/fatigue, cognitive functioning, medication effects and social functioning. The QOLIE-31-P has an additional question for each subscale to ask the overall impact of the issues of the corresponding subscale in addition to the same 31 questions with those in the original QOLIE-31 as well as a final question to ask a responder to rate the importance of all subscales. We obtained prior consent from Joyce A. Cramer who had developed the QOLIE-31-P for its translation into Japanese. Ms. Cramer also gave lots of advice on ways to translate the QOLIE-31-P.

Procedures for Translation and Adaptation into Japanese and Validation of the Japanese Version

In the process of development of the Japanese version of the QOLIE-31-P, we complied with the guidelines and standards for linguistic validation of translation and cultural adaptation that have been well-recognized. The procedures are described below.

Forward Translation (from American English into Japanese)

The original QOLIE-31-P in American English was translated into Japanese by independent two translators. Another translator resolved discrepancies between the independent forward translations and produced one final reconciled forward translation.

Back Translation (from Japanese into American English)

A translator who had not been involved in forward translation or reconciliation developed a translation from Japanese back to American English. The project manager compared and checked the original, forward-translated and backward-translated versions and prepared a version of questionnaire used for review and refinement.

Medical Review (from the Physician Viewpoint)

The questionnaire prepared after back translation as described above was used to review and refine wording in the translation from linguistic (Japanese) and medical standpoints. A modified version of questionnaire reflecting results of the review was prepared, which was again translated from Japanese to American English by a translator who had not been involved in the previous forward/backward translation process to ensure conceptual equivalence with the original version.

Then, another translator who had not been involved in the previous forward/backward translation process compared and checked the modified Japanese version and its backward-translated version, resolved discrepancies if any, and developed a new version to be used in an interview study with patients.

Cognitive Debriefing by Interview with Patients with Epilepsy

The questionnaire translated in the way described above was administered to 10 patients with epilepsy followed by an interview with them to check appropriateness of wording of the questionnaire through patients' viewpoint.

This interview study was conducted in Shizuoka Institute of Epilepsy and Neurological Disorders between April and May 2008. Study participants were patients with epilepsy aged 16 years or older who were native speakers of Japanese, were able to understand the questions and explanation in the QOL questionnaire and responded to the questions, and were able to answer questions by the interviewer (clinical psychologist).

Prior to the interview study, the physician gave explanation and obtained written informed consent from the patients. Then, the patients completed the questionnaire, followed by interview by the responsible interviewer about overall impression of the questionnaire (required scholastic ability level and understandability) or impression of individual questions (e.g., identification of those difficult to understand or difficult to answer). The interviewer tried to promote voluntary speaking of the patients to avoid any bias.

The interview study was reviewed and approved by the Ethics Committee of Shizuoka Institute of Epilepsy and Neurological Disorders and written informed consent was obtained from every patient (as well as the patient's parent/guardian if the patient is a minor) prior to the start of the interview study.

RESULTS

Patients' Demographics

Table 1 shows demographic data of 10 patients participating in the interview study. Five male and five female patients participated in the study. Their mean age was 38.9 years (range: 19 to 69 years).

As for the educational background, two patients finished junior high school, three finished high school, two finished specialized vocational high school, one was in university and two finished university. Five patients had a permanent job, while two had no job, two were full-time housewives and one was a student.

Scoring

Subscale and overall scores of the 10 patients were calculated according to the scoring manual for the QOLIE-31 [10] and summarized as shown in Table 2. The mean overall score was 63.2 and the mean individual subscale score ranged from 38.3 to 72.2 with lower mean subscale score for "medication effects" than the other subscales.

Two patients did not answer one or more of the questions for the "medication effects" subscale and one of them could not answer because of receiving no pharmacotherapy.

Table 1. Patients' demographics

	Patient (n=10)
Gender	
Male	5 (50%)
Female	5 (50%)
Age	
Mean	38.9 years
SD	16.8
Median	34 years
Minimum	19 years
Maximum	69 years
Educational background	
Junior high school	2 (20%)
High school	3 (30%)
Higher professional school	2 (20%)
University (including an university student)	3 (30%)
Current occupation	
Full-time employed	5 (50%)
Unemployed	2 (20%)
Housekeeping	2 (20%)
Student	1 (10%)

SD: Standard deviation.

Table 2. QOLIE-31-P summary scores (n=10)

Subscales	Seizure worry	Overall quality of life	Emotional well-being	Energy/ fatigue	Cognitive	Medication effects	Social function	Overall score
Mean	50.1	67.3	70.4	60.5	72.2	38.3	53.9	63.2
SD	29.2	15.6	18.8	21.3	26.5	29.8	30.7	17.7
Minimum	4	40	40	30	13.3	0	0	32.8
Maximum	100	95	96	90	100	77.8	100	89.3
Missing data (%)	0%	0%	0%	0%	0%	10%	0%	0.8%

Scholastic Ability Level Required for Reading Comprehension

Table 3 summarizes the scholastic ability level that was considered by the patients to require for comprehension of the questionnaire.

Half (five) of the patients answered that high school (16- to 18-year-old) level of scholastic ability was required, while three answered that elementary (7- to 12-year-old) level sufficed.

Table 3. Scholastic level of the questionnaire

School grade/age level	Patient (n=10)
Elementary school level/7-12 year-old level	3
Junior high school level/13-15 year-old level	2
High school level/16-18 year-old level	5

Q. In which educational level (i.e. which school grade/age level) would you rank the expression of this document?

Understandability

Table 4 summarizes understandability (comprehensibility) of the questionnaire perceived by the patients using a visual analog scale (VAS) of 1 to 5 where 1 was "incomprehensible" and 5 was "very easy to comprehend". None of the patients answered that the questionnaire was "incomprehensive", while the response ranged from 3 to 5 in most patients.

Table 4. Comprehensibility of the questionnaire

Comprehension level	Patient (n=10)
1. (incomprehensible)	0
2.	1
3.	3
4.	5
5. (very easy to comprehend)	1

Q. On a scale of 1-5 (5 being ‘very easy to comprehend’ and 1 being ‘incomprehensible’), how would you rate the comprehensibility of this instrument?

Overall Impression

Table 5 summarizes overall impression (tone) of the text in the questionnaire. Some patients had a positive impression ("informative" for two patients and “convincing" for another two patients), while three patients had a passive impression. However, no patient had a "biased" impression. Other specific comments included: "the past 4 weeks" was a too long period to recall, specific examples might be helpful for understanding, and if the physician saw the responses, he/she would help the patient (he/she would be able to understand specific points of the patient's distress).

Modification of Wording

Based on the results of the interview study, words and phrases used in the text of the questionnaire that were objectively considered inappropriate were modified. Table 6 shows all of the modifications actually made and related comments. Although many other comments were given by the patients, they did not lead to modifications since most of them were subjective opinions or personal problems.

Table 5. The overall tone of the text in the questionnaire

The overall tone of the text	Patient (n=10)
Neutral	4
Biased	0
Informative	2
Convincing	2
Passive	3
Other	6

Q. How would you describe the overall tone of the text? (Neutral, biased, informative, convincing, passive) (Multiple answers permitted)

Table 6. Terms or phrases that patients think inappropriate in the text of the questionnaire

Inappropriate Items or phrases	Responses	Resolution
Quality of Life	Respondent 1: "The 'quality' is a difficult term. Respondent 6: "Since 'quality of life' is vague and may differ depending on whether it refers to the financial aspect, mental aspect or the family relationship aspect, it would be convenient when more focused. Respondent 7: "I don't understand the nuance of the word 'quality.'" Respondent 10: "Vague. I cannot find any way to answer."	To support the clarity, the English 'quality of life' was added in parentheses after this term in Japanese at the first time it appears.
No exit	Respondent 6: "I was confused as to what kind of mentality this word implicated."	To support the clarity, the translation was revised to "as bad as or worse than not having an escape path" (in Japanese).
Worn out	Respondent 1: "I would prefer to use "depressed" or "feel melancholy". Respondent 2: "Difference in nuance is hard to understand." Respondent 3: "I was confused about whether these referred to the mental aspect or the physical aspect." Respondent 5: "Would be better to include furigana." Respondent 8: "People may not be able to read these characters." Respondent 10: "Young children may not understand the meaning."	To support the clarity, respondent 5's recommendation of using furigana, the phonemic translation of the kanji was implemented.

Q. Please list any terms or phrases (if any) that you think inappropriate in the texts. Please give a brief summary of why you think it may not be the most appropriate term or phrase.

Japanese Version of the QOLIE-31-P

The Japanese version of the QOLIE-31-P finalized based on the above results of the interview study is provided in Appendix.

DISCUSSION

We used the linguistic validation process for translation and cultural adaptation well-recognized to develop the Japanese version of the QOLIE-31-P developed by Cramer et al. The questionnaire prepared through the process of forward translation from the original version and back translation was reviewed from Japanese linguistic and medical viewpoints. Then, the cognitive debriefing interview was performed to assess the required comprehension level as well as understandability and appropriateness of wording of the questionnaire through a viewpoint of patients with epilepsy.

The demographics of patients participating in the interview study showed no bias and the study could be performed in a wide range of patients in terms of age and the knowledge level. Specifically, there were the same number of males and females, the age ranged from 19 to 69 years, and the educational level ranged from junior high graduate to university graduate.

The scholastic ability level that was considered by the patients to require for comprehension of the questionnaire moderately varied: half (five) of the patients answered that high school (16- to 18-year-old) level of scholastic ability was required, while three answered that elementary (7- to 12-year-old) level sufficed. However, the age or educational level of patients was not related to their response concerning the required scholastic ability level. As for understandability, none of the patients answered that the questionnaire was "incomprehensive", while most (nine) patients showed moderate or higher level of comprehension (3 to 5). The understandability by patients was also not related to their age or educational level. In summary, some questions seemed to be slightly difficult to understand but the patients could answer almost all of the questions by themselves regardless of their age and educational level. Therefore, the finalized Japanese version of the QOLIE-31-P was considered as an appropriate instrument for assessment of the QOL in Japanese adults with epilepsy. Based on the interview study (cognitive debriefing) results, three modifications to wording of the questionnaire were made. The first problem identified was the term "quality of life", which is also included in the title of the questionnaire. Four of the 10 patients answered that this term was difficult to understand. Although the term "quality of life" has recently become widespread in Japan, this result revealed that all individuals has not yet been able to understand its right meaning without supplemental explanation and/or an accompanied English term. Since it is difficult to briefly explain its meaning, we only decided to add the English version of the term. The second issue was a phrase "As bad as or worse than no exit" used in the first question. One patient told that he/she was confused as to what kind of mentality this word implicated. The original English of this phrase is "As bad as or worse than being dead", which was literally translated in the Japanese translation after review of the back translation that was subjected to the medical review. In this review, "being dead" was replaced by a more gentle one, that is, "not having an exit". This rather restrictive expression (no exit) was changed to "no escape" (specifically, "not having an escape path") in the finalized version to make the phrase easier to understand. The third item was the phrase "worn out". In Japanese, "worn out" is written in kanji. Six of the 10 patients answered that this phrase was difficult to understand or they could not read it written in kanji. Since the translation seemed to convey the right meaning, the *furigana* (phonetic translation of the kanji) was used to make it readable. Although there were some other comments from patients concerning inappropriate words and phrases, they were regarded as subjective opinions or personal problems and lead to no modification of the questionnaire. Following these revisions, the Japanese version of the QOLIE-31-P was finalized for use in clinical practice. In the interview study, eight of the 10 patients answered all of the questions in the questionnaire. The remaining two patients also answered all of the questions except for some that they could not answer for a reasonable cause such as no medication. Therefore, the questionnaire was considered to have no problems in terms of the construct.

The overall and subscale scores were calculated for the 10 patients in an exploratory manner. Although it was impossible to correlate these scores with characteristics of epilepsy (e.g., seizure type, seizure frequency, medications used) because of the small sample size, possible reasons for the lower mean subscale score for "medication effects" compared to the other subscales should be further investigated. Kubota et al. [11] also reported the lower mean subscale score for "medication effects" in approximately 600 adult patients with epilepsy whose QOL was assessed using the QOLIE-31.

In the process of development of a new questionnaire, it is necessary to assess its psychometric properties, specifically, the validity (i.e., the ability of the questionnaire to measure and describe what it is supposed to measure and describe) and the reliability (i.e., the consistency with which the same results are achieved). [12] The validity and reliability of this Japanese version have not been verified and their establishment is a further challenge. However, psychometric properties of multi-lingual translation versions of the precedent QOLIE-31 have been determined [13-15] and it has been demonstrated that their validity and reliability levels are as high as those of the original language version. The QOLIE-31-P, the revised version of the QOLIE-31, has some additional questions but is unlikely to be substantially inferior to the QOLIE-31 in terms of the overall validity and reliability. Since the Japanese version of the QOLIE-31-P described here was developed through the linguistic validation process that has been used for development of translations to other languages, it is unlikely that the validity and reliability of the original version substantially changed in the process of translation. Therefore, this Japanese version is expected to demonstrate sufficient levels of validity and reliability.

This questionnaire is designed for use in adult patients with epilepsy (aged 18 years or older) by self-administration. There are few QOL questionnaires in Japanese language for children with epilepsy whose validity and reliability have been demonstrated. [16] Since a decline in QOL is also significant for children as is the case for adult patients, there is a great demand for development of an appropriate QOL questionnaire for children. Assessment of the QOL over time in patients with epilepsy using this Japanese version of the questionnaire allows determination of the responsiveness to the QOLIE-31-P and quantitative monitoring of the QOL of patients. Evaluation of subscale scores may allow analysis of factors contributing to decreased QOL. The questionnaire may also be used as a tool for improving interactive communication and bridging the gap between patient and physician. Since there are a lot of papers reporting QOL assessment results using the QOLIE-31 in the US and Europe, it is possible to compare the QOL between Japanese and non-Japanese patients with epilepsy.

Moreover, the Japanese version of the questionnaire can be used to evaluate indicators of medical technology and pharmacotherapy.

PROVISION AND USE OF THE JAPANESE VERSION OF THE QOLIE-31-P

The copy of the QOLIE-31-P (Japanese) is available from the website of Epilepsy.com, an NPO operated by Ms. Cramer and her colleagues (http://professionals.epilepsy.com/page/qoltools.html) through the courtesy of Ms. Cramer. Healthcare professionals and researchers can use the questionnaire for the research purpose at no charge. Profit-making enterprises that use the questionnaire for a commercial purpose should obtain permission for use from Ms. Cramer and pay a usage fee. The scoring manual for the original QOLIE-31 also applies to scoring of the QOLIE-31-P. This manual is available from the website (http://www.rand.org/health/surveys_tools/qolie/).

APPENDIX: JAPANESE VERSION OF THE QOLIE-31-P QUESTIONNAIRE

Item	Subscale	Contents
OQL		Overall, how would you rate your quality of life? (Circle one number on the scale below.) 10: Best Possible Quality of Life 0: Worst Possible Quality of Life (as bad as or worse than being dead)
Part A		These questions are about how you have been *feeling* during the past 4 weeks. For each question, please indicate the one answer that comes closest to the way you have been feeling. How much of the time during past 4 weeks… (Circle one number on each line) (1: All of the time, 2: Most of the time, 3: A good bit of the time, 4: Some of the time, 5: A little of the time, 6: None of the time)
1	E/F	Did you feel full of pep?
2	E/F	Did you have a lot of energy?
3	E/F	Did you feel worn out?
4	E/F	Did you feel tired?
5	E/F	Reviewing only questions in Part A, consider the overall impact of these issues on your life in the past 4 weeks. (Circle one number.) How much do the above problems and worries about *energy* distress you overall? (1: Not at all, 2: Somewhat, 3: Moderately, 4: A lot, 5: Very much)
Part B		These questions are about how you have been feeling during the past 4 weeks. For each question, please indicate the one answer that comes closest to the way you have been feeling. How much of the time during past 4 weeks… (Circle one number on each line) (1: All of the time, 2: Most of the time, 3: A good bit of the time, 4: Some of the time, 5: A little of the time, 6: None of the time)

Item	Subscale	Contents
6	EWB	Have you been a very nervous person?
7	EWB	Have you felt so down in the dumps that nothing could cheer you up?
8	EWB	Have you felt calm and peaceful?
9	EWB	Have you felt downhearted and blue?
10	EWB	Have you been a happy person?
11	EWB	Reviewing only questions in Part B, consider the overall impact of these issues on your life in the past 4 weeks. (Circle one number.) How much do the above problems and worries about *emotions* distress you overall? (1: Not at all, 2: Somewhat, 3: Moderately, 4: A lot, 5: Very much)
Part C		The following questions are about how you *feel* and about problems you may have with daily *activities* during the past 4 weeks. For each question, please indicate the one answer that comes closest to the way you have been feeling. The following question asks about how you <u>feel</u> and how things have been going for you. How much of the time during the past 4 weeks… (Circle one number on each line)
12	SF	Has your health limited your social activities (such as visiting with friends or close relatives)? (1: All of the time, 2: Most of the time, 3: A good bit of the time, 4: Some of the time, 5: A little of the time, 6: None of the time)
13	SF	The following questions ask about problems you may have with certain *activities.* How much of the time during the past 4 weeks your epilepsy or antiepileptic medication has caused trouble with… (Circle one number on each line) Leisure activities (such as hobbies, going out) (1: A great deal, 2: A lot, 3: Somewhat, 4: Only a little, 5: Not at all)
14	SF	Driving (or transportation) (1: A great deal, 2: A lot, 3: Somewhat, 4: Only a little, 5: Not at all)
15	SF	How much do your work limitations bother you? (1: Not at all bothersome, 5: Extremely bothersome)
16	SF	How much do your social limitations bother you? (1: Not at all bothersome, 5: Extremely bothersome)
17	SF	Reviewing only questions in Part C, consider the overall impact of these issues on your life in the past 4 weeks. (Circle one number.) How much do the above problems and worries about *daily activities* distress you overall? (1: Not at all, 2: Somewhat, 3: Moderately, 4: A lot, 5: Very much)
Part D		These questions are about thinking, reading, concentrating and memory problems you may have had during the past 4 weeks. For each question, please indicate the one answer that comes closest to the way you have been feeling. How much of the time during past 4 weeks… (Circle one number)

Appendix. (Continued)

Item	Subscale	Contents
18	CO	Did you have difficulty reasoning and solving problems (such as making plans, making decisions, learning new things)? (1: All of the time, 2: Most of the time, 3: A good bit of the time, 4: Some of the time, 5: A little of the time, 6: None of the time)
19	CO	In the past 4 weeks, have you had any trouble with your memory? (1: Yes, a great deal. 2: Yes, somewhat. 3: Only a little. 4: No, not at all)
20	CO	In the past 4 weeks, how often have you had … (Circle one number on each line) (1: All of the time, 2: Most of the time, 3: A good bit of the time, 4: Some of the time, 5: A little of the time, 6: None of the time) Trouble remembering things people tell you?
21	CO	Trouble concentrating on reading?
22	CO	Trouble concentrating on doing one thing at a time?
23	CO	How much do your memory difficulties bother you? (1: Not at all bothersome, 5: Extremely bothersome)
24	CO	Reviewing only questions in Part D, consider the overall impact of these issues on your life in the past 4 weeks. (Circle one number.) How much do the above problems and worries about *mental function* distress you overall? (1: Not at all, 2: Somewhat, 3: Moderately, 4: A lot, 5: Very much)
Part E		These questions are about problems you may have related to your epilepsy or antiepileptic medication. During the past 4 weeks … (Circle one number on each line)
25	ME	How much do physical effects of antiepileptic medication bother you? (1: Not at all bothersome, 5: Extremely bothersome)
26	ME	How much do mental effects of antiepileptic medication bother you? (1: Not at all bothersome, 5: Extremely bothersome)
27	ME	How worried are you that medications you are taking will be bad for you if taken for a long time? (1: Very worried, 2: Somewhat worried, 3: Not very worried, 4: Not worried at all)
28	ME	Reviewing only questions in Part E, consider the overall impact of these issues on your life in the past 4 weeks. (Circle one number.) How much do the above problems and worries about *effects of medication* distress you overall? (1: Not at all, 2: Somewhat, 3: Moderately, 4: A lot, 5: Very much)
Part F		These questions are about how you feel about your seizures during the past 4 weeks. For each question, please indicate the one answer that comes closest to the way you have been feeling. How much of the time during past 4 weeks… (Circle one number)
29	SW	Have you worried about having another seizure? (1: All of the time, 2: Most of the time, 3: A good bit of the time, 4: Some of the time, 5: A little of the time, 6: None of the time)

Item	Subscale	Contents
30	SW	How fearful are you of having a seizure during the next month? (1: Very fearful, 2: Somewhat fearful, 3: Not very fearful, 4: Not fearful at all)
31	SW	Do you worry about hurting yourself during a seizure? (1: Worry a lot, 2: Occasionally worry, 3: Don't worry at all)
32	SW	How worried are you about embarrassment or other social problems resulting from having a seizure during the next month? (1: Very worried, 2: Somewhat worried, 3: Not very worried, 4: Not at all worried)
33	SW	How much do your seizures bother you? (1: Not at all bothersome, 5: Extremely bothersome)
34	SW	Reviewing only questions in Part F, consider the overall impact of these issues on your life in the past 4 weeks. (Circle one number.) How much do the above problems and worries about *seizures* distress you overall? (1: Not at all, 2: Somewhat, 3: Moderately, 4: A lot, 5: Very much)
Part G		The following question asks about how you feel about your overall quality of life. Please indicate the one answer that comes closest to the way you have been feeling.
35	OQL	How has the quality of your life been during the past 4 weeks (that is, how have things been going for you)? (Circle one number) (1: Very well: could hardly be better, 2: Pretty good, 3: Good and bad parts about equal, 4: Pretty bad, 5: Very bad: could hardly be worse)
36	OQL	Reviewing only questions 1 and 36 in Part G (on page 1 and this page), consider the overall impact of your quality of life in the past 4 weeks. (Circle one number) How much does the state of your *quality of life* distress you overall? (1: Not at all, 2: Somewhat, 3: Moderately, 4: A lot, 5: Very much)
Part H		
37	–	How good or bad do you think your *health* is? On the scale below, the best imaginable state of health is 100 and the worst imaginable state is zero (0). Please indicate how you feel about your health by circling one number on the scale. Please consider your epilepsy as part of your health when you answer this question. (100: Best imaginable health state, 0: Worst imaginable health state)
Part I		Considering all the questions you have answered, please indicate the areas related to your epilepsy that are most important to you now.
38	–	Number the following topics from '1 to 7' with '1' corresponding to the very most important topic and '7' to the least important one. Please use each number only once. A. Energy (tiredness), B. Emotions (mood), C. Daily activities (work, driving, social), D. Mental activity (thinking, concentrating, memory), E. Medication effects (physical, mental), F. Seizure worry (impact of seizures), G. Overall quality of life

SW: seizure worry, OQL: overall quality of life, EWB: emotional well-being, E/F: energy/fatigue, CO: cognitive, ME: medication effects, SF: social function.

 Supporting information about the Patient-Weighted QOLIE-31-P is available on www.epilepsy.com.

ACKNOWLEDGMENTS

We thank TransPerfect Internationals, Inc. for assistance to the study. This study was supported by grants from GlaxoSmithKline K.K. (GSK). GSK provided financial support to an author for the translation of the manuscript.

REFERENCES

[1] Gilliam F, Kuzniecky R, Faught E, Black L, Carpenter G, Schrodt R. Patient-validated content of epilepsy-specific quality-of-life measurement. *Epilepsia* 1997;38 (2): 233-236.

[2] Vickrey BG, Hays RD, Graber J, Rausch R, Engel J, Brook RH. A health-related quality of life instrument for patients evaluated for epilepsy surgery. *Med. Care* 1992; 30 (4): 299-319.

[3] May TW, Pfäfflin M. Evaluating comprehensive care: description of the PESOS and its psychometric properties. In: Pfäfflin M, Fraser RT, Thorbecke R, Specht U, Wolf P, eds. Comprehensive care for people with epilepsy. Eastleigh: John Libbey, 2001: 319-340.

[4] Cramer JA, Hammèe GV, The N132 Study Group. Maintenance of improvement in health-related quality of life during long-term treatment with levetiracetam. *Epilepsy and Behavior* 2003; 4: 118-123.

[5] Leone MA, Beghi E, Righini C, Apolone G, Mosconi P. Epilepsy and quality of life in adults: A review of instruments. *Epilepsy Res.* 2005; 66: 23-44.

[6] Hayden M, Penna C, Buchanan N. Epilepsy: patient perceptions of their condition. *Seizure* 1992; 1: 191-197.

[7] Cramer JA, Perrine K, Devinsky O, Bryant-Comstock L, Meador K, Hermann B. Development and cross-cultural translations of a 31-item quality of life in epilepsy inventory. *Epilepsia* 1998; 39 (1): 81-88.

[8] PROQOID Patient-Reported Outcome and Quality of Life Instruments Database. (Online) available from <http://www.proqolid.org/instruments/quality_of_life_in_epilepsy_inventory_31_qolie_31>, (accessed 2008-09-30).

[9] Wild D, Grove A, Martin M, Eremenco S, McElroy S, Verjee-Lorenz A, et al. Principles of good practice for the translation and cultural adaptation process for patient-reported outcomes (PRO) measures: Report of the ISPOR task force for translation and cultural adaptation. *Value in Health* 2005; 8: 94-104.

[10] Vickrey BG, Perrine K, Hays RD, Hermann RD, Gramer JA, Meedor KJ, et al. Quality of life in epilepsy QOLIE 31 (version 1.0); scoring manual and patient inventory. Santa Monica, CA: RAND, 1993.

[11] Kubota H, Awaya Y. Factors influencing on quality of life in Japanese patients with epilepsy. Epilepsia 2007; 48 (Suppl. 6): 31-32.

[12] Ikegami N, Fukuhara S, Shimoduma K, Ikeda S. Clinical QOL assessment handbook. Igakushoin, Tokyo, 2001.

[13] May TW, Pfäfflin M, Cramer JA. Psychometric properties of the German translation of the QOLIE-31. *Epilepsy and Behavior* 2001; 2: 106-114.

[14] Picot MC, Crespel A, Daurès JP, Baldy-Moulinier M, Hasnaoui AEL. Psychometric validation of the French version of the quality of life in epilepsy inventory (QOLIE-31): Comparison with a generic health-related quality of life questionnaire. *Epileptic Disord.* 2004; 6: 275-285.

[15] Beghi E, Niero M, Roncolato M. Validity and reliability of the Italian version of the Quality-of-Life in Epilepsy Inventory (QOLIE-31). *Seizure* 2005; 14: 452-458.

[16] Kakinuma H, Nakai A, Honma K, Yagi N, Niida Y, Matsushima A et al. Adaptation of English-written health-related quality of life measure for children. *No To Hattatsu* 2007;39 (1):65-67.

In: The International Psychiatry and Behavioral ...
Editor: Nash Boutros

ISBN: 978-1-62257-566-4

Chapter 12

COTARD'S SYNDROME*

Hans Debruyne[1,2,3#], Michael Portzky[1], Kathelijne Peremans[1] and Kurt Audenaert[1]

[1]University Hospital Ghent, Department of Psychiatry, Ghent, Belgium.
[2]P.C. Dr. Guislain Psychiatric Hospital, Ghent, Belgium
[3]Zorgsaam/RGC, Department of Psychiatry, Terneuzen, The Netherlands

ABSTRACT

Cotard's syndrome is characterised by nihilistic delusions focussed on the individual's body including loss of body parts, being dead or not existing at all. The syndrome as such is neither mentioned in DSM-IV-TR nor in ICD-10. There is growing unanimity that Cotard's syndrome with its typical nihilistic delusions externalizes an underlying disorder. Despite Cotard's syndrome is not a diagnostic entity in our current classification systems, recognition of the syndrome and a specific approach towards the patient is mandatory.

This paper overviews the historical aspects, clinical characteristics, classification, epidemiology and etiological issues and includes recent views on pathogenesis and neuro-imaging. A short overview of treatment options will be discussed.

Keywords: Cotard's syndrome, nihilistic delusion, misidentification syndrome, review

INTRODUCTION: HISTORICAL ASPECTS AND CLASSIFICATION

Cotard's syndrome is named after Jules Cotard (1840-1889), a French neurologist who described this condition for the first time in 1880, a case report of a 43-year old woman.

---

* Original Citation: Debruyne H, Portzky M., Peremans K., Audenaert K.; Mind & Brain, journal of psychiatry 2011; 2:(1); 67-72.

Corresponding author: Hans Debruyne M.D., Debruynehans@yahoo.com

> Mrs. X, affirms she has no brain, no nerves, no chest, no stomach, no intestines; there's only skin and bones of a decomposing body. ... She has no soul, God does not exist, neither the devil. She's nothing more than a decomposing body, and has no need to eat for living, she cannot die a natural death, she exists eternally if she's not burned, the fire will be the only solution for her. (Translation from: Cotard 1880)[1]

Cotard formulated a new type of depression, characterized by anxious melancholia, ideas of damnation or rejection, insensitivity to pain, delusions of non-existence concerning ones own body and delusions of immortality. He categorised this under *lypémanie*, a kind of psychotic depression, based on the analogy with five cases described in 1838 by Esquirol [1]. Later, Cotard introduced *délire des negations* as a new terminology for the syndrome [2]. The eponym *Cotard's syndrome* was introduced in 1887 by Séglas [3]. A few years later Régis stated that the syndrome (he named it *délire de Cotard*) was not only associated with depression, but might be linked to other psychiatric disorders as well [4].

Two components of the syndrome were defined by Tissot: an *affective component* associated with anxiety and a *cognitive component* associated with the presence of delusion [5]. Loudet and Martinez made a first attempt to classify different types of the syndrome. They described a *non-generalised délire de negation*, associated with paralysis, alcoholic psychosis and dementia and the 'real' *Cotard's syndrome*, only found in anxious melancholia and chronic hypochondria [6]. Later, in 1968, Saavedra proposed a classification into three types: *depressive*, *mixed* and *schizophrenic*. He drew a distinction between a 'genuine' Cotard's syndrome occurring during depressive states and what he described as a pseudonihilistic or pseudo-Cotard syndrome, classified as 'co-anaesthetic schizophrenia' [7].

In 1995, for the first time, a classification was made on evidence basis. In a retrospective factor analysis of 100 cases in literature, Berrios and Luque subdivided Cotard's syndrome into three types. A first type included a form of *psychotic depression*, characterized by anxiety, melancholic delusions of guilt and auditory hallucinations. A second type, described as *Cotard's syndrome type I*, was associated with hypochondriac and nihilistic delusions and absence of depressive episodes. The third group was the *Cotard's syndrome type II*, with anxiety, depression, auditory hallucinations, delusions of immortality, nihilistic delusions and suicidal behaviour as characteristic features [8].

Cotard's syndrome is currently not classified as a separate disorder in DSM-IV-TR and ICD-10. In DSM-IV-TR, nihilistic delusions are categorized as mood congruent delusions within a depressive episode with psychotic features [9]. Classifying Cotard's syndrome as a separate entity is an extremely difficult exercise in our current diagnostic classification system.

METHODS

For this article, we started from the search results for 'Cotard syndrome', 'Cotard's syndrome' and 'nihilistic delusion(s)', using PubMed and Web of Science. Relevant articles in English, French, Dutch and German were gathered. Since data on this topic is scarce, we looked every article for relevant cross references. A general internet search on Google was also used. From this last results, we only included articles written in peer reviewed journals. Using this method, we tried to obtain all available peer reviewed data on this topic. This was necessary because there are no controlled studies available. All literature is dominated by case studies and some case series.

PRESENTATION AND COURSE

As described earlier, nihilistic delusions concerning the individual's body are the central features of Cotard's syndrome. In an analysis of 100 cases, the most prominent symptoms in Cotard's syndrome are: depressive mood (89%), nihilistic delusions concerning one's own existence (69%), anxiety (65%), delusions of guilt (63%), delusions of immortality (55%) and hypochondriac delusions (58%) [8]. Some case reports concerning delusional denial of pregnancy despite clear morphologic signs [10] and delusional paralysis in a patient with psychomotor agitation [11] are reported as a special form of Cotard's syndrome. However, the classification of these delusions as nihilistic delusions concerning one's body can be debated. A classical description of the course of Cotard's syndrome is given by Enoch and Trethowan. In it's early stages Cotard's syndrome is characterised by a vague feeling of anxiety, with a varying time-span from weeks to years. This anxious state gradually augments and can result in nihilistic delusions, where denial of life or denial of body parts are the prominent features. The patient looses sense of reality [12].

Despite the delusion of being dead, these patients show an increased tendency to automutilation or suicidal behaviour. Additional symptoms may include analgesia and mutism. The core symptoms always reflect a preoccupation with guilt, despair and death [12]. Delusions can be accompanied by a *délire d'énormité*, a delusion of massive increase of body measures. This has been described as the *manic Cotard's syndrome* [12].

As the syndrome often occurs in association with other psychotic states, symptoms of these specific disorders are likely to be present. As an example, nihilistic delusions grafted on a depressive illness are often associated by other characteristics of a depressive episode such as weight loss and sleeping difficulties and the syndrome associated with organic disease is often associated with other symptoms such as desorientation or neurological signs [12]. The duration of the syndrome can vary from weeks to years, depending the underlying disorder [13].

In 1999, Yamada made a proposal for staging Cotard's syndrome[14]. Based on a case report, he defined three stages: germination stage, blooming stage and chronic stage. The *germination stage* is characterised by important hypochondria, cenesthopathy and depressive mood. A diagnosis of Cotard's syndrome cannot be made in this stage yet. In the *blooming stage*, the characteristic features of Cotard's syndrome (nihilistic delusions, delusions of immortality together with anxiety and negativism) are seen. The last stage, the *chronic stage* is differentiated in two forms: one with persistent emotional disturbances (depressive type) and a second where depressive symptoms are less prominent (paranoid type) [14]. This hypothesis was supported in a second case report [15].

EPIDEMIOLOGY

The prevalence and incidence of this rare syndrome is not known. Only one study reported on prevalence in a selected psychogeriatric population in Hong Kong. In 2 out of 349 patients, Cotard's syndrome was diagnosed suggesting a prevalence of 0.57% in this population. A prevalence of 3.2% was reached when severely depressed elderly were included [16]. A recent study found 0.62% (n=3) of patients in a Mexican sample (screened over a 2 year period) of primary psychiatric patients having Cotard's syndrome [17]. Using the same methodology they found also 0.11% (n=1) having Cotard's syndrome in a sample of neurological patients with mental disturbances [17]. The likelihood of developing Cotard's delusion appears to increase with age [18]. Berrios and Lucque found a mean age of 56 years in their analysis of 100 cases [8]. A more recent study of 138 cases reported a mean age of 47.7 years [19]. Women, appear to be more vulnerable [12]. The syndrome is found in different ethnic groups [18]. Cotard's syndrome is also occasionally described in children and adolescents [19-30]. Diagnosis of Cotard's syndrome in people under 25 years old was described to be associated with bipolar disorder [19].

Since Cotard's syndrome is conceptualised as part of an underlying disorder, several psychiatric and somatic diseases have been associated with the syndrome. Unipolar [10, 12, 16, 31-44] or bipolar [12, 14, 15, 19, 25, 29, 45-49] depression are the most common associated psychiatric disorders, but also co-morbid psychotic disorder [12, 13, 37, 45, 50-53] has been reported. Some studies reported on the occurrence of Cotard's syndrome with more uncommon psychiatric syndromes (hydrophobia [41], lycantrophy [48], folie a deux [54], Capgras delusion [12, 21, 51, 54, 55, 56], Capgras and Fregoli delusion [30], depersonalisation disorder [17]). Also parkinsonian symptoms, disappearing with successful treatment are described [17]. Several organic conditions were also associated: dementia [13, 57], major depressive episode in mild cognitive impairment [46], depression in frontotemporal atrophy [58], severe mental retardation [59], typhoid fever [60], cerebral infarction [61], superior sagittal sinus thrombosis [62], brain tumors [63], temporal lobe epilepsy [61,64], limbic epileptic insults [64], postictal depression [28], cerebral arteriovenous malformation [65], cerebral arteriovenous malformation and epilepsy [61], migraine [64], Laurence-Moon-Bardet-Biedl syndrome [67], multiple sclerosis [65], Parkinson's disease [68,69], brain injury [70,71,72], a non-infectious complication of heart transplantation [73], as a consequence of an adverse drug reaction to aciclovir and its prodrug valaciclovir[74]and in herpetic [77] and non-herpetic [17] encephalitis.

ETIOLOGY AND PATHOGENESIS

Neuro-imaging

The first structural imaging study was performed in 1986, using Computed Tomography (CT). An association of Cotard's syndrome with multifocal brain atrophy and inter-hemispheric enlargement was suggested [75].

Others have described an enlargement of the third and lateral ventricle [50], a specific lesion to the temporoparietal areas [65], and changes in the non-dominant temporoparietal areas, sometimes together with frontal damage [72]. In general, these studies point to an important role for the fronto-temporo-parietal circuitry in the pathophysiology of the syndrome. However, in most cases, gross structural changes on structural brain imaging were absent [70].

Several functional imaging studies in Cotard's syndrome patients were published. A dopamine D2 receptor SPECT study with ^{123}I-iodobenzamide (IBZM), performed in one patient, showed an asymmetric striatal D_2 receptor binding in favour of the left hemisphere. These SPECT-findings persisted after remission.

In this specific patient, no perfusion alterations were found with ^{99m}Tc-hexamethyl-propylenamide oxime (HMPAO) SPECT before treatment [33]. Several, but not all, case studies reported decreased perfusion in several cortical areas measured with the same perfusion SPECT tracer. In one patient a left-sided hypoperfusion in temporal, parietal and frontal lobes was found with full recovery of the left inferior frontal hypoperfusion and minimal remaining hypoperfusion in the left temporal lobe after successful treatment using electroconvulsive therapy (ECT) [50]. A similar recovery of perfusion was found in another patient after ECT-treatment in the medial parietal cortex, medial and dorsolateral prefrontal cortex, the basal ganglia and thalamus [42].

Successful treatment with ECT in a patient with underlying major depressive disorder resulted in recovery of left and right temporal hypoperfusion [40] and normalization of perfusion in the frontal cortex was reported after treatment with antidepressants [36]. In one patient, severe right hemispheric dysfunction on neuropsychological tasks was not accompanied by perfusion abnormalities measured with ^{99m}TC Ethyl Cysteine Dimer (ECD) SPECT [46].

Psychological and Neuropsychological Factors

A depersonalisation phenomenon was reported as an essential step in de development of Cotard's syndrome by Séglas (1887) [3]. Alheid elaborated depersonalisation in the Cotard's syndrome context using the German terminology 'Leib' (body for me) and 'Körper' (body as such). Depersonalization may occur when 'Körper' prevails over 'Leib', and when the body is less associated with the self ('Leib'). However, in depersonalisation, the patient feels like being dead (indifference of affect) while in Cotard's syndrome the patient is convinced to be dead (lack of feeling) [7, 12].

In the development of bizarre psychiatric syndromes related to parietal brain dysfunction, Critchley stated that the role of premorbid personality characteristics is essential [12]. With regard to this premorbid personality characteristics, it is proposed that in Cotard's syndrome, patients with a more internal attributional style (which is often co-occurring with depression) are more vulnerable to develop the syndrome. While patients with a more external attributional style (which is more co-occurring with paranoia) are more prone to develop Capgras' syndrome (a delusion where familiar persons are replaced by identical impostors) [76]. This hypothesis that Cotard's patients have a more internal attribution style was empirically tested in one case [77]. A significant higher score on two attribution bias indices (internalising bias index, internalising bias for negative events) calculated on the IPSAQ (Internal, Personal and Situational Attributions Questionnaire) was found in this patient with

Cotard's syndrome compared to control subjects [77]. However, several authors reported the co-occurrence of both Cotard's syndrome and Capgras's syndromes [12, 21, 51, 54-56]. Vinkers suggested that a combination of attribution styles occur in these patients, in so far that these patients are both depressed and paranoid or that they suffer from delusions about self-identity and about identity of others [78]. Unfortunately, evidence-based proof for this hypothesis is lacking.

The origin of both syndromes (and other delusional misidentification syndromes) is supposed to be related to a dysfunction of an information processing subsystem where face and body recognition is associated with recognition of familiarity. When a feeling of familiarity is absent, the patients may experience a feeling of derealisation and depersonalisation [79]. This hypothesis is supported by several studies for a number of misidentification syndromes and especially for Capgras' syndrome [80-82]. Interestingly, in studies on face recognition tasks with skin conductance as outcome measure the differential autonomic response to familiar faces compared to unknown faces is absent in patients with Capgras' syndrome [80, 81]. Another patient with atypical Capgras' delusion showed impaired interpretation of facial expressions. This leads to mistake differences in expression for differences in identity [82]. For Cotard's syndrome, a lack of differential autonomic response to anything is suggested. This can lead to the delusion of being death, where in Capgras' delusion there is only lack of familiarity to familiar faces, leading to the delusion of familiar persons being replaced by identical impostors. In this hypothesis, the psycho-pathology in Cotard's syndrome is more severe and more generalised [84, 86]. On the other hand, the lack of feeling of familiarity cannot completely explain the pathophysiology of delusional misidentification syndromes. Patients with brain damage of the ventromedial region of the frontal cortex also demonstrate absence of differential autonomic responsivity to familiar faces, despite the absence of delusions. The same is seen in patients suffering from pure autonomic failure. There a lack of differential autonomic responsivity to anything is seen despite the absence of delusions. Therefore, to explain delusions, a second factor is needed. This factor is responsible for the failure to reject the hypothesis (e.g. I'm dead as a explanation for the lack of feeling of familiarity to anything) despite the presence of (often overwhelming) evidence against it [82-87]. Hence, for Cotard's syndrome, a two-factor hypothesis is proposed. Here, the first factor contributes to the total lack of autonomic response to anything (as in pure autonomic failure), the second to not being able to reject the hypothesis 'I'm dead' [84, 86]. In this hypothesis the loss of affect (first factor) is more pronounced and generalised than in Capgras patients [90]. On the other hand, the difference in attributional style could also be an explanation for the different hypothesis formation in the first factor [17].

The importance of the right dorsolateral prefrontal cortex (RDLPFC) for hypothesis evaluating was demonstrated with fMRI [87, 88, 89]. It has also been observed that right frontal damage is commonly occurring in cases of delusional misidentifications (including Cotard's syndrome) [84].

PROGNOSIS AND TREATMENT

Complete recovery may occur as spontaneously and as suddenly as its onset, even in the most severe cases [12]. Enoch and Trettowan link the prognosis to the underlying disorder.

"If the nihilistic delusions are related to an acute psycho-organic syndrome, the prognosis is good and the condition tends to resolve. If, however, it is associated with a depressive illness, it may well persist even when the other symptoms of the depressive illness have cleared. Under this circumstance, and where the condition becomes chronic, the delusional state of negation usually waxes and wanes in intensity, depending on the periodic fluctuations of the depressive disorder. When the phenomenology is part of a schizophrenic illness, it usually improves when the other symptoms respond to therapy, but it can also persist for years as part of a chronic schizophrenic condition" [12].

In general no further statements can be made about prognosis from the available literature. In most publications, prognosis is not discussed. It seems prognosis can widely vary from spontaneous recovery to a very severe chronic condition. An important exclusion for this is when Cotard's syndrome is diagnosed under the age of 25 years. In these cases, there seems to be an association with bipolar disorder [19].

Diagnostic work-up of the underlying disorders should therefore be a guide for treatment. Several reports are published about successful treatments. Pharmacological monotherapy such as amitriptyline [27], aripiprazole [32], duloxetine [91], fluoxetine [17], olanzapine [21, 92], sulpiride [55], lithium [26, 27] has been reported as effective. However usually combination strategies are used (clomipramine/amitriptyline [12], pimozide/amitriptyline [24], haloperidol /clomipramine [22], cyamemazine/paroxetine [29], risperidone/fluoxetine [36], haloperidol/ mirtazapine [44], risperidone/sertraline [46], risperidone citalopram [10], amisulpiride/ clozapine [93], clozapine/fluvoxamine/imipramine [33], paroxetine/pramipexole [43], quetiapine/venlafacine [94], olanzapine/escitalopram/lorazepam [95]. Adding bromocriptine to clomipramine and lithium had a beneficial effect in a patient with bipolar disorder type I [47].

The most reported treatment strategy for Cotard's syndrome is electroconvulsive therapy (ECT) [11-16, 23-25, 29, 31, 34, 37-42, 45, 48, 50, 58, 59, 93, 96-98]. Based on the classification of Berrios and Luque [8], a suggestion was made that ECT is indicated in patients with Cotard's syndrome and psychotic depression, while antipsychotics exert better effects in Cotard's syndrome type I [93]. In one patient, spontaneous recovery after two grand mal seizures was reported illustrating the usefulness of seizure activity in the treatment of Cotard's syndrome [99]. Treatment should initially follow current treatment guidelines of the underlying conditions, since no randomised studies are performed on this Cotard's syndrome. In depressive disorder with psychotic features, ECT (often in combination with farmacotherapy) seems to be the most supported strategy.

Enoch and Trettowan rightly argue that apart from these treatments, special measures can be needed. The severe distress may lead to important suicide risk, especially in patients suffering from major depressive disorder. This may be in contrast with the delusion of being already dead. During recovery this risk may even become more pronounced when the patient becomes more active [12]. They also mention the importance of therapeutic support for these patients. They indeed suffer form severe fright and despair, making contact with caring professionals essential [12].

Discussion

Despite Cotard's syndrome was first described more than a century ago, literature on this topic remains restricted to case reports. Although the syndrome is rare, more larger scale research is needed to further clarify the pathophysiologic underpinnings of the disease and its relation to other delusions of misidentification such as Capgras syndrome.

Promising hypotheses have been formulated, but evidence based support is lacking. To elucidate uncertainties regarding epidemiology, course, associated diseases, treatment options and prognosis, a careful registration of all cases could be of great value. In this regard recognition of this condition is essential. The restriction of publications to case reports is a potential pitfall. Sometimes general conclusions on course, pathophysiology or treatment are made, based on one or a few cases. For this literature on this topic has to be read carefully.

The syndrome as such is not catalogued in our current classification system. It has to be diagnosed as a part of an underlying disorder. Also treatment is guided by this diagnosis.

Although Cotard's syndrome is more like a symptom of its underlying condition, in our opinion recognition of this phenomenological entity remains important.

Its very specific presentation un spite of the extensive list of etiologies, indicating a shared pathological pathway, is intriguing. In the management of these patients a better understanding of the psychopathology and its neuropsychologic mechanisms can be of a great value. Specific safety measures can also be required due to the dramatic symptomatology.

References

[1] Cotard J: Du délire hypocondriaque dans une forme grave de la mélancholie anxieuse. *Ann. Med. Psychol.* 1880; 4: 168-174.

[2] Cotard J: Du délire des négations. *Arch. Neurol.* 1882; 4: 282-428.

[3] Séglas J: Mélancholie anxieuse avec délire des negations. *Progr. Med.* 1887; 46: 417-419.

[4] Régis E: Notre historique et clinique sur le délire de negations. *Gaz. Med. Paris* 1893; 2: 61-64.

[5] Tissot F: Délire des negations terminé par guérison. Cosidérations sur l'hypochondrie et la melancholie. *Ann. Med. Psychol.* 1921; 79: 321-328.

[6] Loudet O, Martinez DL: Sobre la psicoénesis y el valor pronostico del sindrome de Cotard. *Arch. Argent. Neurol.* 1933; 1: 1-12.

[7] Saavedra V: El syndrome de Cotard. Consideraciones psicopathologicas y nosograficas. *Rev. Neuropsiquiatr.* 1968; 11: 175-211.

[8] Berrios GE, Luque R: Cotard's syndrome: analysis of 100 cases. *Acta Psychiatr. Scand.* 1995; 91: 185-188.

[9] American Psychiatric Association: Diagnostic and statistical manual of mental disorders, fourth edition, text revision (DSM-IV-TR). Washington: *APA*, 2000: 413.

[10] Walloch JE, Klauwer C, Lanczik M, Brockington IF, Kornhuber J. Delusional denial of pregnancy as a special form of Cotard's syndrome. *Psychopathology* 2007; 40: 61-64.

[11] Reif A, Murach WM, Pfuhlmann B: Delusional paralysis: an unusual variant of Cotard's syndrome. *Psychopathology* 2003; 36: 218-220.

[12] Enoch D, Trethowan W: Cotard's syndrome. In Uncommon psychiatric syndromes (3rd ed.). Oxford: Butterworrh and Heinemann; 1991:162-183.

[13] Hansen ES, Bolwig TG: Cotard syndrome: an important manifestation of melancholia. *Nord. J. Psychiatry* 1995; 36: 218-223.

[14] Yamada K, Katsuragi S, Fujii I: A case study of Cotard's syndrome: stages and diagnosis. *Acta Psychiatr. Scand.* 1999; 100: 396-399.

[15] Duggal HS, Jagadheesan K, Haque Nizamie S: Biological basis and staging of Cotard's syndrome. *Eur. psychiatr.* 2002; 17: 109-109.

[16] Chiu HFK: Cotard's syndrome in psychogeriatric patients in Hong Kong. *Gen. Hosp. Psychiatr.* 1995; 17: 54-55.

[17] Ramirez-Bermudez J, Aguilar-Venegas LC, Crail-Melendez D, Espinola-Nadurille M, Nente F, Mendes MF: Cotard syndrome in neurological and psychiatric patients. *J. Neuropsychiatry Clin. Neurosci.* 2010; 22: 409-416.

[18] Edelstyn NMJ, Oyebode F: A review of the phenomenology and cognitive neuropsychological orgins of the Cotard delusion. Neurology psychiatry and brain research 2006; 13: 9-14.

[19] Consoli A, Soultanian C, Tanhuy M, Laurent C, Perisse D, Luque R, Berrios GE, Cohen D: Cotard's syndrome in adolescents and young adults is associated with an increased risk of bipolar disorder. *Bipol. disorders* 2007; 9: 665-668.

[20] Allen JR, Pfefferbaum B, Hammond D, Speed L: A disturbed child's use of a public event: Cotard's syndrome in a ten-year-old. *Psychiatry* 2000; 63: 208-213.

[21] Butler PV: Diurnal variation in Cotard's syndrome (copresent with Capgras delusion) following traumatic brain injury. *Aust. N. Z. J. Psychiatry* 2000; 34: 684-687.

[22] Camarero M, Real V: Sindrome de Cotard en adolescente. *Psiquiatria Biologica* 1997; 4: 213-214.

[23] Cohen D, Cottias C, Basquin M: Cotard's syndrome in a 15-year old girl. *Acta Psychiatr. Scand* 1997; 4: 164-165.

[24] Dugas M, Haflon O, Badoual AM, Golse B, Huet S: Le syndrome de Cotard chez l'adolescent. *Neuropsychiatr. Enf.* 1985; 33: 493-498.

[25] Fillastre M, Fontaine A, Depecker L, Degiovanni A: Cinq cas de syndrome de Cotard de l'adolescent et de l'adulte jeune. *Encéphale* 1992; 18: 65-66.

[26] Haflon O, Mouren-Simeoni MC, Dugas M: Le syndrome de Cotard chez l'adolescent. *Ann. Med. Psychol.* 1985; 149: 876-879.

[27] Liebowitz MC, McGrath PJ, Bush SC: Mania occurring during treatment for depersonalisation: A report of two cases. *J.Clin.Psychiatry* 1980; 41: 33-34.

[28] Mendhekar DN, Gupta N: Recurrent posticatal depression with Cotard delusion. *Indian J. Pediatr.* 2005; 72: 529-531.

[29] Soultanian C, Perisse D, Révah-Levy A, Luque R, Mazet P, Cohen D: Cotard's syndrome in adolescents and young adults: a possible onset of bipolar disorder requiring a mood stabilizer? *J. Child Adolesc. Psychopharmacol.* 2005; 15: 706-711.

[30] Yalin S, Varol Tas F, Güvenir T: The coexistence of Capgras, Fregoli and Cotard's syndromes in an adolescent case. *Arch. Neuropsychiatry* 2008; 45: 149-151.

[31] Christensen RC: Cotard's syndrome in a homeless man. *Psychiatric services* 2001; 52: 1256-1257.

[32] De Berardis, Serroni N, Campanella D, Marasco V, Moschetta FS. A case of Cotard's syndrome successfully treated with aripiprazole monotherapy. Prog. Neuro-Psychopharmacol. *Biol. Psychiatry* 2010; 37; 1348.

[33] De Risio S, De Rossi G, Sarchiapone M, Camardese G, Carli V, Cuomo C, Satta MA, Di Giuda D: A case of Cotard syndrome: 123I-IBZM SPECT imaging of striatal D2 receptor binding. *Psychiatry Res.* 2004; 27: 719-721.

[34] Hagen S, Voss SH. Cotard's syndrome in depression and maintenance electroconvulsive therapy. Ugeskr Leager 2002; 164: 3452-3453 (abstract).

[35] Hamon JM, Ginestet D: Délire des négations: à propos de quatre observations. *Ann. Med. Psychol.* 1994; 152: 425-443.

[36] Hashioka S, Monji A, Sasaki M, Yoshida I, Baba K, Tashiro N. A patient with Cotard syndrome who showed an improvement in single photon emission computed Tomography findings after successful treatment with antidepressants. *Clin. Neuropharmacol.* 2002; 25: 276-279.

[37] Ko SM. Cotard's syndrome – Two case reports. *Sing. Med. J.* 1989; 30: 277-278.

[38] Kucia K, Delkowski RS. ECT treatment of Cotard's syndrome in a patient with combined valvular heart disease and persistent atrial fibrillation. *Wiad Lek* 2004; 57: 290-292 (abstract).

[39] Leistedt S, Coumans N, Ladha K, Linkowski P. La négation du corps: à propos de trois observations concernant les délires de Jules Cotard. Ann. Med. Psychol. 2009, 167: 669-676.

[40] Lohmann T, Nishimura K, Sabri O, Klosterkötter J. Succesful electroconvulsive therapy of Cotard syndrome with bitemporal hypoperfusion. *Nervenartz* 1996, 67: 400-403.

[41] Nejad AG: Hydrophobia as a rare presentation of Cotard's syndrome: a case report. *Acta Psychiatr. Scand.* 2002; 106: 156-158.

[42] Petracca G, Migliorelli R, Vazquez S, Starkstein SE: SPECT findings before and after ECT in a patient with major depression and Cotard's syndrome. *J. Neuropsychiatry Clin. Neurosci.* 1995; 7: 505-507.

[43] Takahashi T, Nibuya M, Nomura S. Delusion of Cotard's syndrome successfully treated with a dopamine agonist. *J. Neuropsychiatry Clin. Neurosci.* 2010, 22: E27.

[44] Wani ZA, Khan AW, Baba AA, Khan HA, Wani QA, Taploo R: Cotard's syndrome and delayed diagnosis in Kashmir, *India. Int. J. Ment. Health Syst.* 2008; 2: 1-4.

[45] Baeza I, Salva J, Bernardo M: Cotard's syndrome in a young male bipolar patient. *J. Neuropsychiatry Clin. Neurosci.* 2000; 12: 119-120.

[46] Debruyne H, Portzky M, Van den Eynde F, Audenaert K: Cotard's syndrome: a review. *Current psychiatric reports* 2009; 11: 197-202.

[47] Kondo S, Hayashi H, Eguchi T, Oyama T, Wada T, Otani K. Bromocriptine augmentation in a patient with Cotard's syndrome. Prog Neuro-Psychopharmacol. *Biol. Psychiatr.* 2003; 27: 719-721.

[48] Nejad AG, Toofani K: Co-existence of lycantrophy and Cotard's syndrome in a single case. Acta Psychiatr Scand 2005; 111: 250-252

[49] Silva JA, Leong GB, Weinstock R, Gonzales CL: A case of Cotard's syndrome associated with self-starvation. *J. Forensic. Sci.* 2000; 45: 188-190.

[50] Caliyurt O, Vardar E, Tuglu C: Cotard's syndrome with schizophreniform disorder can be successfully treated with electroconvulsive therapy: case report. *Rev. Psychiatr. Neurosci.* 2004; 29: 138-141.
[51] Joseph AB: Cotard's syndrome in a patient with coexistent Capgras' syndrome in schizophrenia. *Prog. Neuropsychopharmacol. Biol. Psychiatry* 2004; 28: 607-609.
[52] Matsukura S, Yoshimi H, Sueoka S, Chihara K, Fujita T, Tanimoto K: β-endorphin in Cotard's syndrome. *Lancet* 1981; 17: 162-163.
[53] Nejad AG, Kerdegari M, Reihani-Kermani H: Self-mutilation of the nose in a schizophrenic patient with Cotard syndrome. *Arch. Iranian Med.* 2007; 10: 540-542.
[54] Wolff G, McKenzie K: Capgras, Fregoli and Cotard's syndromes and Koro in folie à deux. *Brit. J. Psychiatry* 1994; 106: 842.
[55] Shiraishi H, Ito M, Hayashi H, Otani K: Sulpiride treatment of Cotard's syndrome in schizophrenia. Prog. Neuro-Psychopharmacol. *Biol. Psychiatry* 2004; 28: 607-609.
[56] Wright S, Young AW, Hellawell DJ: Sequential Cotard and Capgras delusions. *Br. J. Clin. Psychol.* 1993; 32: 345-349.
[57] Conchiglia G, Della Rocca G, Grossi D: When the body image becomes 'empty': Cotard's delusion in a demented patient. *Achta Neuropsychiatrica* 2008, 20: 283-284.
[58] Fazzari G, Benzoni O, Sangaletti A, Bonera F, Nassini S, Mazzarini L, Pacchiarotti I, Sani G, Koukopoulos AE, Sanna L, Gasparotti R, De Rossi P, Lazano S, Savoja V, Giraldi P: Improvement of cognition in a patient with Cotard's delusions and frontotemporal atrophy receiving electroconvulsive therapy (ECT) for depression. *Int. Psychiogeriatrics* 2009; 21: 600-603.
[59] Kearns A: Cotard's syndrome in a mentally handicapped man. *Brit. J. Psychiatr.* 1987; 150: 112-114.
[60] Campbell S, Volow MR, Cavenar JO: Cotard's syndrome and the psychiatric manifestations of typhoid fever. *Am. J. Psychiatr.* 1981; 138: 1377-1378.
[61] Drake MEJ: Cotard's syndrome and temporal lobe epilepsy. P*sychiatr. J. Univ. Ott.* 1988; 13: 36-39.
[62] Hu WT, Diesing TS, Meissner I: Cotard's syndrome in a patient with superior sagittal sinus thrombosis. *Biol. Psychiatr.* 2006; 56: 263S.
[63] Bathia MS: Cotard syndrome in parietal lobe tumor. *Indian Pediatrics* 1993; 30: 1019-1021.
[64] Greenberg DB, Hochberg FH, Murray GB: The theme of death in complex partial seizures. *Am. J. Psychiatr.* 1984; 141: 1587-1589.
[65] Gardner-Thorpe C, Pearn J: The Cotard syndrome. Report of two patients: with a review of the extended spectrum of 'délire des négations'. *Eur. J. Neurology* 2004; 11: 563-566.
[66] Bathia MS, Agrawal P, Malic SC: Cotard's syndrome in migraine (a case report). *Indian Journal of Medical Sciences* 1993; 47: 152-153.
[67] Lerner V, Bergman J, Greenberg D, Bar El Y: Laurence-Moon-Bardet-Biedl syndrome in combination with Cotard's syndrome. Case report. *Isr J. Psychiatr. Relat. Sci.* 1995; 32: 291-294.
[68] Cannas A, Spissu A, Floris GL Congia S, Saddi MV, Melis M, Mascia MM, Pinna F, Tuveri A, Solla P, Milia A, Giagheddu M, Tacconi P: Bipolar affective disorder and Parkinson's disease: a rare, insidious and often unrecognised association. *Neurol. Sci.* 2002; 23: S67-S68.

[69] Factor SA, Molho ES. Treating auditory hallucinations and Cotard syndrome in Parkinson disease. *Clin. Neuropharmacol.* 2004, 27: 205-207.
[70] Kundlur SNC, George S, Jaimon M: An overview of the neurological correlates of Cotard syndrome. *Eur. J. Psychiat.* 2007; 21: 99-116.
[71] Paulig M, B¨ttger S, Sommer M, Prosiegel M: Depersonalisationssyndrom nach erworbener Hirnschädigung. Überblick anhand von 3 Fallbeispielen und Literatur sowie Diskussion ätiologischer Modelle. *Nervenartzt.* 1998; 69: 1100-1106.
[72] Young AW, Robertson IH, Hellawell DJ: Cotard delusion after brain injury. *Psychol. Med.* 1992; 22: 799-804.
[73] Munoz P, Valerio M, Palomo J, Fernandez-Yanez J, Fernandez-Cruz A, Guinea J, Bouza E: Infections and non-infectious neurologic complications in heart transplantations recepients. *Medicine* 2010; 89: 166-175.
[74] Hellden A: Death Delusion, report two cases of Cotard's syndrome as an adverse drug reaction to aciclovir and its prodrug valaciclovir. *BMJ* 2007; 335: 1305.
[75] Joseph AB, O'Leary DH: Brain atrophy and interhemispheric fissure enlargement in Cotard's syndrome. *J. Clin. Psychiatr.* 1986; 47: 518-520.
[76] Gerrans P. Refining the explanation of Cotard's delusion. *Mind and Language* 2000; 15: 111-122.
[77] McKay R, Cipolotti L: Attributional style in a case of Cotard delusion. *Conscious Cogn.* 2007; 16: 349-359.
[78] Vinkers DJ: Reactie op 'Het syndroom van Cotard. Een overzicht'. *Tijdschr Psychiatr.* 2008; 50: 391-392.
[79] Young AW, Leafhead KM: Betwixt life and death: case studies of Cotard delusion. In Method in madness: case studies in cognitive neuropsychiatry. Edited by Halligan PW, Marshall JC. Hove, East Sussex: *Taylor and Francis;* 1996: 147-171.
[80] Ellis HD, Young AW, Quayle AH, de Pauw KW: Reduced automatic responses to faces in Capgras delusion. *Proc. Biol. Sci.* 1997; 264: 1085-1092.
[81] Hirstein W, Ramachandran VS: Capgras syndrome: a novel probe for understanding the neutral representation of the identity and familiarity of persons. *Proc. Biol. Sci.* 1997; 264: 437-444.
[82] Breen N, Caine D, Coltheart M: The role of affect and reasoning in a patient wiht a delusion of misidentification. *Cognitive neuropsychiatry* 2002; 7: 113-137.
[83] Davis M, Coltheart M, Langdon R, Breen N: Monothematic delusions: Towards a two-factor account. *Philosophy, Psychiatry and Psychology* 2001; 8: 133-158.
[84] Coltheart M: The 33rd Sir Frederick Barlett Lecture Cognitive neuropsychiatry and delusional belief. *The Quarterly Journal of Experimental Psychology* 2007; 60: 1041-1062.
[85] Coltheart M, Langdon R, McKay R: Schizophrenia and monothematic delusions. *Schizophrenia bulletin* 2007; 33: 642-647.
[86] Coltheart M: The neuropsychology of delusions. *Ann. N. Y. Acad. Sci.* 2010; 1191: 16-26.
[87] Corlett PR, Aitken MR, Dickinson A, Shanks DR, Honey GD, Honey RA, Robbins TW, Bullmore ET, Fletcher PC: Prediction error during retrospective evaluation of causal associations in humans: fMRI evidence in favor of an associative model of learning. *Neuron* 2004; 44: 877-888.

[88] Fletcher PC, Anderson JM, Shanks DR, Honey R, Carpenter TA, Donovan T, Papadakis N, Bullmore ET: Responses of human frontal cortex to surprising events are predicted by formal associative learning theory. *Nat. Neursosci.* 2001; 10: 1043-1048.

[89] Turner DC, Aitken MR, Shanks DR, Sahakian BJ, Robbins TW, Scharzbauer C, Fletcher PC: The role of the lateral frontal cortex in causal associative learning: exploring prevantative and super-learning. *Cereb. Cortex* 2004; 14: 872-880.

[90] Gerrans P. Delusions as performance failures. *Cognitive neuropsychiatry* 2001; 6: 161-173.

[91] Kozian R: Duloxetin bei Cotard Syndrom. *Psychiatr. Prax* 2005; 32: 412-413.

[92] Jitsuiki H, Sasaki T, Wada K, Takaishi Y, Mifune Y: Two cases of senile mood disorders successfully treated with olanzapine. *Intl. Clin. Psychopharmacol.* 2006; 24: A6.

[93] Madani Y, Sabbe BGC: Het Cotardsyndroom. Differentiële behandling volgens subclassificatie. *Tijdschr. Psychiatr.* 2007; 49: 49-53.

[94] Chan JH, Chen CH, Robson D: Case report: effective treatment of Cotard's syndrome: quetiapine in combination with venlafaxine. *Psychiatry Clin. Neurosci.* 2009; 63: 125-126.

[95] Ruminjo A, Mekinulov B: A case report of Cotard's syndrome. *Psychiatry* (Edgmont) 2008; 5(6): 28-29.

[96] Bourgeois M: Le syndrome de Cotard aujourd'hui. *Ann. Med. Psychol.* 1969; 127: 534-544.

[97] Mahgoub NA, Hossain A: Cotard's syndrome and electroconvulsive therapy. *Psychiatr. Serv.* 2004; 55: 1319.

[98] Montgomery JH, Vasu D: The use of electroconvulsive therapy in atypical psychotic presentations: a case review. *Psychiatry* (Edgmont) 2007; 4 (10): 30-39.

[99] Malone K, Malone JP: Remarkable resolution of an uncommon psychosyndrome – epilepsy-induced remission of Cotard's syndrome. *Irish Journal of Psychological Medicine 1992*, 9: 53-54.

CHILD AND ADOLESCENT

In: The International Psychiatry and Behavioral ...
Editor: Nash Boutros

ISBN: 978-1-62257-566-4

Chapter 13

Child Abuse and Its Long-Term Consequences: An Exploratory Study on Egyptian University Students*

***Khalid Mansour*#1, *Eman Roshdy*[2], *Peter E. Langdon*[3], *Omaima A. Daoud*[4], *Mahmood El-Saadawy*[5], *Ali Al-Zahrani*[6] and *Abdulshafi Khashaba*[7]**

[1]Basildon Hospital, Basildon, Essex, UK
[2]Faculty of Medicine, Zagazig University, Egypt
[3]School of Medicine, Health Policy and Practice, Faculty of Health, University of East Anglia, Norwich, UK
[4]Psychiatry, Faculty of Medicine, Zagazig University, Egypt
[5]Occupational Medicine, Faculty of Medicine, Zagazig University, Egypt
[6]Psychology, Faculty of Medicine, Taif University, Saudi Arabia
[7]Psychiatry, Faculty of Medicine, Zagazig University, Egypt

Abstract

Introduction: child abuse and its long term consequences in adulthood have been recently gaining increased attention in the Arab world. This study is an extension of a similar study in Saudi Arabia, and aims to explore some epidemiological characteristics of the problem in Egypt.

Aims: to study the prevalence of child abuse and associated psychological problems in adulthood, as presented in a sample of university students in Egypt.

Method: 963 students, from three different colleges of Zagazig University (Medicine, Education and Arts and Literature) answered multi-questionnaires including: General health Questionnaire (GHQ), Child Traumatic Questionnaire (CTQ) and Psychological Problem Scale (PPS).

---

* Original Publication: Mansour et al. The Arab Journal of Psychiatry (2010) Vol.21 No.2. Page (137-163).

Correspondence: Dr Khalid A Mansour, E-mail: kmansour@btinternet.com

Results: Students reported having suffered Emotional neglect (19%), Emotional abuse (8.9%), Physical neglect (44%) and Physical abuse (6%) and Sexual abuse (13%). Moderate to severe childhood abuse was correlated with various combinations of psychological problems (Low Self-Esteem, Dissociation, Self Harm, Impulsivity and Aggression) in adulthood. Gender and situational stresses, as indicated by GHQ, did not seem to influence the results as much as low income and big family size.

Conclusion: a large proportion of our sample reported both child abuse and several long term pathological consequences of abuse in adulthood. The problem seems to be serious in this middle class sample and it remains possible that these problems could be worse in lower social classes.

Keywords: Child abuse, Arab World, Child Traumatic Questionnaire (CTQ), Psychological Problem Scale (PPS), sexual abuse, physical neglect

INTRODUCTION

The subject of child abuse and its long-term implications in adulthood has been widely studied in the literature in different areas of the world and across different cultures. (Dunn, 2009 [1]; Bouchard et al, 2008 [2]; Finkelhor et al, 2005 [3]; Arias, 2004 [4]; Briere and Elliott, 1994 [5]; Turner et al, 2006 [6]; Widom, 1999 [7]). The effects of child abuse vary depending on the circumstances of the abuse or neglect, personal characteristics of the child, and the child's environment. Consequences may be mild or severe; disappear after a short period or last a lifetime. Consequences could affect the individual physically, psychologically, behaviourally, or a combination of all three ways. Ultimately, due to related costs to society such as the health care, social services and educational systems, abuse and neglect impact not just on the child and family, but rather the whole of society (Child Welfare Information Gateway, 2008 [8]; Gilbert et al, 2009 [9]).

It is unfortunate that this area of research has not received much attention in Arabic literature for a long time. It has been only recently, within the last 10 – 15 years that this subject started to be covered in the media and by social and political establishments (BBC, 2004 [10]). During this period, the subject of child abused started to be covered by five main establishments; (1) the independent satellite TV channels and internet web-sites, (2) political organisation especially those interested in the recent Middle East wars, (3) Middle East academics, (4) the international organisations concerned with children rights and (5) governmental agencies. It is probably the emergence of the new independent media sector in the Middle East during the last 25 years, which has been the main factor for breaking the taboos about child abuse and sexual harassment in the Arab world (BBC, 2004[10]).

A fairly large number of satellite TV channels and a much larger number of internet websites started to compete to engage the public by producing this brave and new coverage of a long tabooed problem and bring it to the open. Dozens, if not hundreds, of websites (including e-bloggers, chat room and e-forums), have been discussing such subjects freely in an unprecedented way. However they have been focused mainly on the subjects of child sexual abuse and sexual harassment of adult women. This has clearly been associated with a significant increase in public interest and awareness as well as an increase in the interests of other agencies. The second major source of interest in child abuse has been the organisations concerned with victims of wars and political crises in the Middle East (e.g. human rights organisations and some political parties). In this regard, the literature about the children suffering in the wars like in Lebanon, Palestine and Iraq have been the most prominent (Baker and Shalhoub-Kevorkian, 1999 [11]; Khamis, 2000 [12]; Macksoud and Aber, 1996 [13]).

During the same period, a relatively large number of scientific publications have been produced by different scientific disciplines (e.g. public health sociology, mental health and paediatric departments). Between 1995 to 2009, the Child Abuse and Neglect Journal (the Official Publication of the International Society for Prevention of Child Abuse and Neglect) has published about 40 psychiatric and psychological articles about child abuse in the Middle East and Arab world (e.g. Abu Baker and Dwairy, 2003 [14]; Youssef et al, 1998-aandb [15,16]; Shalhoub-Kevorkian, 1999 [17]). Many studies have been produced in Arabic (e.g. Al-Sayed, 1993 [18]; Essali, 2008 [19]). Publications from Paediatrics departments about child abuse have been mainly about physical abuse and physical complications of child abuse (e.g. , Al-Mahroos, 2007 [20]; Al-Moosa et al, 2003 [21]).

International organisations working in the Middle East (e.g. UNICEF [22], UNRWA [23], WHO [24], ISPCAN [25], Save the Children [26] and Human Rights Watch [27]) have also been working mainly with governmental agencies to combat child abuse in the area and provide some services. They have also been organising conferences and publishing research (see web sites of these organisations). These organisations have played a significant role in increasing the awareness of the problem. Some Arabic governments have since started to develop specialised organisations to combat child abuse (e.g. National Commission for Childhood of Saudi Arabia [28]). The recent emergence of interest in child abuse has freed the subject from some old taboos but has also attached some new ones. The new controversies would perhaps influence the debate about child abuse for some time to come. The subject of child abuse has been covered by political opposition and independent parties in the context of their criticism of the living conditions in the Arab countries (ikhwan-web [29], Syrian Women Observatory [30], Egyptian Centre for Women's Rights [31], IslamOnLine.net [32]). Child abuse has also been a subject used in the local Middle Eastern war propagandas. Most of the independent Arabic views highlight the children suffering in the war zones in an attempt to condemn Israel and its American and western allies. On the opposite side, many Israeli and western media agencies in the area, supported by some local voices, express the view that traditional Arab and Islamic culture could be facilitating abuse of women and children. One example of these new sensitivities is the scepticism about the publications about child abuse in Palestine produced by Palestinian academic and others who worked at the time in Israeli universities. These papers constitute probably more than half of the Child Abuse and Neglect Journal publications mentioned above.

Research Design

In this study, we have followed a fairly similar methodology as in the Saudi study (Al-Zahrani, 2005 [33]). Two of our authors have been involved in that study. 1500 questionnaires (see appendix) were distributed to students in three colleges in Zagazig University (Medicine, Education and Arts and Literature). 963 responses were received (458 from College of Education, 341 from College of Art and Literature and 164 from College of Medicine). Some of the responses were partially incomplete and subsequently the missing parts have not been included in the statistical analysis. The three colleges were chosen to represent different levels of functioning and socioeconomic status among Egyptian students. In accordance with general public attitude in Egypt, students from Faculty of Medicine have usually been considered to be of higher academic status, more motivated and have relatively higher economic and social status compared to other students. It is also widely assumed that student from colleges of Art and Literature are from relatively lower economic and social status, while students from the colleges of Education lie in-between.

The following psychological tools have been included in the questionnaires:

The Arabic version of General health Questionnaire-12 (GHQ – 12) (Daradkeh et al, 2001 [34]): The General Health Questionnaire (Goldberg, 1978 [35]) has been extensively used in different settings and different cultures. The GHQ focuses on two major areas – the inability to carry out normal functions and the appearance of new and distressing psychological phenomena such as depressive symptoms, social dysfunction, sleep disturbance, anxiety, and dysphoria in people in community and medical settings. The GHQ assesses the respondent's current state (state-stress) and asks if that differs from his or her usual trait-stress. The questionnaire was originally developed as a 60-item instrument but at present a range of shortened versions of the questionnaire including the GHQ-30, the GHQ-28, the GHQ-20, and the GHQ-12 are available. The scale asks whether the respondent has currently been experiencing a particular symptom or behaviour difficulties. Each item is rated on a four-point scale (less than usual, no more than usual, rather more than usual, or much more than usual). Child Traumatic Questionnaire (CTQ) (Bernstein and Fink, 1998[36]): The CTQ is a 28-item self-report inventory that provides brief screening for histories of abuse and neglect. The CTQ is appropriate for adolescents (aged 12 and over) and adults.

The CTQ inquires about five types of maltreatment: emotional, physical, and sexual abuse and emotional and physical neglect with five items representing each type. The CTQ also includes a 3-item minimization/Denial Scale for detecting false-negative trauma reports. Each item consists of 5 options such as; never true; rarely true; sometimes true; often true; and very often true. Al-Zahrani's (2005) [33] study condensed the five questions in the CTQ that originally dealt with sexual abuse to one, in order to avoid cultural sensitivities especially considering that participants may not be accustomed to these kind of questions.

The Arabic translation of the questionnaire has been standardised to the Saudi Arabic dialect. Psychological problem scale: Al-Zahrani (2005) [33] collected several questions from different scales in order to explore the various areas of psychological problems caused by child abuse. The Arabic translation of the questionnaire has been standardised to the Saudi Arabic dialect. The questions are related to the feelings of the subjects during the last few weeks. They consist of 13 questions intended to explore the following:

1. Low self-esteem: (Q13 and Q14) (Rosenberg, 1965 [37]).
2. Dissociation: (Q15 and Q16) (Vanderlinden et al, 1993 [38]).
3. Post-traumatic Stress disorder: (Q17 and Q18) (Joseph et al, 1997 [39]).
4. Self-harm: (Q19): (First et al ,1997 [40]).
5. Impulsiveness: (Q20 and Q 21) (First et al, 1997 [40]).
6. Eating Disorder: (Q22 and Q23) (The Centre for Eating disorder. Com; Al-Zahrani, 2005 [33])
7. Aggression (Q24 and 25) (Briere and Runtz, 1990 [41]).

Data Preparation and Analysis

All data were stored and analysed using SPSS for Windows® Version 18.0.0. (2009). Initially, given the large sample size, data were inspected for significant departures from normality by examining appropriate histograms. Examination revealed difficulties with skewness and/or kurtosis for the psychological variables and the abuse variables.

As a consequence, it was decided to make use of appropriate non-parametric statistics. Comparisons were made between male and female participants across demographic, psychological and abuse variables using χ^2 or the Mann Whitney U test. Differences between colleges were examined using the Kruskal Wallis Test and post hoc tests were calculated using the Conover-Inman method. Finally, participants were grouped according to the level of abuse reported, and two groups were formed: those who reported none to minimal abuse, and those who reported moderate to extreme abuse. These two groups were compared using Mann Whitney U tests.

Results

Males vs. Females (table 3): Analysis of the demographic data revealed that males were significantly older in age than females ($z=2.724$, $p=0.006$), while there was no significant difference between males and females regarding paternal or maternal age, or number of siblings (Table 3). There was no significant difference between males and females in terms of maternal education (χ^2 (2)=1.32, $p=0.52$), but there was for paternal education (χ^2 (2)=8.87, $p=0.012$). A higher proportion of males had fathers who attended university in comparison to females. There was no significant difference between males and females regarding parental income (χ^2 (2)=2.89, $p=0.24$), parental martial status (χ^2 (2)=1.30, $p=0.52$), or area of residence (χ^2 (2)=3.76, $p=0.153$).

There was a significant sex difference regarding the type of college attended. Males tended to study medicine and art and literature more so than females, while females tended to study education more so than males (χ^2 (2)=242.82, $p<0.001$).

Comparing males and females across the psychological variables revealed that females had a significantly higher mean score on the GHQ ($p<0.001$), and significantly lower self esteem ($p=0.043$). There were no other significant differences between males and females across the psychological variables (Table 3). Considering abuse, males reported experiencing significantly highly levels of physical abuse ($p<0.001$), emotional abuse ($p<0.001$), emotional neglect ($p<0.001$) and sexual abuse ($p=0.018$) than females (Table 3). However, females reported significantly higher levels of denial than did males ($p=0.001$).

Colleges (table 4): Comparing across groups of colleges revealed that there was a significant difference between education, art and literature and medicine in terms of participants' age (χ^2 (2, N=903)=303.44 $p<0.001$), maternal age (χ^2 (2, N=892)=55.42, $p<0.001$), paternal age (χ^2 (2, N=845)=29.42, $p<0.001$), and number of siblings (χ^2 (2, N=921)=20.76, $p<0.001$; Table 4). Further inspection of these differences using post hoc tests revealed that all types of colleges were significantly different from each other across these variables (Table 4). There was also a significant difference between colleges in terms of parental income.

Table 1. Demographic Characteristics and Descriptive Data

(NB: all statistical tests regarding demographic data and descriptive data are two-tailed):

Variable	%	N=
Sex		
Male	31.6	304
Female	63.9	615
Missing	4.6	44
College		
Education	47.6	458
Art and Literature	35.4	341
Medicine	17.0	164
Parental Marital status		
Divorced	2.8	27
Widowed	11.7	113
Married	82.6	795
Missing	2.9	28
Area of Residence		
Urban	34.9	336
Rural	60.0	578
Abroad	2.1	20
Missing	3.0	29
Parental Income		
Less than Average	6.7	65
Average	64.7	623
More than Average	24.6	237
Missing	3.9	38
Maternal Education		
Primary School	25.1	242
Secondary School	29.6	285
University	31.9	307
Missing	13.4	129
Paternal Education		
Primary School	18.6	179
Secondary School	24.3	234
University	48.9	471
Missing	8.2	8.2
Variable	*M* (SD)	N=
Age	19.25 (1.73)	903
Maternal Age	44.45 (6.04)	894
Paternal Age	51.12 (6.09)	845
Number of Siblings	3.65 (1.81)	921

Fewer than the number of expected students attending education and medicine came from families with less than average income, while more than the number of expected students attending art and literature came from families with less than average income (χ^2 (4)=25.54, p<0.001). Considering psychological problems overall, there was a significant difference between colleges on the PPS total score (χ^2 (2, N=875)=9.08 p=0.011) and Self-Harm (χ^2 (2, N=948)=16.99 p<0.001).

Table 2. Gender * College Cross-tabulation

		College			Total
		Faculty of education	Faculty of arts and literature	Faculty of Medicine	
Gender	Male	31	178	95	304
	Female	397	152	66	615
Total		428	330	161	919

Examination of these differences revealed that those attending art and literature colleges reported a significantly ($p<0.05$) higher PPS total score and self-harm score than those attending education or medicine colleges, while there was no significant difference between those attending education and medicine colleges ($p>0.05$) on these two variables. There was a significant difference between the colleges regarding physical neglect (χ^2 (2, N=849)=10.25 p=0.006), physical abuse (χ^2 (2, N=857)=66.14 p<0.001), emotional neglect (χ^2 (2, N=846)=48.10 p<0.001), emotional abuse (χ^2 (2, N=816)=18.78 p<0.001), and sexual abuse (χ^2 (2, N=867)=24.06 p<0.001).

Considering physical neglect, those attending art and literature colleges reporting a significantly ($p<0.05$) lower score on physical neglect than those attending medicine, while there was no difference between art and literature and education ($p<0.05$) or medicine and education ($p<0.05$). With the exception of physical neglect, consistently across all of the abuse and neglect variables, those attending art and literature colleges reported significantly greater levels ($p<0.05$) of abuse and neglect than those attending education and medicine, while there was no significant difference between education and medicine ($p<0.05$). In the meantime, participants from education and medical colleges scored significantly higher on the denial scale compared to participants from the Art and Literature colleges (χ^2 (2, N=856)=37.76 p<0.001).

Prevalence of Abuse (table 5): Examining the prevalence of different kinds of abuse within this sample revealed that 3.9% of the sample indicated that they had experienced moderate to extreme emotional abuse, while 6.0% indicated that they had experienced moderate to extreme emotional neglect. The prevalence of physical abuse and neglect categorised as moderate to extreme was 4.0% and 9.0% respectively. Sexual abuse that was categorised as moderate to extreme was found to exist within 9% of the sample (Table 5). Psychological impact of different types of abuse (table 6): Those who reported none to minimal abuse were compared to those who reported moderate or higher levels of abuse (Table 6).

Those who reported suffering moderate to extreme levels of emotional abuse were significantly younger in age (p=0.017), and reported significantly higher scores on the GHQ (p=0.020), and PPS total (p<0.008). This group also reported significantly lower self esteem (p=0.043), higher self-harm (p<0.001) and higher aggression (p=0.001; Table 6). Those reporting moderate to extreme emotional neglect were significantly younger age (p=0.005) and had more siblings (p=0.001) than those reporting none to minimal emotional neglect. Those reporting moderate to extreme emotional neglect also had significantly a higher self harm score (p=0.005) and a higher total PPS score (p=0.042; Table 6).

Table 3. Demographic and descriptive data regarding males and females (p<0.01 - *p<0.05)**

Variable	Male		Female		
	M (SD)	*N=*	*M(SD)*	*N=*	*Mann Whitney U p= two tailed)*
Age	19.52** (2.34)	294	19.11 (1.32)	599	0.006
Maternal Age	44.39 (6.19)	283	44.70 (5.48)	586	0.442
Paternal Age	51.22 (6.68)	281	51.12 (5.78)	542	0.470
Number of Siblings	3.68 (2.03)	298	3.62 (1.69)	598	0.651
General Health Questionnaire (GHQ)	14.71 (6.79)	280	16.03** (5.82)	592	<0.001
Psychological Problems Scale Total (PPS)	4.69 (2.14)	268	4.84 (2.31)	566	0.616
Self Esteem	0.42 (0.64)	296	0.53* (0.74)	606	0.043
Dissociation	0.86 (0.61)	299	0.86 (0.56)	604	0.969
Post Traumatic Stress	1.09 (0.66)	293	1.05 (0.66)	603	0.472
Self-Harm	0.11 (0.31)	297	0.14 (0.35)	607	0.18
Impulsivity	1.12 (0.79)	294	1.17 (0.77)	598	0.353
Eating Disorders	0.41 (0.59)	296	0.44 (0.57)	609	0.353
Aggression	0.70 (0.73)	298	0.62 (0.68)	606	0.203
Childhood Trauma Questionnaire (CTQ)					
Physical Neglect	7.25 (2.64)	256	7.02 (2.16)	563	0.632
Physical Abuse	2.43** (3.84)	266	1.31 (3.22)	551	<0.001
Emotional Neglect	6.33* (4.90)	258	5.55 (4.74)	548	0.016
Emotional Abuse	3.80** (4.19)	250	2.64 (3.58)	527	<0.001
Sexual Abuse	0.68* (1.28)	270	0.44 (1.02)	557	0.018
Denial	6.20 (2.87)	274	6.91** (2.92)	544	0.001

Table 4. Descriptive data across the three colleges

Variable	Education	Art and Literature	Medicine		
	M (SD)	*M(SD)*	*M (SD)*	χ^2 (df, N=)	*Post Hoc Tests*
Age	19.22 (1.163)	18.36 (1.23)	20.56 (0.82)	χ^2 (2, N=903)=303.44 p<0.001	AL<M*; AL<E*; M>E*
Maternal Age	44.49 (5.50)	42.73 (6.51)	46.73 (4.74)	χ^2 (2, N=892)=55.42, p<0.001	AL<M*; AL<E*; M>E*
Paternal Age	51.72 (5.88)	49.45 (6.68)	52.61 (4.87)	χ^2 (2, N=845)=29.42, p<0.001	AL<M*; AL<E*; M>E*
Number of Siblings	3.59 (1.69)	3.99 (2.04)	3.32 (1.69)	χ^2 (2, N=921)=20.76, p<0.001	AL>M*; AL>E*; M<E*
General Health Questionnaire (GHQ)	15.52 (5.64)	14.72 (6.47)	15.45 (5.63)	χ^2 (2, N=914)=1.33, p=0.515	AL<M; AL<E; M<E
Psychological Problems Scale Total (PPS)	4.54 (2.14)	5.03 (2.43)	4.40 (2.21)	χ^2 (2, N=875)=9.08 p=0.011	AL>M*; AL>E*; M<E
Self Esteem	0.47 (0.70)	0.52 (0.74)	0.45 (0.67)	χ^2 (2, N=946)=2.68 p=0.262	AL>M; AL>E; M<E
Dissociation	0.84 (0.54)	0.87 (0.64)	0.81 (0.58)	χ^2 (2, N=947)=3.25 p=0.197	AL>M; AL>E; M<E
Post Traumatic Stress	1.06 (0.62)	1.07 (0.69)	1.02 (0.69)	χ^2 (2, N=939)=1.28 p=0.529	AL<M; AL>E; M>E
Self-Harm	0.09 (0.29)	0.16 (0.37)	0.09 (0.30)	χ^2 (2, N=948)=16.99 p<0.001	AL>M*; AL>E*; M<E
Impulsivity	1.09 (0.77)	1.41 (0.70)	0.98 (0.87)	χ^2 (2, N=935)=1.97 p=0.374	AL>M; AL>E; M<E
Eating Disorders	0.39 (0.54)	0.47 (0.61)	0.38 (0.56)	χ^2 (2, N=947)=0.19 p=0.374	AL>M; AL>E; M<E
Aggression	0.59 (0.68)	0.70 (0.73)	0.54 (0.64)	χ^2 (2, N=947)=5.53 p=0.062	AL>M; AL>E; M<E

Table 4. (Continued)

Variable	Education	Art and Literature	Medicine		
	M (SD)	*M(SD)*	*M (SD)*	χ^2 (df, N=)	*Post Hoc Tests*
Childhood Trauma Questionnaire (CTQ)					
Physical Neglect	7.13 (1.58)	7.09 (3.01)	7.58 (1.84)	χ^2 (2, N=849)=10.25 p=0.006	AL<M*; AL<E; M<E
Physical Abuse	0.96 (2.19)	2.87 (4.78)	0.86 (2.54)	χ^2 (2, N=857)=66.14 p<0.001	AL>M*; AL>E*; M>E
Emotional Neglect	4.97 (4.01)	7.82 (5.69)	4.59 (3.67)	χ^2 (2, N=846)=48.10 p<0.001	AL>M*; AL>E*; M<E
Emotional Abuse	2.33 2.92)	4.10 (4.83)	2.42 (4.26)	χ^2 (2, N=816)=18.78 p<0.001	AL>M*; AL>E*; M>E
Sexual Abuse	0.34 (0.83)	0.80 (1.40)	0.41 (1.02)	χ^2 (2, N=867)=24.06 p<0.001	AL>M*; AL>E*; M>E
Denial	7.26 (2.73)	6.23 (3.06)	7.22 (2.63)	χ^2 (2, N=856)=37.76 p<0.001	AL<M*; AL<E*; M<E

(E=Education; AL=Art and Literature; M=Medicine; *p<0.05).

Table 5. Prevalence of Abuse

Variable	None to Minimal		Low to Moderate		Moderate to Severe		Severe to Extreme	
	N=	%	N=	%	N=	%	N=	%
Total Emotional Abuse N=816	743	91.1	41	5.0	17	2.1	15	1.8
Males (N=250)	218	87.0	18	7.0	7	3.0	7	3.0
Females (N=527)	490	93.0	20	4.0	10	2.0	7	1.0
Missing (N=39)	35	90.0	3	8.0	0	0.0	1	2.0
Total Emotional Neglect N=846	683	81.0	103	12.0	36	4.0	24	3.0
Male (N=258)	198	77	37	14	13	5	10	4
Female (N=548)	452	82	59	11	23	4	14	3
Missing (N=40)	33	83	7	17	0	0	0	0
Total Physical Abuse N=857	809	94.0	15	2.0	9	1.0	24	3.0
Male (N=266)	241	90.5	10	4.0	4	1.5	11	4.0
Female (N=551)	529	96.0	4	1.0	5	1.0	13	2.0
Missing (N=40)	39	98	1	2	0	0	0	0
Total Physical Neglect N= 859	484	56.0	302	35.0	57	7.0	16	2.0
Male (N=256)	140	55.0	85	33.0	22	8.5	9	3.5
Females (N=563)	314	56.0	209	37.0	33	6.0	7	1.0
Missing (N=40)	30	75	8	20	2	5	0	0
Total Sexual Abuse N=867	751	87.0	33	4.0	35	4.0	48	5.0
Male (N=270)	221	82.0	12	4.0	14	5.0	23	9.0
Female (N=557)	495	89.0	20	4.0	17	3.0	25	4.0
Missing (N=40)	35	88	1	2	4	10	0	0

Table 6. Comparisons across psychological and family related variables according to severity of abuse

	Emotional Abuse				Emotional Neglect				Physical Abuse			
	None to Minimal (N=507)		Moderate to Extreme (N=83)		None to Minimal (N=678)		Moderate to Extreme (N=131)		None to Minimal (N=543)		Moderate to Extreme (N=63)	
	M=	SD	M=	SD	M=	SD	M=	SD	M=	SD	M=	SD
Age	19.22	1.39	19.16*	1.28	19.33	1.82	18.91**	1.31	19.24	1.36	18.92**	1.33
Maternal Age	44.55	5.99	44.31	5.37	44.66	5.54	44.32	6.54	44.68	5.92	43.56**	6.05
Paternal Age	51.46	5.68	51.42	6.95	51.25	5.66	50.55	7.77	51.44	5.62	50.46**	6.85
No of Siblings	3.54	1.62	3.89	2.20	3.49	1.66	4.10**	2.07	3.56	1.61	3.98**	2.36
GHQ	15.08	5.82	15.92*	5.38	15.16	6.01	16.15	6.82	15.22	5.80	15.80	6.15
Self-Esteem	0.48	0.68	0.53*	0.70	0.47	0.69	0.44	0.71	0.46	0.69	0.59	0.77
Dissociation	0.81	0.57	0.92	0.52	0.84	0.57	0.86	0.56	0.84	0.56	0.90	0.55
PTSD	1.05	0.66	1.13	0.69	1.03	0.65	1.05	0.68	1.06	0.67	1.17	0.66
Self Harm	0.11	0.31	0.23***	0.42	0.11	0.31	0.19**	0.39	0.11	0.31	0.23*	0.42
Impulsivity	1.10	0.78	1.30	0.76	1.13	0.78	1.18	0.79	1.13	0.78	1.22	0.77
Aggression	0.60	0.68	0.81**	0.72	0.63	0.70	0.74	0.75	0.61	0.69	0.77*	0.67
Eating Disorders	0.40	0.54	0.55	0.65	0.41	0.57	0.46	0.61	0.41	0.56	0.50	0.63
Total Psychological Problems	4.51	2.15	5.47**	2.40	4.59	2.23	5.05*	2.30	4.62	2.21	5.38	2.30

	Physical Neglect				Sexual Abuse			
	None to Minimal (N=318)		Moderate to Extreme (N=87)		None to Minimal (N=507)		Moderate to Extreme (N=53)	
	M=	SD	M=	SD	M=	SD	M=	SD
Age	19.29	1.44	18.92*	1.20	19.24	1.38	18.96*	1.18
Maternal Age	44.97	5.56	43.71**	6.42	44.58	5.97	44.90	5.36
Paternal Age	51.56	5.22	50.73	7.04	51.37	5.79	51.29	5.52
No of Siblings	3.73	1.76	3.92	2.05	3.55	1.72	4.19*	1.72
GHQ	15.48	6.01	16.47	5.78	15.17	5.81	17.09**	6.11
Self-Esteem	0.50	0.72	0.61	0.76	0.46	0.69	0.67	0.80
Dissociation	0.85	0.56	0.94	0.52	0.83	0.57	1.02****	0.58
PTSD	1.10	0.67	1.11	0.69	1.06	0.67	1.17	0.73
Self Harm	0.11	0.31	0.26**	0.44	0.12	0.32	0.21*	0.41
Impulsivity	1.15	0.76	1.24	0.74	1.13	0.78	1.38	0.64
Aggression	0.60	0.67	0.81**	0.69	0.61	0.69	0.78*	0.73
Eating Disorders	0.39	0.52	0.53	0.67	0.42	0.55	0.58	0.68
Total Psychological Problems	4.70	2.15	5.50*	2.36	4.63	2.20	5.78***	2.46

(* $p<0.05$ ** $p<0.01$ *** $p<0.001$).

Considering those who reported experiencing moderate to extreme physical abuse, they were significantly younger in age (p=0.002), had significantly more siblings (p=0.003), and reported that their mother (p=0.005) and father (p=0.019) were younger (parental ages) than those who reported experiencing none to minimal physical abuse. Those reporting moderate to extreme physical abuse reported engaging in significantly higher levels of self harm (p=0.015) and aggression (p=0.029). There were no significant differences between the two groups across the remaining variables for physical abuse (Table 6). Considering physical neglect, those reporting moderate to extreme levels were significantly younger in age (p=0.012) and reported that their mothers were also significantly younger (p=0.007) than those who reported experiencing none to minimal physical neglect. Those reporting moderate to extreme physical neglect also reported significantly higher self harm (p<0.001), aggression (p=0.003), and PPS total (p=0.032) than did those reporting none to minimal physical neglect. Finally, comparing those who reported moderate to extreme sexual abuse to those who reported none to minimal revealed that the moderate to extreme group were younger in age (p=0.027) had significantly more siblings (p=0.001), and significantly higher GHQ (p=0.003) and PPS total scores (p<0.001). They also had significantly higher levels of dissociation (p=0.002), self-harm (p=0.015) and aggression (p=0.046). The difference between the two groups on the measure of self-esteem (p=0.080), impulsivity (p=0.057), and eating disorders (p=0.057) all approached significance at the two tailed level. There were no other significant differences between these two groups (Table 6).

DISCUSSION

Limitations of the Study

In this study, there is a lack of formal randomisation in allocating participants. The questionnaires are too brief and the translation used has not been standardised on Egyptian dialects. This may lead to possible errors in understanding questions. There has been only one question used to identify history of sexual abuse.

We made it this way, as in the Saudi study, to minimise any cultural sensitivities among our participants. The Al-Zahrani questionnaires (Al-Zahrani, 2005 [33]), used in this study, have been designed to be brief, to avoid exhausting participants with too many questions. This has meant that some of the other important long term consequences of child abuse not being included, e.g. “Misuse of Psychoactive Substances” (Dube et al., 2001 [42]; Swan, 1998 [43]), “Revictimisation” (Coid et al, 2001 [44]), physical health implications (Flaherty et al., 2006 [45]; Springer et al, 2007 [46]), offending and abusive behaviour (Siegel, 2003 [47]; English et al, 2004 [48]) and others.

There are other limitations that need to be considered when interpreting results from this study. There is the possibility that “recall” bias and selection bias may have affected the participants’ responses. There are no clinical assessments based on direct interviews to verify the results of the questionnaires. The high numbers of female subjects compared to male subjects could be due to selection error. The sample in this study is not fully representative of Egyptian society, and it is quite possible that the prevalence of abuse is much higher in uneducated and poorer social classes. The data about "parents' employment" and "parents' income" may lack validity and reliability because the questions were relatively brief.

Demographic and Descriptive Data Regarding Males and Females (Table 3)

In the table it was demonstrated that Female subjects are significantly; younger in age and have higher mean scores on the GHQ and on PPS-self-esteem difficulties scale. These results are consistent with the general perception that females in Arabic modern cultures are under more pressure due various added challenges (i.e. the expectation to do well in both education and work on top of their traditional role a wives and mothers).

However, it came as a surprise that the male participants have had significantly higher scores on the CTQ regarding physical abuse, sexual abuse, emotional abuse and the emotional neglect subscales. They are also descriptively higher on the physical neglect subscale. This is different from the stereotypes that boys receive preferential treatment from their parents compared to girls. However, middle class Arabic families also tend to be more protective towards girls than boys. However, it remains possible that these results were affects by the higher scores on the CTQ-denial subscale.

These results might be explained by the observation that middle class Egyptian families tend to underestimate the adverse experiences their boys go through during childhood while giving most their attention towards protecting girls. These families are usually less protective about boys outside home which can increase risks of some types of abuse including sexual abuse, away from parents' supervision. It is also known that Egyptian parents can use more physical punishment as a mean of disciplining boys as compared with girls, as it is the case in schools (Youssef et al, 1998-aandb [15,16]), which slightly increase risks of physical and emotional abuse among boys compared to girls.

Demographic and Descriptive Data Across the Three Colleges (Table 4)

Total GHQ score is descriptively higher in participants from Education and Medical colleges compared to college of Art and Literature. This probably indicates higher situational-stresses among the first group more than trait-stresses. It is well known that studying in Medical and Education colleges is harder than it is in college of Art and Literature.

Participants from the Art and Literature colleges are higher in all scores on the PPS though statistically significant only in total score PPS and "self harm" score. They are also scored significantly higher on the physical abuse, emotional abuse, emotional neglect and sexual abuse subscales of the CTQ as compared to participants from both colleges of Medicine and Education. However the "denial" score is significantly higher in participants from Medical and Education colleges. This could mean that participants from these two colleges are underreporting child abuse. Unfortunately, difficulties with skewness and kurtosis within the data prevented the use of parametric statistical analysis where Denial could have been entered as a covariate (e.g., ANCOVA). However, these participants reported higher scores, on emotional neglect subscale than participants from the Arts and Literature colleges. The differences between the participants from the college of Art and Literature compared to the participants from the other two colleges may be associated with the fact that they have less parental income, less parental education and higher number of siblings.

Prevalence of Abuse (Table 5)

Comparing the prevalence findings from this study to other studies is difficult. Different studies use different samples in each country, and have made use of differing questionnaires from the current study. Results can also vary widely in the same country at different times. The most relevant outcome from the current study is that childhood abuse and its psychological implications are far more prevalent in our societies than mental illnesses without abuse. Childhood abuse is also a major trigger of mental illness in later adulthood (Gilbert et al, 2009 [9]). This means that mental health services need to further develop resources and facilities to detect and manage this kind of problems. Social, educational and legal establishments need to give similar attention to this phenomenon.

In our study, the prevalence of physical abuse (6%) seems to be an underestimation as corporal punishment is a widespread phenomenon in Egyptian families and in Egyptian schools. Youssef et al (1998-aandb [15,16]) did a survey of corporal punishment in a number of preparatory and secondary schools in Alexandria in 1998. Their studies revealed that 37.47% of children were disciplined physically, by their parents, in the form of beating and a few were also burned or tied. In 25.83% of them, this harsh discipline led to physical injuries of variable degrees of severity amounting to fractures, loss of consciousness, and permanent disability. The study also revealed that a substantial proportion of boys (79.96%) and girls (61.53%) incurred physical punishment at the hand of their teachers. Teachers were using their hands, sticks, straps, shoes, and kicks to inflict such punishment without sparing a part of their students' body. Physical injuries were reported by a significantly higher percentage of boys, the most common being bumps and contusions followed by wounds and fractures. Among boys, serious injuries such as loss of consciousness and concussion were encountered.

The lower prevalence of physical abuse in our study may be due to errors in reporting, or associated with a "normalisation" of physical abuse within Egyptian society, considering that it is commonly used within home and schools.

The participants could have also been underreporting physical abuse due to "denial", and corporal punishment may be considered by some as something different from abuse (e.g. "discipline", "educational motivator", "harsh form of care", etc"). It is also possible that the reporting of physical abuse has been affected by recall bias. In a society where corporal punishment is the norm, when participants are asked about "physical abuse in childhood" they tend to report only exceptional incidents of corporal punishment which hurt them more than usual.

Long Term Impact of Abuse (Table 6)

In this study, as shown in table 6, we have separated each type of abuse and considered their associations with other psychological difficulties. However, this is an artificial separation, as in real life, child abuse is more likely to occur in more than one form than not. So it is better to interpret results in this context.

The results of this study are consistent with the international literature about the link between childhood abuse and a number of psychological problems in adulthood as listed in the PPS questionnaire. Descriptively, all types of abuse, have been found to be associated with higher scores on PPS and many are statistically significant (table 6). However, this association is not dependent on the scores of the GHQ (indicative of current stress level) and seems to be due to "trait" problems and not "state" problems. However, certain points need to be considered while interpreting these results. One example is the influence of demographics data on the results e.g. income, number of siblings and parents level of education. It is possible that poverty, and large size families, could be a confounding factor for both the occurrence of abuse as well as the high scores on the PPS. In the results of table 6, it seems that "Self harm" is the most sensitive psychopathological variable to different types of childhood abuses. These results suggest that a special attention needs to be given to history of self harm and its possible connection to abuses during childhood.

Table 7. Prevalence studies of child abuse in different countries

Country	Authors	Year	Number of cases	Breakdown of cases (%)
United kingdom	May-Chahal and Cawson[49]	2005	2,869	Total abused (16%), Physical abuse (7%), Sexual abuse (11), Emotional abuse (6%), Emotional Neglect (6%), absence of care (6%), Absence of supervision (5%)
USA	Briere and Elliott [50]	2003	935	Physical abuse (20.9%: 22.2% of males and 19.5% of females), Sexual abuse (23.3%: 14% of males and 32% of females),
USA	Hussey, Chang and Kotch [51]	2006	15 197	Supervision neglect (41.5%), Physical assault (28.4%), Physical neglect (11.8%), Sexual abuse (4.5%)
Canada	MacMillan et al [52]	1997	9953	Physical abuse (31.2% of males and 21.1% of females), Severe physical abuse (10.7% of males and 9.2% of females), Sexual abuse (4.3% of males and 12.8% of females),
Saudi Arabia	Al-Zahrani [33]	2005	832	Emotional neglect (26.6%) Emotional abuse (22.8%) Sexual abuse (22.7%) Physical neglect (18.4%) Physical abuse (12.2%)
Egypt	This study (Mansour et al)	2010	963	Emotional neglect (19%) Emotional abuse (8.9%) Sexual abuse (13%) Physical neglect (44%) Physical abuse (6%)

This is also consistent with the literature (Glassman et al, 2007 [53]; Yates et al, 2008 [54]). "Aggression" is also highly related to childhood abuse in our study. This could be one of the mechanisms how the abused could turn into abusers (Widom, 1989 [55]; Widom and Maxfield, 2001 [56]). In contrast with the international literature (Goldman et al, 2003 [57]), our study has revealed that the scales of "Post Traumatic Stress Disorder", Eating Disorder, "Impulsivity" and to some extent "Dissociation" have not been statistically correlated with any form of abuse ("Dissociation" is statistically related to "sexual Abuse") despite that they have been descriptively higher in all forms of abuse. This could be explained as because of the lack of awareness of these concepts in Egyptian and Arabic cultures. There is also the factor of vague wording of the Arabic translation of the questions of these subscales, which may have contributed to these results.

Conclusion

This study aims at drawing attention to the phenomenon of child abuse in Arabic societies. Our study and the Saudi study suggest that it is a fairly wide spread problem which affects many individuals. The prevalence of child abuse found, suggests that it is more prevalent than most of the well known mental disorders like depression and schizophrenia (without abuse). We hope that clinicians in the Arab world will make more effort to identify these problems, provide effective therapies and increase public awareness. We hope that resources can be provided by Arab governments to make this possible. We also hope that our research would encourage other Arab researchers to produce more studies in this field.

References

[1] Dunn SE. Childhood Maltreatment and Adult Post-Traumatic Stress Disorder Symptomatology in Abused, Suicidal, Low-Income, African American Women: A Moderated Mediational Model (2009). http://etd.gsu.edu/theses/available/etd-07172009-104106/unrestricted/dunn_sarah_e_200908_phd.pdf.

[2] Bouchard EM, Tourigny M, Joly J, Hébert M, Cyr M. Psychological and health sequelae of childhood sexual, physical and psychological abuse, *Rev. Epidemiol. Sante Publique* 2008; Oct; 56(5):333-44.

[3] Finkelhor D, Ormrod R, Turner HA, and Hamby SL. The victimization of children and youth: A comprehensive, national survey. *Child Maltreatment* 2005; 10, 5-25.

[4] Arias I. Report from the CDC. The Legacy of Child Maltreatment: Long-Term Health Consequences for Women. *Journal of Women's Health*. June 2004, 13(5): 468-473.

[5] Briere JN, and Elliott DN. Immediate and long-term impacts of child sexual abuse. *The Future of Children* 1994; 4, 54-69.

[6] Turner HA, Finkelhor D, and Ormrod R. The effect of lifetime victimization on the mental health of children and adolescents. *Social Science and Medicine* 2006; 62,13-27.

[7] Widom CS. Posttraumatic stress disorder in abused and neglected children grown up. *American Journal of Psychiatry* 1999; 156, 1223-1229.

[8] Child Welfare Information Gateway. Long-Term Consequences of Child Abuse and Neglect: Factsheet. www.childwelfare.gov. U.S. Department of Health and Human Services; Administration for Children and Families, Administration on Children, Youth and Families, *Children's Bureau.* Washington, DC 2008.
[9] Gilbert R, Kemp A, Thoburn J, Sidebotham P, Radford L, Glaser D and MacMillan, HL. Child maltreatment one. Burden and consequences of child maltreatment in high-income countries. *The Lancet* 2009; Vol. 373 No. 9657 pp 68-81.
[10] BBC. Arab meeting tackles child abuse (2004). http://news.bbc.co.uk/1/hi/world/middle_east/3487806.stm
[11] Baker A and Shalhoub-Kevorkian N. Effects of political and military traumas on children: The Palestinian case. *Clinical Psychology Review* 1999; Volume 19, Issue 8, Pages 935-950.
[12] Khamis V. Child psychological maltreatment in Palestinian families. Child Abuse and Neglect 2000; Volume 24, Issue 8, Pages 1047-1059.
[13] Macksoud MS and Aber JL. The War Experiences and Psychosocial Development of Children in Lebanon. *Child Development* 1996; 67, 70-8.
[14] Abu Baker K and Dwairy M. Cultural norms versus state law in treating incest: a suggested model for Arab families. Child Abuse and Neglect 2003 ; Volume 27, Issue 1, Pages 109-123.
[15] Youssef RM, Attia MS and Kamel MI. Children experiencing violence I: parental use of corporal punishment - A review of the past 10 years. Child Abuse and Neglect 1998; Volume 22, Number 10, pp. 959-973.
[16] Youssef RM, Attia MS and Kamel MI. Children experiencing violence II: prevalence and determinants of corporal punishment in schools. Child Abuse and Neglect 1998 ; Volume 22, Issue 10, Pages 975-985.
[17] Shalhoub-Kevorkian N. The politics of disclosing female sexual abuse: a case study of Palestinian society. Child Abuse and Neglect 1999; Volume 23, Issue 12, Pages 1275-1293.
[18] Al-Sayed SH. Children Abuse; Clinical Study (in Arabic); Psychological Studies 1993 ; volume 3; Number 4: pp 499-524.
[19] Essali MA. Protecting children from abuse and neglect in Syria (in Arabic). APN e.Book. Arabpsynet (2008). http://www.arabpsynet.com/apneBooks/eB13/eB13AMContandPref.pdf
[20] Al-Mahroos FT. Child abuse and neglect in the Arab Peninsula. *Saudi Med. J.* 2007; Vol. 28 (2): 241-248.
[21] Al-Moosa A, Al-Shaiji J, Al-Fadhli A, Al-Bayed K and Adib SM. Paediatricians' knowledge, attitudes and experience regarding child maltreatment in Kuwait. *Child Abuse and Neglect 2003*; Volume 27, Issue 10, Pages 1161-1178.
[22] UNICEF Arabic website. http://www.unicef.org/arabic/
[23] UNRWA. http://www.un.org/unrwa/
[24] WHO Arabic website. http://www.who.int/ar/
[25] ISPCAN in the Middle East. The First Arab ISPCAN Regional Conference on Child Abuse and Neglect, 2004, Jordan: Violence against Children, Breaking the Silence; Strengthening Responses. http://www.ispcan.org/PastConferences.htm
[26] Save The Children. http://www.savethechildren.org.uk
[27] Human rights Watch in Arabic. http://www.hrw.org/ar.

[28] National Commission for Childhood of Saudi Arabia. www.childhood.gov.sa
[29] Ikhwan-web.http://www.ikhwanweb.com/article.php?id=17415andref=search.php
[30] Syrian Women Observatory. www.nesasy.org/
[31] Egyptian Centre For Women's Rights. http://ecwronline.org/
[32] IslamOnLine.net. http://www.islamonline.net/Arabic/index.shtml
[33] Al-Zahrani AH. Child Abuse and Neglect; Its Causes and Consequences in the Kingdom of Saudi Arabia. Ali Hassan Al-Zahrani, Riyadh, Saudi Arabia 2005. ISBN: 9960-47-454-2.
[34] Daradkeh TK, Ghubash R and El-rufaie OE. Reliability, validity, and factor structure of the Arabic version of the 12-item General Health Questionnaire. *Psychol. Rep.* 2001;89:85–94.
[35] Goldberg D. The general health questionnaire. Nfer-Nelson, Windsor, Berkshire 1978.
[36] Bernstein DP and Fink L. Childhood Trauma Questionnaire: A retrospective self-report manual San Antonio, TX: *The Psychological Corporation* 1998.
[37] Rosenberg MS. Rosenberg Low self-esteem Scale. In M. Johnston; S. Wight; and J. Weinman (Eds), Measures in health psychology: a user's portfolio, individual and demographic differences, *NFER-NELSON: UK* 1965.
[38] Vanderlinden J, Van Dyck R, Vandereyken W, Vertommen H and Verkes RJ. The Dissociation Questionnaire (DIS-Q): Development and Characteristics of a new self-report questionnaire. *Clinical Psychology and Psychotherapy* 1993; 1: 21-27.
[39] Joseph S, Williams R, Yule W. Understanding Post-traumatic Stress: A Psychosocial Perspective on PTSD and Treatment. John Wiley and Sons Ltd: England 1997.
[40] First MB, Gibbon M, Spitzer RL, Williams JBW and Benjamin LS. Structured Clinical Interview For DSM-IV AXIS II Personality Disorders, SCID- II, American Psychiatric Press, Inc: Washington, DC 1997.
[41] Briere J and Runtz M. Differential adult symptomatology associated with three types of child abuse histories. Child Abuse and Neglect: *The International Journal* 1990; 14, 357-364.
[42] Dube SR, Anda RF, Felitti VJ, Chapman D, Williamson DF and Giles WH. Childhood abuse, household dysfunction and the risk of attempted suicide throughout the life span: Findings from the Adverse Childhood Experiences Study. *Journal of the American Medical Association* 2001; 286, 3089-3096.
[43] Swan N. Exploring the role of child abuse on later drug abuse: Researchers face broad gaps in information. NIDA Notes 1998; 13(2). Retrieved April 27, 2006, from the National Institute on Drug Abuse website: www.nida.nih.gov/NIDA_Notes/NNVol 13N2 /exploring.html
[44] Coid J, Petruckevitch A, Feder G, Chung W, Richardson J and Moorey S. Relation between childhood sexual and physical abuse and risk of revictimisation in women: a cross-sectional survey. *The Lancet* 2001; Volume 358, Issue 9280, 450 – 454.
[45] Flaherty EG, Thompson R, Litrownik AJ, Theodore A, English, DJ, Black MM, et al. Effect of early childhood adversity on health. *Archives of Pediatrics and Adolescent Medicine* 2006 ; 160, 1232-1238.
[46] Springer KW, Sheridan J, Kuo D, and Carnes M. Long-term physical and mental health consequences of childhood physical abuse: Results from a large population-based sample of men and women. *Child Abuse and Neglect* 2007; 31, 517-530.

[47] Siegel J. The Relationship Between Child Sexual Abuse And Female Delinquency And Crime: A Prospective Study. *Journal of Research in Crime and Delinquency* 2003; Vol. 40, No. 1, 71-94.

[48] English DJ, Widom CS, and Brandford C. Another look at the effects of child abuse. *NIJ journal* 2004; 251, 23-24.

[49] May-Chahal C and Cawson P. Measuring child maltreatment in the United Kingdom: A study of the prevalence of child abuse and neglect. *Child Abuse and Neglect* 2005; Volume 29, Issue 9, Pages 969-984.

[50] Briere J, Elliott DM. Prevalence and psychological sequelae of self-reported childhood physical and sexual abuse in a general population sample of men and women. *Child Abuse Negl.* 2003; 27(10):1205-22.

[51] Hussey JM, Chang JJ and Kotch JB. Child Maltreatment in the United States: *Prevalence, Risk Factors, and Adolescent Health Consequences. Pediatrics* 2006;118(3):933–942.

[52] MacMillan HL, Fleming JE, Trocme N, Boyle MH, Wong M, Racine YA et al. Prevalence of child physical and sexual abuse in the community. Results from the Ontario Health Supplement. *Journal of the American Medical Association* 1997; 278(2): 131-135.

[53] Glassman LH, Weierich MR, Hooley JM, Deliberto TL and Nock MK. Child maltreatment, non-suicidal self-injury, and the mediating role of self-criticism. *Behaviour Research and Therapy* 2007 ; 45(10): 2483-2490.

[54] Yates TM, Carlson EA and Egeland B. A prospective study of child maltreatment and self-injurious behavior in a community sample. *Development and Psychopathology* 2008; 20:651-671.

[55] Widom CS. The cycle of violence. *Science* 1989; 244, 160-166.

[56] Widom CS and Maxfield MG. An update on the "cycle of violence." Washington, DC: U. S. Department of Justice, Office of Justice Program, *National Institute of Justice* 2001.

[57] Goldman J, Salus MK, Wolcott D and Kennedy KY. A Coordinated Response to Child Abuse and Neglect: The Foundation for Practice. U.S. Department of Health and Human Services, Administration for Children and Families, Administration on Children, Youth and Families, Children's Bureau, *Office on Child Abuse and Neglect* 2003.

In: The International Psychiatry and Behavioral ... ISBN: 978-1-62257-566-4
Editor: Nash Boutros

Chapter 14

THE EFFECT OF PUPPET PLAY THERAPY INTERVENTION ON THE COMMUNICATIVE SKILLS OF AUTISTIC CHILDREN*

Seyyed Mohsen Asghari Nekah[1*], Gholam-Ali Afrooz[2], Abbas Bazargan[2] and Mohsen Shokoohi Yekta[2]

[1]Psychology and Educational Sciences, Ferdowsi University of Mashhad, Iran
[2]Psychology and Educational Sciences, Tehran University, Tehran, Iran

ABSTRACT

Introduction: The quintessential characteristic of autism spectrum disorders (ASD) is having difficulty with basic skills. Due to this, those diagnosed need special intervention. The purpose of this article is to investigate the effect of the puppet play therapy intervention on communicative skills of autistic children.

Materials and Methods: This research has been implemented as quasi-experimental designs with a pre-post test and control group as a design based action research method. The preschool age autistic children of Mashhad city was a statistical population of this study, in which ten persons have cleaved in control and samples, and the intervention group participated in puppet play therapy intervention. The Early Social-Communication Scales (ESCS) were performed in the past and before the intervention. The data was analyzed by The Mann-Whitney U and the wilcoxon's Signed-Ranks Tests were also analyzed.

Results: Findings indicate that in terms of total score, the ESCS (P=.009) intervention has been significant. Also on subscales, in the eye contact area of initiating behavioral requests (P= .012) and on low-level behavioral requests (P= .012), responding to social interaction (P=.015), total initiating behavioral requests (P=.011), and sub-tests

---

* Original Citation: Asghari Nekah, S. M., Afrooz, G. A., Bazargan, A., & Shokoohi Yekta, M. (2011). The effect of puppet play therapy intervention on communicative skills of autistic children. Journal of Fundamentals of Mental Health, 13(49), 2-57.

* Corresponding author : Seyyed Mohsen Asghari Nekah, Assistant professor of Ferdowsi University .Faculty of psychology and educational sciences, Department of educational sciences, Ferdowsi University of Mashhad, Azadi Sq., Mashhad, Iran, Fax: +98511-8783012 Phone: +98511-8803616, Asghari-n@um.ac.ir

of request implementation skills in retail applications (P=.005), puppet play therapy intervention has been significant. In addition, in achievement sub-objects (P=.335), to initiating requests (P=.214), pointing to objects (P=1.00), and objects given (P=.74) presented in puppet play therapy intervention has been not significant. Qualitative findings from the parental report also indicate intervention to be effective.

Conclusion: The results indicate that puppet play therapy has been effective for communicative skills of autistic children, and the results of the study can be used to strengthen the effectiveness of education placed - therapeutic interventions.

Keywords: Autistic child, play therapy, puppet play therapy, communicative skills, design based action research

INTRODUCTION

Autism is the most prominent kind of developmental disorder from spectrum disorders of Pervasive Developmental Disorder that put autistic children and their families in special conditions. Mothers of children with autism experience a constant and endless challenge [1]. The prevalence of autism is increasing for different reasons. In the beginning of the recent decade, it was estimated that the prevalence of autism was 1 in 335 [2]. But according to the Center for Prevention and Disease Control, this rate has been rising in recent years.

Especially considering autism spectrum disorders, it has increased to 1 in 150 [3], and it has attracted specialist attention in various branches of science and World Health planners to the extent that the World Health Organization dedicating a day for global information about this disorder, and has demanded a comprehensive effort to recognize and implement early detection and intervention [4].

Lack of eye contact, social smile limitation, little interest, slight tendency to other's countenances, unpleasantness towards physical contact, verbal communication failure, limitations in understanding the views of others, failing to share joy, and failure and limited partnership in games are part of the restrictions and defects [5]. Also, development of play skills in autistic children are associated with some defects and damages. Failing in object probing, failure in a variety of playing with objects, lack of initiative and innovative games, and a failure and delay in symbolic games are among the damages and shortcomings in these children [6].

Several intervention programs for autistic children are proposed and implemented that are based on the extent of the goal, variation in intervention, the intervention rate per week, and the duration of intervention can be divided into two categories of comprehensive programs and specific interventions [7]. Some interventions have proposed comprehensive programs that include different growth areas such as sensory, motor, speech, communication, behavioral, and emotional areas. However, such programs often require systematic and formal interventions that are usually presented in the context of educational programs and in schools and medical training clinics [8]. It is worth noting that in these interventions, different tools are used in attempts to provide motivation, change behavior, and facilitate communication and interpersonal interaction. Some of these educational and rehabilitative interventions include instruments such as common toys, books and pictures, computers, audio - visual equipment [9], musical instruments [10], and appropriate robots for playing or establishing communication with autistic children [11], and tools and equipment used in occupational therapy.

In addition, the review of rehabilitative and therapeutic interventions for autistic children such as activities by Davis [12], Matson [8], Luiselli [13] and Lu, Petersen, and Lacroix and Rousseau [14], introduce play therapy as a safe treatment, consistent with the developmental characteristics of autistic children, that has frequently played a role in educational, psychological, and rehabilitative interventions. For this reason, doing research in this area is a kind of investment associated with multidimensional scientific achievement for children, families, and professionals [8, 12,14].

Although the process of development and understanding nonverbal communication skills in normal children is developed in childhood, in autistic children, developing communication skills is associated with deficiency and restriction. Therefore, they need a therapeutic and educational intervention [15, 16]. Meanwhile, beginning and answering the joint attention is one of the major defects of nonverbal communication skills in autistic children [17] and it is a diagnostic criterion considered to be one of the goals and priorities for interventions for autistic children. However, the progress and effectiveness of these interventions is carried out more slowly, but more subtle interventions are more effective [18]. Play therapists have considered diverse and creative interventions in working with autistic children. For example, Lu et al. using an action research project studied the use of playing with sand as a means to motivate autistic children and to direct them towards make believe plays. The results revealed that autistic children showed a considerable increase in verbal expression, and establishment and continuation of social interaction, and an increase in make believe and spontaneous games 10 weeks after the program [14].

In a case study, during 16 sessions of play therapy, a six and a half year old boy with severe autism showed progress in the areas of make-believe play, attachment, social interaction, and improvement towards change, but changes in faith behavior were less [19]. In a research which was introduced in order to plan a play therapy program for 12 autistic children aged from 6 to 12 years old in a primary school, during 12 thirty-minute sessions with a random selection and a single group design with pre-test and post-test, the analysis of parental questionnaire findings suggested that play therapy was significantly effective in the four areas of social communication (verbal, nonverbal, social interaction, and challenging behaviors) [12]. Using hand puppets for autistic children can be considered art therapy and complementary therapy programs in the area of autistic children's emotions [20]. Hand dolls and simple dolls have been used in training empathy and emotional understanding skills for children with autism. In a research with four autistic children ages 5 to 8 years old, using hand dolls with different emotional states, some games were played in four to five sessions per week in 20 minute sessions. After 30 sessions of intervention for all autistic children, a systematic increase was revealed in sympathetic responses to the stimulus and cues in intervention sessions [21].

Puppet play therapy for autistic children and adolescents facilitates communication with other children and adolescents and increases positive emotions . Researchers using an approach which is called relation therapy with the help of hand puppets began to work with children and adolescents with Asperger and autism. They needed to help their dolls to develop a good attitude and feelings toward everyday life situations. Parents reported that participants in puppet therapy had more happy and positive emotions [22].

Review of theories and research in the field of autism suggest that communication problems and deficiencies are the most fundamental and main features of this disorder and a major priority in the design of therapeutic interventions. However, defects in playing skills, especially shortages in make-believe playing and innovative plays are one of the main characteristics of autistic children [6]. However, given the capacity of play in stimulating the child's senses, play-oriented interventions for autistic children can provide an interaction ground and enrich communication activities. Play works as a launching pad for the autistic child. Moreover, a review of researches and written texts about interventions for autistic children shows that play is always one of the tools or methods used in a part of the intervention process [8, 13]. Therefore, a mixture of design and implementation of play-oriented interventions, with the direction of the communication considered a special priority, has possible theoretical effectiveness.

A review of therapeutic and educational interventions and programs for autistic children shows that considering the multidimensional nature and complexity of the autism disorder, most programs have been designed and implemented as a comprehensive measure and they involve presentation of large and compact meetings using behavioral approaches and there has been less attention paid toward subtle and more specific programs such as play therapy [8, 11, 13].

Research reports and theories offered show that puppets have been used mostly in consulting activities with normal children with emotional and behavioral problems, especially for children affected by sexual abuse or to prepare children to cope with negative emotions before surgery, or to establish communication with affected children [23,25,24], and their main goal is facilitating communication, catharsis and emotional recognition, and expression during interviews [26]. Although the theoretical foundations, early assumptions, and experiences of those involved in rehabilitation and treatment of autistic children indicate consistent and probable benefits of using puppets in play therapy with autistic children [27], though direct and independent use of puppets has not been reported and these activities have used puppets as a means of creating positive emotions [22] and in teaching empathy and emotional understanding skills and the like [21]. The current research is intended to study the effectiveness of puppet play therapy intervention on communicative skills in autistic children using an action research design-oriented method.

METHODS

This study seeks to develop and expand a proposed early intervention, to complete it and to assess the effectiveness of the puppet play therapy intervention designed for autistic children. To achieve these objectives, we attempted to run an action research design-oriented cycle with the participation of the mothers in accordance with Table (1). A quasi-experimental design was used with the experimental group and control group of autistic children with pre-tests and post-tests, to estimate the effectiveness of the final model. The use of such a plan would allow the researcher to select the groups randomly and to use pre-tests and post-tests to implement intervention using action research based on real participant problems, and to implement the intervention in a step by step manner to revise and complete it [28,29]. At the beginning of the research implementation, the autistic children in official services (autism clinic and school in Mashhad) were 53 total; 12 of them were 3 to 6 year-old children.

Table 1. The action research design-oriented process

Process Group	Before	While Action Research	After
experimental	Pre-test Early social communication scale	Intervention programs based on participatory action research	Post-test Early social communication scales
control	Pre-test Early social communication scales	---------------------	Post-test Early social communication scales
Participants	autistic children	Researcher(therapist), therapist assistants, mothers	autistic children

Since one child was from another city and came temporarily and occasionally, the researcher considered 5 children, used simple random sampling, thus ten pre school autistic children in the clinic were randomly divided into two groups of experimental and control groups.

To respect the rights of subjects, the parents' satisfaction was obtained and the research process was explained to them and all questions answered. The right for withdrawal of the plan in individual interviews at any time was explained. After the pre-tests, the intervention was presented in a 4 × 6 meter room on the second floor of a public clinic (Smile Clinic in Mashhad). The floor of the room was covered with carpet, and it was equipped with two closets for supplies, a desk and some chairs for children, and three other chairs for companions. Interventions were presented every day from 8 to 12, from the middle of Aban (November) until the last week of Esfand (March), based on the proposed plan and considering experiences and exchanging views about previous sessions and the possible presence of parents. One graduate student in psychology and education of exceptional children and a student of psychology helped the therapist in implementing the interventions.

Different parts of the interventions were filmed and recorded randomly by one of the assistants. Tapes were reviewed as one of the sources providing feedback for improving the presentation of the play therapy process. Also, the assistants would insert their views and ideas and their overall assessment and interpretations about the child on a worksheet in each session. Most times, mothers were invited to the room as observers between the sessions. But under certain circumstances, such as heavy reliance or stereotyped behaviors which were reinforced by mothers, their presence was not possible in the play therapy room. Although the researcher tried to equalize puppet play therapy sessions for all children, because of problems such as illness or family problems, the number of children attending the sessions varied. The number of sessions ranged from 16 to 29 . On the whole, all of the 5 participants got on average 22 sessions of intervention, so that one child experienced 16 sessions, one 19 sessions, two 23 sessions, and one 29 sessions of the puppet play therapy.

To consider professional ethics, the researcher did not deprive the control group and their families from pursuing therapeutic educational activities and both groups benefited from training and ongoing rehabilitative programs. While the experimental group participated in the puppet play therapy programs, the control group took part in ongoing activities at the clinic or were engaged and entertained by parents and caregivers and this was the only difference between the two groups.

A compensation program (a program similar to the intervention for the control group) can be run simultaneously with the main intervention (puppet play therapy), so it can be considered a quasi-intervention group or the placebo group. Unfortunately due to time constraints, holidays, and scattering of the control group members in different districts, the program did not provide for the control group after the intervention phase.

After implementing the puppet play therapy sessions and the completion of the intervention period, post-tests were performed for the two groups. For getting mothers' comments and their opinions about the effectiveness of treatment, some reports were gathered in the form of open questions and interviews or short conversations with them, during the sessions and especially at the end of the intervention program.

The questions were about qualitative data follow-ups, about the effectiveness of the activities and the child's behavior at home. Finally, by analyzing the process and the achieved experiences through organizing the findings and interactions with colleagues and mothers, the researcher developed a proposed program for puppet play therapy. In the present research, Early Social Communication Scale (ESCS) was applied as a pre-test and post-test which is a means of assessing nonverbal communication skills and it is done by observing the structured visual records of multiple assignments and its implementation takes 15 to 25 minutes. The version used in this study is adapted from Mundy [30].

This test has 25 semi-structured situations (or stimulus recall) [30]. As a result of observing the video recordings from performing the Early Social Communication Scale, the behavior of the children can be categorized into three early social communication behaviors: behaviors related to joint attention, behaviors related to requested manner, and behaviors related to social interaction. Based on operational instruction, the test is used for normal children aged 8 to 30 months or for abnormal children with developmental retardation. Regarding the children's verbal status, the present sample matches the instruction of this scale. Scale reliability and validity of the Early Social Communication Scale are presented in four articles about the process of collecting performing guidelines for the test by Mundy et al. The content validity and its appropriateness with theoretical foundations of early social communication and matching its scores with age changes and developmental conditions have been reported in very desirable levels [31].

Based on random selection of video recordings the test reliability of the Early Social Communication Scale has been reported ($r = 94.0$) for areas of joint attention, and $r = 75.0$ for social interaction [31]. In another report, the calculated agreement coefficient has been estimated as $r = 90.0$ for joint attention, $r = 86.0$ for behavioral requests, and $r = 87.0$ for social interaction. In addition, Laing et al. have mentioned the reliability of the Early Social Communication Scale in subtests from $r = 88.0$ to $r = 98.0$ [32]. Other researchers have estimated subtest reliability at $r = 80.0$ for initiating joint attention and $r = 76.0$ for responding to joint attention [33]. Grading is based on the observing of the video recordings and it is scored zero and one based on the performing state of the behavior. Since the test is based on observation and recording the frequency of behavior, it is not a normative test, and its implementation has not been observed in Iranian study yet.

RESULTS

Demographic status of autistic children as part of the results shows that these children ranged from two years and five months to seven years and four months (a mean of 66 months and a standard deviation of 84.1), and early diagnosis of children was done according to the clinical examination method and clinical signboard of autism symptoms. Nine of these children became aware of this disorder by direct referral of parents to a specialist and one of them had an initial diagnosis by a speech-language pathologist and was referred to a specialist. Speaking status of these children as another description of autism showed that eight children couldn't speak and two of them could only say a few words (less than ten meaningful words). Regarding order of birth, seven children in our sample were the first born and the only child, two children were the second child, and only one child was the third born . It should be noted that all the children were boys. Reviewing the effectiveness of interventions requires four general kinds of comparison that are: (a) - between group comparisons in pre-tests and post-tests regarding the general condition of communication skills (status of each group compared with the other group), (b) - within-group comparisons of pre-tests and post-tests regarding the general condition of communication skills (status of each group compared to itself), (c) - Comparison between both groups' pre-tests regarding the areas of communication skills and ESCS subtests, and (d) - Comparison between both groups' post-tests in the areas of communication skills and ESCS subtests. In the following section, the obtained data and statistical calculations will be presented and discussed based on groups and types of tests in all kinds of comparisons, along with more detailed comparisons. In comparing both groups' pre-tests and post-tests regarding the general condition of communication skills:

Evaluation and comparison of the starting condition of two groups in communication skills (dependent variable), and data obtained from taking the Early Social Communication Scale (ESCS) and calculating the overall score for the two groups with the Mann-Whitney U test indicates the following statistical calculations:

A reviewing table 2 in regards to the pretest shows that considering $z= -1.358$ and $p= 0.175$, it can be concluded that there is no significant difference between the communication skills of autistic children in the control group and experimental group before the intervention.

The scores of the post-test in the above table also shows that since the Z value of the test is -2.619 and $p= 0.009$, it can be concluded that there is a significant difference between the communication skills of autistic children in the control group and experimental group after the intervention. Comparing the control group and experimental group pre-tests regarding the general condition of communication skills:

Verifying the lack of difference between the general condition of communication skills of the control group requires the use of appropriate tests for two dependent samples of a small size ($n =5$). Therefore, comparing the control group pre-test and post-test was done by using the Wilcoxon signed ranks test, and performing the following statistical operations yielded the following findings (Table 3):

Table 2. The pre-test and post-test total score of the groups

phase	group	mean of ranks	Total of ranks	Mann-Whitney U	z	p
pre-test	control	4.20	21.00	6.000	-1.358	0.175
	experimental	6.80	34.00			
post-test	control	3.00	15.00	0.000	-2.619	0.009
	experimental	8.00	40.00			

Table 3. The pre-test and post-test total score of each group compared to itself

group	status of mean of ranks	number of means	mean of ranks	Total of ranks	z	p
control	Increase (positive rank)*	3	3.00	9.00	-0.412	0.680
	decrease (negative rank) **	2	3.00	6.00		
experimental	Increase (positive rank) *	5	3.00	15.00	-2.032	0.042
	decrease (negative rank) **	0.00	0.00	0.00		

*post-test > pre-test **post-test < pre-test.

Table 3 shows in a comparison between the pre-test and post-test in the control group, since z = -0.412 and p = 0.680, there is no significant difference between the mean of ranks in the pre-test and post-test control group. In addition, since z = -2.032 and p = 0.042, no significant difference is observed between the mean of ranks in the pre-test and post-test experimental group. Comparison between the pre-tests of the two groups considering communication skills and subtests in ESCS are explained below.

It is worth noting that the Early Social Communication Scale includes several areas of communication skills, such as initiative joint attention, initiative behavioral requests, reaction to behavioral requests, initiative social behavior, and reaction or response to social interaction; each of these domains of communication skills includes several sub tests which are presented in Table (4).

According to Table (4) and considering the absolute amount of z and p for sub tests before the intervention, there is no significant difference between communication skills of the two groups. Therefore, on account of existing significant differences between the experimental group and control group, we will proceed with differences existing or not existing between the experimental group and control group after implementing the intervention. The obtained data for the post-tests of the two groups about ESCS sub tests are presented in Table (5).

As seen in Table (5), considering the absolute value of z and its corresponding p value, in refusal with eye contact (p=0.018), in eye contact (p=0.012), in initiative behavioral requests at a low level (p=0.012), in overall initiative behavioral requests (p=0.011), in doing a social action (p=0.015), and in compliance (p=0.005), there is a significant difference between two groups. But in other sub tests, no significant difference is observed, therefore it can be said that implementing puppet play therapy could have a considerable effect in already mentioned sub tests.

DISCUSSION AND CONCLUSION

Puppet play therapy is one of the recommended play therapy interventions for autistic children during which the therapist or parent, using a hand puppet, tries to create incentives in the child, activate him, communicate with him, and guide his behaviors. This study was intended to plan, implement, and evaluate some kind of play therapy intervention aimed at facilitating relations, and shaping and enhancing communication skills, so that it could be used alone or along with other therapeutic interventions in the educational and rehabilitative programs. Therefore, the therapist and his designing and implementing of puppet play therapy was reviewed for its effectiveness in a communicative designed based action research.

To verify the overall effectiveness of the pre-tests and post-tests, the two groups (experimental and control) were compared. As Table (2) indicates, there was no significant difference between the scores of the two groups before the intervention (p=0.75). In other words, both groups had a similar situation in terms of communication skills before the intervention, and this is a desirable condition and it is necessary to verify the effectiveness of an intervention.

Table 4. Results of comparison between the pre-tests of the two groups in ESCS domains and its sub tests

domain	sub test	mean of ranks		total of ranks		Mann-whitney U	Z	P
		experimental	control	experimental	control			
Initiative joint attention	Initiative joint eye contact	7.10	3.90	35.50	19.50	4.500	-1.697	0.090
	Initiative joint exchange of looks	5.30	5.70	26.50	28.50	11.500	-0.211	0.833
	Initiative joint pointing	5.50	5.50	27.50	27.50	12.500	0.000	1.000
	Initiative joint showing	5.50	5.50	27.50	27.50	12.500	0.000	1.000
Initiative social behavior	Refusal without eye contact	6.50	4.50	32.50	22.50	7.500	-1.500	0.134
	Refusal with eye contact	7.00	4.00	35.00	20.00	5.000	-1.928	0.054
Initiative behavioral requests	Eye contact	6.50	4.50	32.50	22.50	7.500	-1.061	0.289
	Accessing	4.80	6.20	24.00	31.00	9.000	-0.783	0.434
	Request	5.00	6.00	25.00	30.00	10.000	-1.000	0.317
	Initiative behavioral requests at low level	6.40	4.60	32.00	23.00	8.000	-0.973	0.331
	Pointing	5.50	5.50	27.50	27.50	12.500	0.000	1.000
	Giving	7.00	4.00	35.00	20.00	5.000	-1.683	0.092
	Overall initiative behavioral requests	7.00	4.00	35.00	20.00	5.000	-1.671	0.095
Reaction to social interaction	Doing a social action	5.50	5.50	27.50	27.50	12.50	0.000	1.000
Reaction to behavioral requests	Compliance	6.00	5.00	30.00	25.00	10.000	-0.655	0.513
	Lack of compliance	5.50	5.50	27.50	27.50	12.500	0.000	1.000
	Lack of compliance with facial expressions	4.80	6.20	24.00	31.00	9.000	-0.780	0.435

Table 5. Comparison between the post-tests of the two groups in sub tests of ESCS

domain	sub test	mean of ranks		total of ranks		Mann-whitney U	Z	P
		experimental	control	experimental	control			
Initiative joint attention	Initiative joint eye contact	5.40	5.60	27.00	28.00	12.000	-0.105	0.916
	Initiative joint exchange of looks	6.20	4.80	31.00	24.00	9.000	-0.764	0.445
	Initiative joint pointing	5.50	5.50	27.50	27.50	12.500	0.000	1.000
	Initiative joint showing	5.00	6.00	25.00	30.00	10.000	-1.000	0.317
Initiative social behavior	Refusal without eye contact	6.70	4.30	33.50	21.50	6.500	-1.423	0.155
	Refusal with eye contact	3.50	7.50	17.50	37.50	2.500	-2.362	0.018
Initiative behavioral requests	Eye contact	7.90	3.10	39.50	15.50	0.500	-2.522	0.012
	Accessing	6.40	4.60	32.00	23.00	8.000	-0.964	0.335
	Request	6.60	4.40	33.00	22.00	7.000	-1.234	0.217
	Initiative behavioral requests at low level	7.90	3.10	39.50	15.50	0.500	-2.522	0.012
	Pointing	5.50	5.50	27.50	27.50	12.500	0.000	1.000
	Giving	7.90	3.10	35.50	19.50	4.500	-1.789	0.074
	Overall initiative behavioral requests	7.90	3.10	39.50	15.50	0.500	-2.530	0.011
Reaction to social interaction	Doing a social action	7.60	3.40	38.00	17.00	2.000	-2.425	0.015
Reaction to behavioral requests	Compliance	8.00	3.00	40.00	15.00	0.000	-2.825	0.005
	Lack of compliance	4.50	6.50	22.50	32.50	7.500	-1.500	0.134
	Lack of compliance with facial expressions	4.00	7.00	20.00	35.00	5.000	-1.928	0.054

In contrast, the comparison of both groups' post-tests revealed that, considering the mean of final scores of the Early Social Communication Scale, there is a significant difference (p=0.009). This difference indicates the overall effectiveness of the puppet play therapy program, and shows that implementing this program has resulted in improvement and enhancement in communication skills of autistic children in the experiment. In other words, puppet play therapy led to considerable improvement in communication skills of autistic children in the experimental group.

Additional follow-up of comparisons of the pre-test and post-test of each group indicates that there was no significant difference between pre-test and post-test in control group (p=0.068), but a significant difference was found between pre-test and post-test in experimental group (p=0.042). Thus the lack of difference in the pre-tests of both groups confirms the effectiveness of puppet play therapy on communication skills of the experimental group.

After obtaining the overall effectiveness, a more detailed study of the effectiveness of the sub tests in initiative joint attention and a review of Table (5) shows that significant differences are observed in none of the sub tests of initiative joint eye contact (p=0.90), exchange of looks (p=0.83), pointing (1.00), and showing (p=1.00). In other words, puppet play therapy and the intervention have failed to improve and increase the sub tests of initiative joint attention.

As it was said in the review of research literature, researchers and scholars such as Mukaddes et al. [34] and Elsabbagh and Johnson [35] in pointing to the nature of the disorder, mention initiative joint attention as one of the main factors that damage communication performance. This is in congruence with a lack of effectiveness in short-term interventions on improving joint attention and decreases its rapid change expectation. On the other hand, it needs more follow up research to show if puppet play therapy can provide a more effective intervention for areas of initiative joint attention.

Another issue is that the present intervention program is concentrated on establishing relationships and activating the child. This can affect the early effectiveness in the domain of initiative joint attention, so it is probable that the findings and ideas of Hwang and Hughes about breaking a skill into minor components and dividing it to more simple skills for increasing joint attention behaviors should be the focus of the intervention in future research [37].

The comparison of the two groups in the initiative social behavior domain which was carried out in two sub tests of refusal without eye contact and refusal with eye contact, shows that puppet play therapy intervention has not been significant and effective (p= 0.155). However, it was significant and effective in refusal with eye contact (p= 0.018). That is, puppet play therapy intervention made autistic children in the experimental group establish eye contact with the therapist even when they refused and refrained from doing something such as throwing an object. In other words, child's refusal to perform an activity as an initiative social behavior and interaction has been improved due to puppet play therapy and it was done with eye contact.

Since resistance and refusal in autistic children is of high frequency and very common, considering the significant efficacy of puppet play therapy in the sub tests, it seems that expanding puppet play therapy activities can lead to direct refusing in autistic children. Because refusing is considered as an initiative interaction by the child and it can be used to begin more interaction with him, puppet play therapy can benefit from refusal as a window for more relationships and more interaction with the child.

The comparison of the post-tests of the two groups in initiative behavioral requests reveals that providing puppet play therapy intervention was not effective in sub tests of accessing objects (p=0.355), initiative requests (p=0.214), pointing (p=1.000), and giving objects to others (p=0.074). However, it was effective in communication sub skills of eye contact in initiative behavioral requests (p=0.012), initiative requests at a low level (p=0.12), and initiative behavioral requests (p=0.011). In other words, these sub skills have improved. Lack of effectiveness in accessing, initiative requests, pointing, and giving objects to others may be interpreted as both the difficult nature of these sub skills and in the type of intervention assignments and activities. In other words, intervention activities have focused on eye contact and interpersonal interaction. Comparing the two groups in responding to a social interaction with a significant difference (p=0.015) indicates that puppet play therapy has been effective in creating opportunities for autistic children to develop social activities. This is also confirmed by the qualitative findings, the therapist's observations and mothers' reports, because the definition of social interaction in the test instruction points to activities such as a child's social smiling, nodding, and facial expressions responding to the therapist's actions, behaviors, and puppets. Numerous observations and reports indicate that during the puppet play therapy sessions, children have shown positive emotional interactions in response to the therapist activities and the doll, and the children's purposeful laughter and smiles were frequent in the sessions.

According to Table (5), comparing the post-tests of the two groups in responding to behavioral requests shows that puppet play therapy has not been effective in sub skills of lack of compliance (p=0.134) and lack of compliance with facial expressions (p=0.054), however, puppet play therapy intervention could significantly improve compliance (p=0.005).

The findings reveal that puppet play therapy was not effective in reducing the children's disobedience or in breaking down their resistance in lack of compliance, but it was successful in encouraging the autistic children to do the therapist's requests. This is congruent with the characteristics of autistic children, that is to say, too much resistance and lack of compliance. As a result of the treatment plan and behavior modification, it is likely that focusing on encouraging children to comply can take priority over breaking down a child's resistance or his disobedience, and this will probably increase the program's effectiveness.

On the whole, in analyzing and drawing a conclusion from the given data from the intervention phase and estimating the effectiveness of puppet play therapy for autistic children's communication skills, it can be said that puppet play therapy generally has been effective in enhancing and improving the communication skills of autistic children and in more detail, puppet play therapy intervention has been significantly effective in sub skills of refusal with eye contact, eye contact in initiative behavioral request domain, behavioral requests at a low level or without eye contact, in overall initiative behavioral requests, in performing a social function and in complying behavior. But this intervention generally has not been effective in initiative joint attention, refusal without eye contact, accessing, compliance, pointing, giving objects, and lack of compliance.

Evaluating the qualitative effectiveness of treatment can be considered a supplement and an expansion of the quantitative findings. Referring to the parents' views and their understanding of the effectiveness of intervention, it is one of the evaluation factors that have been suggested by some researchers [12]. Therefore, recorded observations by the therapist and his colleagues and parents' reports about activities outside the treatment room and their observations in the play therapy room have provided considerable evidence for the efficacy of the therapeutic intervention. Analyzing and concluding from some of these seems to be useful. In this regard, the observations of the therapists and mothers reveal that in many sessions and in many activities during the puppet play therapy, children showed unique positive emotions which were unexpected even for mothers.

The emotional effectiveness of puppet play therapy is consistent with the findings of research that used hand puppets for counseling and therapeutic interventions such as Bernier's art therapy experiences [36], Depa's activities in sexually abused children [24], and Athanassiaadou et al. in changing children's attitude and excitement toward the operating room [25].

The attractiveness of such a program and children's interest and selectivity, especially in autistic children, is considered as one criteria of the effectiveness of the program. The qualitative findings and the reports of the autistic children's families clearly show that the attractiveness criterion and the children's tendency toward attending the play room have been established. The mothers reported that during the program and even a few weeks after the intervention performance, if children were to enter the clinic, they immediately walked to the game room and tried to open the door, after they realized that the play therapy room was closed, they became willing to proceed to their own programs in other rooms (speech therapy, occupational therapy, or general play room).

More detailed analysis of this type of behavior in an autistic child is obtained when the characteristics of autism, lack of attention to stimulus, and lack of interest in activities are also considered as the main features of the disorder. In addition, maintaining an autistic child's interest and tendency toward the puppet play room and space after a few weeks can be interpreted as an indicator of the effectiveness of puppet play therapy. This all suggests that the autistic child has seen some benefits and privileges for himself in the puppet play therapy program, or the characteristics of the game have reinforced the child because upon arriving at the clinic, he would leave main programs and went to the puppet play therapy room.

It is worth noting that since the treatment and rehabilitation of autistic children is often individualized, and its process is difficult and slow, this research was restricted to one sex and age group (pre-school children) in selecting the study sample. Moreover, due to some seasonal diseases and several problems of some parents, the number of intervention sessions for each child was different from others, and in spite of the permanent interest of the parents, the researcher's expectation was not completely met. In addition, since puppet play therapy intervention was designed and implemented in this study, it is recommend that medical and educational centers and universities, welfare organizations, and the department of exceptional children education provide the possibility of expanding this program and further research in this area by developing play therapist teaching programs in the field of teaching puppet play therapy.

REFERENCES

[1] Meirsschaut M, Roeyers H, Warreyn P .Parenting in families with a child with autism spectrum disorder and a typically developing child: Mothers' experiences and cognitions .*Res. Autism. Spectr. Disord.*9-661 :(4)4 ;2010

[2] Yeargin-Allsopp M, Rice C, Karapurkar T, Doernberg N, Boyle C, Murphy C. Prevalence of autism in a United States metropolitan area. *J. Am. Med. Assoc.* 2008; 121(3): 547-54.

[3] Center for Disease Control and Prevention (CDC). New data on autism spectrum disorders from multiple communities in the United States. [cited 2008 Sep 8]. Available from: URL; http://www.cdc.govod/oc/media/pressrel/2007/r070208.html

[4] Hassanzadeh S. Letter to the editor: About international day of information about autism. *J. Res. Excep. Children* 2008; 1(27): 1.

[5] Prelock PA, Prendeville J, Unwin G. Peer play interventions to support the social competence of children with autism spectrum disorders (ASD). *Semin Speech Lang.* 2006; 27(1): 32-46.

[6] Landa R. Eaerly communication development and intervention for children with autism. *Mental Retard Dev. Disabil. Res. Rev.* 2007; 13: 16-25.

[7] Callahan K, Henson R. Social validation of evidence-based practices in autism by parents, teachers, and administrators. *J. Autism Dev. Disord.* 2008; 38: 678-92.

[8] Matson JL. Clinical assessment intervention for autism. Philadelphia: *Elsevier;* 2008: 15.

[9] Nikopoulos CK, Keenan M. Effects of video modeling on training and generalization of social initiation and reciprocal play by children with autism. *Eur. J. Behav. Anal.* 2004; 5: 1.

[10] Kissinger L, David W. Using the harp as a communication channel with children with autism. *Int. J. Spec. Educ.* 2008; 23(3): 156-9.

[11] Billard A, Robins B, Nadel J, Dautenhahn K. Building robota, a mini-humanoid robot for the rehabilitation of children with autism. *Tech. J.* 2007; 19(1): 37-49.

[12] Davis NO, Carter AS. Parenting stress in mothers and fathers of toddlers with autism spectrum disorders: Associations with child characteristics. *J. Autism Dev. Res.* 2008; 38: 1278-91.

[13] Luiselli K, Russo DC, Walter P, Wilcyznski C, Wilcyznski SM. Effective practices for children with autism-educational and behavioral support interventions that work. Oxford: *Oxford University;* 2008: page?

[14] Lu L, Petersen F, Lacroix L, Rousseau C. Stimulating creative play in children with autism through sandplay. Arts Psychother 2010; 37: 56-64.

[15] Gray DE. Ten years on: A longitudinal study of families of children with autism. *Intellect Dev. Disabil.* 2002; 27(3): 215-22.

[16] Ingersoll B, Schreibman L. Teaching reciprocal imitation skills to young children with autism using a naturalistic behavioral approach: Effects on language, pretend play, and joint attention. *J. Autism Dev. Disord.* 2006;36: 487-505.

[17] Siller M, Sigman MD. The behaviors of parents of children with autism predict the subsequent development of their children's communication. *J. Autism Dev. Disord.* 2002; 32: 77-89.

[18] Goldstein H. Communication intervention for children with autism. A review of treatment efficacy. *J. Autism Dev. Disord.* 2002; 32(5): 373-96.

[19] Josefi O, Ryan Y. Non-directive play therapy for young children with autism: A case study. Clin. Child Psychol. Psychiatr. 2004; 9: 533-51.

[20] Autism Society of Canada. What is autism spectrum disorder? Brochure. [cited 2006 Mar 18]. Available from: URL; http://www.autismsocietycanada.ca/

[21] Schrandt J, Buffington A, Townsnd D, Poulson CL. Teaching empathy skills to children with autism. J. Appl. Behav. Anal. 2009; 42: 17-32.

[22] Welch J. The playful healer. The newsletter of the Florida Association for Play Therapy. 2004, V10, N4. [cited 2004]. Available from: URL; http://www.floridaplay therapy.org/"www.floridaPlaytherapy.org

[23] McLeod J. Qualitative research in counselling and psychotherapy. London: *Sage;* 2001: 102.

[24] Depa M, Astramovich R. Using puppets in a variety of therapeutic interventions to help children who have been harmed by sexual abuse: Strategies for play therapists. Play Therapy TM. [cited 2008]. Available from: URL; http://www.a4pt.org/"www.a4pt.org

[25] Athanassiadou E, Tsiantis J, Christogiorgos S, Kolaitis G. Evaluation of the effectiveness of psychological preparation of children for minor surgery by puppet play and brief mother counseling. *Psychother. Psychosom.* 2009; 78(1): 62-3.

[26] Roth JH, Dadds MR, McAloon J. Evaluation of a puppet interview to measure young children's self-reports of temperamt. *Behav. Change* 2005; 21(1): 37-56.

[27] National Research Council. Educating children with autism. Washington. DC: *National Academy;* 2001: 41.

[28] Stringer ET. Action research: A handbook for practitioners. 3rd ed. Thousand Oaks, CA: *Sage*; 2007: 25.

[29] Kelly A, Richard L, Beak J. Handbook of design research methods in education. London: *Routledge* 2008: 518.

[30] Mundy P, Delgado C, Block J, Venezia M, Hogan A, Seibert J. A manual for the abridged early social communication scales (ESCS). Available through the University of Miami, Psychology department, Coral Gables, Florida. Available from: URL; http://www.pmundy@miami.edu

[31] Strid K. Memory, attention and interaction in early development: Exploring individual differences among typical children and children with autism. Sweden: Göteborg University, *Department of psychology;* 2007: 34.

[32] Laing E, Laing E, Longhi A. Atypical development of language and social communication in toddlers with Williams syndrome. *Deve. Sci.* 2002; 5(2): 233-46.

[33] Dawson G, Meltzoff AN, Osterling J, Rinaldi J, Brown E. Children with autism fail to orient to naturally occurring social stimuli. *J. Autism Dev. Disord.* 1998; 28(6): 479-85.

[34] Mukaddes NM, Kilincaslan A, Kucucyazici G, Sevketoglu T, Truncer S. Autism in visually impaired individuals. *Psychiatr. Clin. Neurosci.* 2007; 61: 39-44.

[35] Elsabbagh M, Johnson MH. Infancy and autism progress, prospects, and challenges. *Progress Brain Research* 2008; 164: 355-83.
[36] Bernier MG. Puppetry as an art therapy technique with emotionally disturbed children. MS. Dissertation. Creative arts in therapy. [cited 1983]. Available from: URL; http://www.takey.com/Thesis_7.pdf
[37] Hwang, B., and Hughes, C. The effects of social interactive training on early social communicative skills of children with autism. *Journal of Autism and Developmental Disorders*, 2000;30: 331-343.

SUBSTANCE USE

In: The International Psychiatry and Behavioral ...
Editor: Nash Boutros

ISBN: 978-1-62257-566-4

Chapter 15

THE ASSOCIATION STUDY OF THE RELATIONSHIP BETWEEN FOURTEEN CANDIDATE GENE POLYMORPHISMS AND DISPOSITIONS TO ALCOHOLISM*

Omar Šerý*#, Jan Lochman, Kateřina Gláslová[1], Radim Štaif, Miroslav Novotný[1], Vladimír Kmoch[1] and Petr Zvolský[1]

Laboratory of Neurobiology and Molecular Psychiatry,
Institute of Biochemistry, Masaryk University,
Faculty of Science, Brno, Czech Republic
[1]Department of Psychiatry, Charles University,
1st Medical Faculty, Praha, Czech Republic

ABSTRACT

The disposition to alcohol dependence is affected by multiple environmental and genetic factors. Modern molecular genetics techniques allow the analysis of specific genes involved in the pathophysiology of complex diseases such as alcohol dependence. Between strategies for susceptibility gene identification are association studies. We carried out the association study of fourteen candidate gene polymorphisms and alcohol dependence. The association study was performed on 847 persons. We found associations between alcohol dependence and COMT, MAO-B, IL6, IL2, LILRA1 and PSG11 genes. All associated genes influence the neurodevelopment of the central nervous system. We suppose the relationship between genes involved in the neurodevelopment of CNS and dispositions to alcohol dependence.

---

* Original Publication: Šerý, O., Lochman, J., Gláslová K., Štaif, R., Novotný M., Kmoch, V., Zvolský P. The association study of the relationship between fourteen candidate gene polymorphisms and dispositions to the alcoholism. Czech and Slovak Psychiatry, 105, 2009, pp. 153-162.

Correspondence: Doc. RNDr. Omar Šerý, Ph.D., Laboratory of neurobiology and molecular psychiatry, Institute of Biochemistry, Faculty of Science, Masaryk University, Kotlářská 2, 611 37 Brno, Czech Republic. E-mail: omarsery@sci.muni.cz, tel. + 420 549 497 312, fax. + 420 542 213 827

Keywords: alcohol dependence, association study, polymorphism, gene, COMT, IL6, IL2, MAO, DAT1, DRD2

Introduction

The first study that observed the relationship between genetic polymorphism and alcohol dependence was published 18 years ago [2]. In that time, the authors of the paper "Allelic association of human dopamine D2 receptor gene in alcoholism" were well ahead of their time. In the following years, the relationships between other genes and alcohol dependence were successfully observed, mainly by using association studies. Japanese researchers devoted their observations primarily to polymorphisms and mutations of receptors of the dopamine system, while European and American researchers begun to study candidate genes from the area of neurotransmitter metabolism that are included in the brain reward system. There were no major breakthroughs resulting from these approaches. Even though no mutation of dopamine receptors causing the dispositions to alcoholism was discovered, it was possible to prove the relationship of polymorphisms of candidate genes from the cascade of enzymes, participating in the metabolism of neurotransmitters as COMT or MAO. Nevertheless, none of the effects of the candidate polymorphisms to this time have been shown to be essential for the dispositions to alcoholism. We hypothesize that the disposition to alcohol dependence is multifactorial and according to our hypothesis, a large number of factors and a big array of genes underlie the disposition to alcoholism. At the time being, we may see a successive introduction of the newest technologies of DNA analysis into psychiatric research (e.g., DNA chips). These chips enable about one million polymorphisms in 96 subjects to be analyzed and reveal to compare the effects of interactions of many polymorphisms on the phenotype in the frame-one analysis, lasting about two days. DNA chip technology is therefore the future for psychiatric research as well, when we could think about the discovery of quite new polymorphisms, which are of essential importance affecting the disposition to alcohol dependence, or we could expect the discovery of unknown haplotypes and genetic interactions that influence the dispositions to alcohol dependence.

The aim of our study was the search of DNA polymorphisms that participate in the disposition to alcohol dependence. These polymorphisms were chosen from genes that also participate in the development, differentiation and modulation of dopamine or opioid systems in the Central Nervous System (CNS). In our study, we have included two new candidate polymorphisms with yet unknown function that were uncovered with the help of whole genome association study of alcohol dependence [9].

Methods

Patients and control subjects were 25 to 50 years of age. The sample of alcohol-dependent patients consisted of 444 subjects. These patients were selected from anti-alcoholic departments of the Faculty General Hospital in Prague, Apolinarska Street and from female departments at Lojovice, from the Anti-alcoholic Departments of the Psychiatric Hospital at Praha 8 – Bohnice, at the Psychiatric Hospital in Jihlava and at the Anti-alcoholic Psychiatric

Department at Cerveny Dvur. The patients signed informed consents before they were included in the study. Every subject from the alcohol-dependent group had an interview with the psychiatrist, in frame of which personal and family anamnesis were evaluated and the diagnosis was ascertained according to ICD 10 [F10.2], DSM IV [303.90] and MAST [Michigan Alcoholism Screening Test]. The control group included 403 subjects that were without alcohol or other dependences (except of coffee). This sample of subjects was collected at various somatic departments of Faculty General Hospital in Prague, at the Transfusion Department in Prague and Brno, at University Departments and different Institutions in cooperation with the Military Authority, during the selections of new military adepts. When these subjects signed the informed consent and filled in the structured questionnaire for the control group (short personal anamnesis with MAST), the information was verified by the member of research group in a personal interview.

The subjects in the control group fulfilled further conditions for the selection into the study; it means non-smoking (at present and in the past), no use of psychoactive drugs (at present and in the past) and an exclusion of present or former abuse of alcohol. The psychiatric and psychological tests of control subjects were performed as well (Lüschers clinical diagnostic, MINI / Minimal International Neuropsychiatric Interview). With the help of questionnaires of CAGE and CSEMY, the relation to alcohol in the last 12 months was evaluated.

After the informed consent was signed, establishment of diagnosis and questionnaires completed, five milliliter samples of venous blood of all subjects were taken by the medical doctor and/or qualified psychiatric nurse. The blood samples were frosted at minus 20 degrees of Celsius and transferred in a thermo box to the laboratory. Particular samples of genomic DNA were isolated from the blood with the use of commercially available isolation kit UltraClean BloodSpin Kit (MoBio, USA).

In our project, we studied subsequent polymorphisms of candidate genes:

- TaqI A polymorphism of the DRD2 gene (dopamine receptor D2), [7]
- Val158Met polymorphism of COMT gene (catechol-O-metyl transferase), [10]
- I/D polymorphism of ACE gene (angiotensin convertase), [17]
- -174 polymorphism of IL-6 gene (interleukin 6), [24]
- delta 32 polymorphism of CCR5 gene (chemokine receptor 5), [3]
- -308 polymorphism of TNF alpha (tumor necrosis factor alpha) – method see below
- M235T polymorphism of AGT gene (angiotensinogen), [18]
- A/G polymorphism in 13th intron of MAO-B gene (monoamino oxidase B), [6]
- -330 polymorphism of IL-2 gene (interleukin 2) – method see below
- A118G (Asn40Asp) polymorphism of Mu opioid receptor gene, [21]
- 196 G/A (Val66Met) polymorphism of BDNF gene (Brain derived neurotrophic factor), [22]
- 40-bp VNTR polymorphism of DAT1 gene (dopamine transporter), [19]
- polymorphism tsc1189131 – method see below
- polymorphism tsc0598556 – method see below

The detection of -308 polymorphism of TNF alpha gene was made according to the method proposed in our laboratory. For PCR reaction primers: 5‘- AGG CAA TAG GTT

TTG AGG GGC AT – 3‘ a 5‘ - CGG GGA AAG AAT CAT TCA ACC AG – 3‘ were used. Amplification reaction was performed in the thermal cycler Techne Touchgene. After initial denaturation lasting 2.5 minutes at 94°C, the DNA was amplified in three step cycles: denaturation 30 seconds at 66°C, extension 30 sec at 72°C. After 35 cycles, the final extension for 5 minutes at 72°C was used. The amplification was followed by restriction analysis: 20 microliters of PCR product was mixed with 2 U of restriction endonuclease *NcoI* (Fermentas, Lithuania). Then the incubation in water bath followed at 37°C for 16 hours. Gel electrophoresis of fragments was performed on 2% agarose gel (EliPhore), stained by ethidium bromide at 80 V for 2 hours. The following fragments were detected: 264 bp that marked genotype "11“, 264 bp and 284 bp that characterized genotype “12”, 284 bp that identified genotype “22”.

The detection of –330 polymorphisms of IL-2 gene was performed according to the method proposed by our laboratory. For PCR reaction of IL-2 gene polymorphism, the primers used were: 12-25‘ – CAA GAC TTA GTG CAA TGC AAG – 3‘ and 12-2 5‘ – TCA CAT GTT CAG TGT AGT TTCA – 3‘. After an initial denaturation lasting 2.5 minutes at 94 °C, DNA was amplified in three step cycles: denaturation 30 sec at 94 °C, annealing 30 s at 56,5 °C, extension 30 s at 72 °C. After 35 cycles, the final extension was done for 5 min at 72 °C. The total length of amplified fragment was 450 bp. The restriction analysis was then performed: 20 uL of the PCR product was mixed with 5 U of restriction endonuclease Hsp92 II (Promega) a further with 1,7 uL of buffer K (Promega). Then the incubation in water bath followed at 37°C for 7 hours. The detection of restriction fragments was performed by ion-exchange chromatography on HPLC system HP1200 series on column TSK- gel DEAE NPR (Supelco). For the washing out of the DNA from the column, the gradient natrium chloride was used. There following fragments were detected: 107 bp for genotype GG, 107 bp and 90 bp for genotype TG and 90 bp for genotype TT. The detection of polymorphism tsc1189131 (the sequence AC004784, the gene nearby the pregnancy beta-1- glycoprotein gene) was performed according to the method proposed by our laboratory. For the detection, an automatic system ABI7300 (Applied Biosystems) was used. For RealTime PCR detection of polymorphism tsc1189131 the primers: 5‘ – ACT TGA ACC AGT GAC CTC TAA – 3‘ and 5′– CTA TCC CCT TCA CTC TTC CT – 3‘were used. For the detection of alleles following TaqMan probes: TAQProbeC – AGC AGA GCG CAA CGA ATG ATC (Yakima Yellow) and TaqProbeT – AGC AGA GTC CAA CGA ATG ATC (FAM) were used. After initial denaturation for 10 minutes at 95°C, DNA was amplified in three step cycles 40 times: denaturation for 20 s at 95°C, annealing 20 s at 56°C, extension 32 s at 72°C. The different genotypes were detected by analysis of the amplification curves that was very different between both alleles. The detection of polymorphism tsc059856 (the sequence AC009892) was performed according to the method proposed in our laboratory. For the detection, an automatic system ABI7300 (Applied Biosystems) was used. For qPCR reaction of polymorphism TS0598556 the primers: 5‘ - GCA CAG GGC TCA GTG ACT TCT – 3‘ and 5‘- AGG GCG TTT TCC TGC ACT CT – 3‘ were used. For the detection of alleles following TaqMan probes: TaqProbeC – TTC CCT TGC AGA TCC TGA GCT (Yakima Yellow) and TaqProbeT – TTC CTT TGC AGA TCC TGA GCT (FAM) were used. After an initial denaturation of 10 minutes at 95°C; DNA was amplified in the three step cycles 40 times: denaturation 20 s at 95°C, annealing 20 s at 59°C and extension 32 s at 72°C. The different genotypes were identified on the base of amplification curves analysis.

Statistical evaluation of the results was performed with the help of software CSS Statistica (Version 7). Contingency tables with the number of subjects for particular studied genotypes were constructed. On the basis of these tables, we proceeded to account for the number of genotype allelic frequencies of observed polymorphisms. For a clear overview of relations, which were followed, the Spearman correlation coefficient was used.

RESULTS

The differences between genotype frequencies were calculated on the basis of several parameters (age, gender, and gene polymorphisms that were followed and genetic predisposition of concrete subjects that cannot be quoted because of ethical reasons).

The results of genotype and allelic frequencies together with the results of statistical comparison are mentioned in Tables 1 – 15. In these tables, there are described research groups with the allelic and genotype frequencies, and the results of evaluation by statistical tests (Fisher exact test for the counting of allelic frequencies and X2 test for counting of genotype frequencies). For repetitive 40-b VNTR, polymorphism of DAT1 gene are devoted two tables from that the first one quotes the number of observed repetitions in the samples of studied subjects and the second table shows the division of repetition into three intervals (long, medium and short repetition) for the use of further statistical elaboration. By the comparison of allelic frequencies with the Fisher exact test, the statistically significant differences were observed in the frequency of the M allele of the COMT gene polymorphism ($p = 0.012$) in the male group, where the dependent subjects had the frequency of M allele 0.48 and men from the control group had the frequency 0.57 (see Table 2). We observed the difference between genotype frequency of –174 polymorphism of IL-6 gene between the whole group of alcoholics and control group ($p=0.035$), (see Table 4). On the contrary, there was evidence for a significant difference between allelic frequencies, if the group was divided according to gender. Opposite to genotype frequency, a significant difference between allelic frequencies of the whole group of alcoholics and the control group ($p=0.09$), male groups ($p=0.082$) and female groups ($p=0.784$) were not observed.

In our study, a significant difference in allelic frequency of A allele of MAO-B gene polymorphism in males was observed (see Table 8). Since A/G polymorphism of MAO-B gene is located on X chromosome, it was analyzed only in the male part of a research group. A statistically significant difference was observed in the frequency of T allele of IL-2 gene polymorphism where T allele in the control group had a frequency of 0.74, and in the dependent subjects, the frequency was 0.65 ($p=0.016$, see Table 9). Genotype frequencies compared by X^2 test show a statistically significant difference ($p=0.024$) as well. Sex difference was not observed by Fisher exact test or by X^2 test ($p > 0.05$). Further, in our study, the relationship between the tsc1189131 polymorphism and alcohol dependence (Fisher exact test $p = 0{,}026$, X^2 test $p = 0{,}051$) in our research group was observed. When the group of persons was divided on the basis of sex in females and males, a difference in allelic frequency was observed. In the group of control persons and in overall population, C allele is present in higher frequency in comparison with G allele (see Table 14).

Table 1. Results of TaqI A polymorphism genotyping for DRD2 gene (C – Controls, A – Alcoholics)

group	number of subjects with given genotype			Total	genotype frequency v %			frequency allele A1	Fisher exact test	X^2 test
	A1A1	A1A2	A2A2		A1A1	A1A2	A2A2			
C	22	102	279	403	5,5	25,3	69,2	0,18		
A	16	137	291	444	3,6	30,9	65,5	0,19	0,672	0,114
C - male	11	44	95	150	7,3	29,3	63,3	0,22		
A - male	12	90	201	303	4,0	29,7	66,3	0,19	0,296	0,303
C -female	11	58	184	253	4,3	22,9	72,7	0,16		
A - female	4	47	90	141	2,8	33,3	63,8	0,20	0,224	0,072

Table 2. Results of Val158Met polymorphism genotyping for COMT gene (C – Controls, A – Alcoholics)

group	number of subjects with given genotype			Total	genotype frequency v %			frequency allele M	Fisher exact test	X^2 test
	MM	MV	VV		MM	MV	VV			
C	104	203	93	400	26,0	50,8	23,3	0,51		
A	104	224	115	443	23,5	50,6	26,0	0,49	0,306	0,557
C - male	48	74	28	150	32,0	49,3	18,7	0,57		
A - male	68	152	83	303	22,4	50,2	27,4	0,48	0,012	0,035
C -female	56	129	65	250	22,4	51,6	26,0	0,48		
A - female	36	72	32	140	25,7	51,4	22,9	0,51	0,43	0,679

Table 3. Results of I/D polymorphism genotyping for ACE gene (C – Controls, A – Alcoholics)

group	number of subjects with given genotype			Total	genotype frequency v %			frequency allele I	Fisher exact test	X^2 test
	II	ID	DD		II	ID	DD			
C	95	202	106	403	23,6	50,1	26,3	0,49		
A	88	228	128	444	19,8	51,4	28,8	0,45	0,214	0,381
C - male	32	81	37	150	21,3	54,0	24,7	0,48		
A - male	63	151	89	303	20,8	49,8	29,4	0,46	0,499	0,562
C -female	63	121	69	253	24,9	47,8	27,3	0,49		
A - female	25	77	39	141	17,7	54,6	27,7	0,45	0,344	0,232

Table 4. Results of -174 polymorphism genotyping for IL-6 gene (C – Controls, A – Alcoholics)

group	number of subjects with given genotype			Total	genotype frequency v %			frequency allele G	Fisher exact test	X^2 test
	GG	CG	CC		GG	CG	CC			
C	126	215	62	403	31,3	53,3	15,4	0,58		
A	132	213	99	444	29,7	48,0	22,3	0,54	0,09	0,035
C - male	53	71	26	150	35,3	47,3	17,3	0,59		
A - male	88	143	72	303	29,0	47,2	23,8	0,53	0,082	0,203
C -female	73	144	36	253	28,9	56,9	14,2	0,57		
A - female	44	70	27	141	31,2	49,6	19,1	0,56	0,784	0,298

Table 5. Results of Delta32 polymorphism genotyping for CCR5 gene (C – Controls, A – Alcoholics)

group	number of subjects with given genotype			Total	genotype frequency v %			frequency allele I	Fisher exact test	X^2 test
	II	ID	DD		II	ID	DD			
C	312	86	5	403	77,4	21,3	1,2	0,88		
A	339	96	9	444	76,4	21,6	2,0	0,87	0,614	0,661
C - male	113	35	2	150	75,3	23,3	1,3	0,87		
A - male	230	68	5	303	75,9	22,4	1,7	0,87	1,04	0,949
C -female	199	51	3	253	78,7	20,2	1,2	0,89		
A - female	109	28	4	141	77,3	19,9	2,8	0,87	0,606	0,493

Table 6. Results of -308 polymorphism genotyping for TNF alpha gene (C – Controls, A – Alcoholics)

group	number of subjects with given genotype			Total	genotype frequency v %			frequency allele 1	Fisher exact test	X^2 test
	11	12	22		11	12	22			
C	285	103	15	403	70,7	25,6	3,7	0,83		
A	330	103	11	444	74,3	23,2	2,5	0,86	0,188	0,381
C - male	107	40	3	150	71,3	26,7	2,0	0,85		
A - male	225	70	8	303	74,3	23,1	2,6	0,86	0,714	0,667
C -female	178	63	12	253	70,4	24,9	4,7	0,83		
A - female	105	33	3	141	74,5	23,4	2,1	0,86	0,256	0,287

Table 7. Results of M235T polymorphism genotyping for AGT gene (C – Controls, A – Alcoholics)

group	number of subjects with given genotype			Total	genotype frequency			frequency	Fisher exact test	X^2 test
					v %			allele T		
	MM	MT	TT		MM	MT	TT			
C	116	206	80	402	28,9	51,2	19,9	0,54		
A	132	216	81	429	30,8	50,3	18,9	0,56	0,582	0,819
C - male	42	78	30	150	28,0	52,0	20,0	0,54		
A - male	87	149	57	293	29,7	50,9	19,5	0,55	0,804	0,933
C -female	74	128	50	252	29,4	50,8	19,8	0,55		
A - female	45	67	24	136	33,1	49,3	17,6	0,58	0,474	0,717

Table 8. Results of A/G polymorphism genotyping for MAO-B gene (C – Controls, A – Alcoholics)

group	number of persons with given allele		Total	allelic frequency		Fisher exact test
				v %		
	A	G		A	G	
C	79	51	130	60,8	39,2	
A	135	137	272	49,6	50,4	0,023
C - male	79	51	130	60,8	39,2	
A - male	135	137	272	49,6	50,4	0,023
*C –female	x	x	x	x	x	
*A -female	x	x	x	x	x	x

*A/G polymorphism was detected only in male.

Table 9. Results of -330 polymorphism genotyping for IL-2 gene (C – Controls, A – Alcoholics)

group	number of subjects with given genotype			Total	genotype frequency			frequency	Fisher exact test	X^2 test
					v %			allele T		
	TT	TG	GG		TT	TG	GG			
C	103	53	19	175	58,9	30,3	10,9	0,74		
A	59	58	19	136	43,4	42,6	14,0	0,65	0,016	0,024
C - male	37	22	8	67	55,2	32,8	11,9	0,72		
A - male	43	45	17	105	41,0	42,9	16,2	0,62	0,098	0,187
C -female	66	31	11	108	61,1	28,7	10,2	0,75		
A - female	16	13	2	31	51,6	41,9	6,5	0,73	0,758	0,357

Table 10. Results of A118G polymorphism genotyping for Mu receptor gene (C – Controls, A – Alcoholics)

group	number of subjects with given genotype			Total	genotype frequency			frequency	Fisher exact test	X^2 test
					v %			allele A		
	AA	AG	GG		AA	AG	GG			
C	313	84	6	403	77,7	20,8	1,5	0,88		
A	105	34	1	140	75,0	24,3	0,7	0,87	0,746	0,564
C - male	117	31	2	150	78,0	20,7	1,3	0,88		
A - male	233	63	6	302	77,2	20,9	2,0	0,88	0,836	0,881
C -female	196	53	4	253	77,5	20,9	1,6	0,88		
A - female	105	34	1	140	75,0	24,3	0,7	0,87	0,824	0,589

Table 11. Results of 196G/A polymorphism genotyping for BDNF gene (C – Controls, A – Alcoholics)

group	number of subjects with given genotype			Total	genotype frequency			frequency	Fisher exact test	X^2 test
					v %			allele A		
	AA	AG	GG		AA	AG	GG			
C	9	124	269	402	2,2	30,8	66,9	0,18		
A	9	134	300	443	2,0	30,2	67,7	0,17	0,834	0,957
C - male	5	47	97	149	3,4	31,5	65,1	0,19		
A - male	5	88	210	303	1,7	29,0	69,3	0,16	0,31	0,410
C -female	4	77	172	253	1,6	30,4	68,0	0,17		
A - female	4	46	90	140	2,9	32,9	64,3	0,19	0,436	0,584

Table 12. Results of 40-bp VNTR polymorphism for DAT1 gene – observed genotypes/repeats 40 bp (C – Controls, A – Alcoholics)

group	number of subjects with given genotype								Fisher exact test	X^2 test
	9/9	10/10	11/11	9/10	9/11	10/11	others	total		
C	17	232	0	141	3	4	3	400	0,417	
A	22	252	0	158	0	6	3	441		0,957
C -male	7	85	0	50	3	3	2	150	0,155	
A -male	18	172	0	106	0	4	2	302		0,410
C -female	10	147	0	91	0	1	1	250	0,218	0,584
A -female	4	80	0	52	0	2	1	139		

Others = in the study, the rare genotypes 8/8, 8/10 and 8/11were found which are found rarely in population; these genotypes were not used for statistical analysis.

Table 13. Results of 40-bp VNTR polymorphism for DAT1 gene – distribution according to "long" and "short" genotype (repetition), (C – Controls, A – Alcoholics)

group	number of subjects with given genotype			Total	genotype frequency v %			frequency allele L	Fisher exact test	X^2 test
	LL	LS	SS		LL	LS	SS			
C	236	145	19	400	59,0	36,3	4,8	0,77		
A	82	53	4	139	59,0	38,1	2,9	0,78	0,818	0,572
C - male	88	53	9	150	58,7	35,3	6,0	0,76		
A - male	176	106	20	302	58,3	35,1	6,6	0,76	0,936	0,203
C -female	148	92	10	250	59,2	36,8	4,0	0,78		
A - female	82	53	4	139	59,0	38,1	2,9	0,78	0,958	0,775

Short genotype SS – genotype 9/9, medium long genotype LS – 9/10 and 9/11, long genotypes LL - 10/10, 10/11 and 11/11

Table 14. Results of tsc1189131polymorphism genotyping (C – Controls, A – Alcoholics)

group	number of subjects with given genotype			Total	genotype frequency v %			frequency allele C	Fisher exact test	X^2 test
	CC	CT	TT		CC	CT	TT			
C	127	200	76	403	31,5	49,6	18,9	0,56		
A	117	215	110	442	26,5	48,6	24,9	0,51	0,026	0,068
C - male	53	76	21	150	35,3	50,7	14,0	0,61		
A - male	87	149	65	301	28,9	49,5	21,6	0,54	0,053	0,111
C -female	74	124	55	253	29,2	49,0	21,7	0,54		
A - female	30	66	45	141	21,3	46,8	31,9	0,45	0,018	0,051

Table 15. Results of tsc0598556polymorphism genotyping (C – Controls, A – Alcoholics)

group	number of subjects with given genotype			Total	genotype frequency v %			frequency allele C	Fisher exact test	X^2 test
	CC	CT	TT		CC	CT	TT			
C	209	167	23	399	52,4	41,9	5,8	0,73		
A	248	169	27	444	55,9	38,1	6,1	0,75	0,494	0,532
C - male	78	56	15	149	52,3	37,6	10,1	0,71		
A - male	168	120	15	303	55,4	39,6	5,0	0,75	0,214	0,121
C -female	131	111	8	250	52,4	44,4	3,2	0,75		
A - female	80	49	12	141	56,7	34,8	8,5	0,74	0,946	0,025

Female groups tested for genotype frequencies of tsc0598556 polymorphism by X^2 test revealed a statistically significant difference (p=0.026). Other significant relationships of this polymorphism was not observed (see Table 15).

In allelic frequencies, the comparison by Fisher exact test and in the comparison of genotype frequencies by X^2 test, no statistically significant difference was found in other analyzed polymorphisms of candidate genes, not even after the set dividing to males and females (p>0,05). Next, double genotypes frequencies were studied in the relationship to the alcohol dependence.

Namely, the relationship of two genotypes combinations was studied. In the combination, tsc1189131 polymorphism and IL6 gene polymorphism revealed a statistically significant difference between the alcohol-dependent subjects and controls (p<0.01, p=0.006). tsc1189131/IL6 genotypes TTCC and CTCC dispose to the alcohol dependence – they were significantly often observed in subjects with alcohol dependence.

In our study, we found the relationship between two gene polymorphism combinations and the disposition to the alcoholism in combinations of genes TNF alpha and angiotensinogen, COMT and DAT1, COMT and MAO B, COMT and BDNF, and BDNF and Mu receptor (see Table 16).

In the group of alcohol-dependent subjects, the relationship between genes IL-2 and angiotensinogen, COMT and BDNF, COMT and MAO B, BDNF and MAO B, was found (see Table 17). In the total group of persons, the relationships between IL-6 gene polymorphism and tsc1189131 polymorphism, BDNF gene polymorphism and Mu receptor gene polymorphism, Mu receptor gene polymorphism and tsc0598556 polymorphism w found (see Table 18).

Table 16. Alcohol - Linkage probability between two polymorphisms within the set of all subjects

Double genotype/color sense	Linkage probability (p)
IL-6 x TSC0598556	0,051
TNFA x AGT	0,025
COMT x DAT1	0,003
COMT x MAO-B	0,003
COMT x BDNF	0,016
Mu x BDNF	0,007

Table 17. Alcoholics - Linkage probability between two polymorphisms within the set of alcoholics

Double genotype/color sense	Linkage probability (p)
IL-2 x ANG	0,02
IL-2 x tsc0598556	0,104
COMT x BDNF	0,039
COMT x MAO-B	0,004
MAO-B x BDNF	0,006

Table 18. Controls - Linkage probability between two polymorphisms within the set of controls

Double genotype	Linkage probability (p)
IL-6 x tsc1189131	0,001
IL-2 x tsc0598556	0,235
BDNF x Mu	0,018
Mu x tsc0598556	0,024

Discussion

Within the association study, the relationship of 14 polymorphisms in a group of 847 subjects was studied. Within the framework of our study, previously observed relationships between the Val158Met polymorphism of COMT gene and alcohol dependence was verified but only in the male part of the research group (for allelic frequencies $p < 0.02$, for genotype frequencies $p < 0.04$). We suppose that this relationship is mediated by the role of COMT in the brain development. As is known, the COMT enzyme catalyzes methylation of katechol estrogens to methoxy estrogens – e.g. 2-methoxy estradiol which is an anti-proliferative metabolite. The role of COMT in neuronal development should be studied in the future. In our previous publication, this relationship is described in more detail [23].

The relationship between the -174 polymorphism of IL-6 gene and disposition to the alcoholism on our total research group was observed (for allelic frequencies $p = 0.09$, for genotype frequencies $p < 0.04$). We assume that the relationship of this polymorphism to alcohol dependence is connected with the effect of IL-6 on neurons surviving and the neurite growth in the time of CNS development. In our previous publication, the relation between the IL-6 and dispositions to alcohol dependence is discussed in more detail [20].

The relationship between the alcohol dependence and studied polymorphism of MAO B gene but only in the male part of the persons was observed. We suppose that a key impact of MAO B to alcohol dependence will be influenced by the fenylethylamine (PEA) level. In the Chinese population, the relationship between the MAO B polymorphism and alcohol dependence has not been observed [13].

For the first time, in the total group of subjects, the relationship between the IL2 gene and alcohol dependence was observed (allelic frequencies $p=0.02$, genotype frequencies $p<0.03$). Marcos et al. [14] in alcohol-dependent subjects determined the relationship between this polymorphism and liver cirrhosis. In previous studies, the higher IL2 production by T lymphocytes in subjects with GG genotypes contrary to TG and TT genotypes was found [8]. IL2 promotes the surviving of cultivated neurons and elongation of their axons and affects the hypothalamo-hypophyseal system as well [16].

Chiu et al. [9] used DNA chip technology utilizing Affymetrix platform to study the relationship between 11120 polymorphisms and alcohol dependence in a group of 1614 subjects. Overall, he founded 20 polymorphisms with more significant relationships to alcohol dependence. Two of these polymorphisms - tsc1189131 (rs1963786) and tsc0598556 (rs272411) we have also selected for our study and we tried to repeat the previously founded association. Within our study, the relationship of tsc1189131 polymorphism to alcohol dependence was confirmed in both cases – in the whole group of subjects (allelic frequencies p=0.03, genotype frequencies p<0.068) and the female group, respectively (allelic frequencies p=0.02, genotype frequencies p<0.051). This polymorphism is located in intron of gene for pregnancy-specific beta-1-glycoprotein 11 (PSG11). As was found before, in the mean time of pregnancy, among others, PSG11 influences the secretion of IL6 and it is mainly produced by placental syncytiotrophoblast. These facts support the relationship between the IL-6 and alcohol dependence and outline once again the possible relationship between alcohol dependence dispositions and the CNS neurodevelopment. Moreover, during the study of interactions between the polymorphisms in a set of controls, a relationship between the polymorphism of IL-6 and tsc1189131 polymorphism was observed. It means a more often incidence of some double genotypes in the control set than it would be expected in normal population. As we mentioned in previous studies, the selection of non-abusing controls subjects seems to be more effective criteria than criteria for alcohol dependence itself. A group of control subjects without the tobacco, drugs abuse and alcohol addiction, creates in comparison with a group of alcoholics determined according to DSMIV criteria the second imaginary part of addiction distribution in the population. Just interaction between the IL6 and tsc1189131 in the non-abusing part of the population can be the guidance in further research with a goal to find a combination of polymorphisms protecting against alcohol dependence.

In the female group, the relationship between the tsc0598556 polymorphism and alcohol dependence was observed (genotype frequencies p<0.03). This polymorphism is located in the intron of the gene for leukocyte immunoglobulin-like receptor (LILRA1). LILTRA1 serves as an immunoreceptor on monocytes and B cells and in minor amounts in dendritic cells and NK cells. It can be supposed that also in this case, this polymorphism affects the disposition to alcohol dependence through the influence of CNS development.

In our study, no relationship between alcohol dependence and genes involved in rennin-angiotensin system (ACE and AGT) was observed. A separate cause is a hypothetic relationship between TaqI A polymorphism of DRD2 gene (newly, this polymorphism was placed in ANKK1 gene - ankyrin repeat and kinase domain containing 1 gene) and alcohol dependence that was not proved during our study. In our previous work, this relationship is discussed in more detail [11].

Dopamine transporter DAT plays a key role in homeostatic regulation of dopaminergic neurotransmissions. Köhnke et al. [12] in his association study compared a group containing 216 subjects with alcohol dependence with 102 controls. He observed a higher frequency of 9 alleles in subjects with alcohol dependence (0.48) in comparison to the controls (0.32). On the other hand, in the study done by Wernicke et al. [26], the relationship of genotype 10/10 to alcohol dependence was proved. On the contrary, a study published by Foley et al. [4] did not confirm the relationship of VNTR polymorphism to alcohol dependence. Also, our study together with studies of other authors does not validate the association of DAT1 gene VNTR polymorphism with alcohol dependence.

Neurotrophins are specific growth factors cooperating on local regulation of synaptic plasticity. During the last years, one of the most often studied neurotrophins is BDNF. BDNF was studied in the connection of pathogenesis of many psychic diseases as mental disorders, depression, anxiety, and schizophrenia and drug dependence. Val66Met polymorphism of BDNF gene was studied in the relationship to alcohol dependence as well. Within the study done by Tsai et al. [25], a relationship of this polymorphism with alcohol-dependent aggression and assault was studied with negative results. In our study, we did not prove the relationship between Val66Met polymorphism of BDNF gene and alcohol dependence ($p > 0.05$).

The relationship of opioid receptors to the origin of alcohol dependence is assumed. An uptake of alcohol can result from a hereditary deficit of the endogenous opioid system. Alcohol interferes with the opioid system and influences the mesolimbic system. Alcohol has an impact on binding properties of opioid receptors and it modulates synthesis of opioid peptides. Alcohol stimulates the release of dopamine in the brain through the regulation of OP1 and OP2 opioid receptors. In the case of the inhibition of these receptors, a human becomes unable to derive enjoyment from alcohol. Polymorphism A118G (Asn40Asp) belongs to the most often studied polymorphisms of Mu opioid receptor gene. Within the year 2006, a meta-analysis of this polymorphism in relationship to alcohol and drug dependence was done. Meta-analysis covered, in total, 8000 subjects, results from 22 publications and 28 types of groups of subjects. In this meta-analysis, the relationship between alcohol and drug dependence and A118G (Asn40Asp) polymorphism was not found. Our study confirms results of this meta-analysis.

CONCLUSION

In our nine-year-long study, we have taken advantage of pieces of knowledge about the molecular causation of alcohol dependence origin and in addition to classical candidate genes, we included in our study two newly determined polymorphisms by whole-genome association study. Furthermore, we contributed to the effort to find the disposition to alcohol dependence by propagation of theory that disposition to alcohol dependence is, to a certain extent, a neurodevelopment disorder and so we tested the influence of candidate genes originated from the group of central nervous system developing modulators such as IL-6, IL-2; a BDNF to this process. As was demonstrated, our assumptions were correct and moreover, the influence of COMT to alcohol dispositions should be deduced rather from its role in CNS development as well as from its relation to the metabolism of neurotransmitters. Overall results from our study indicate interesting interactions between the studied polymorphisms and supported the hypothesis of multigenic basis of alcohol dependence disposition and complex functional relations of candidate genes. For practice, our results showed that the disposition to alcohol dependence could be formed during CNS development and it does not need to have relation to direct effect of alcohol on the CNS. While impact of genes on alcohol dependence disposition cannot be affected directly; by the influencing of the environment, we can eliminate an arising of the alcohol dependence in persons with genetic disposition. This influence of environment mainly covers the protection of emotional background in the time of adolescence and life-time abstinence from alcohol and other drugs.

Acknowledgments

This project was supported by an internal grant agency of Ministry of Health of the Czech Republic - IGA MZ ČR č. NR9298-3/2007 and further by the project of Ministry of education, youth and sport of Czech Republic - MSM0021622413.

References

[1] Arias, A., Feinn, R., Kranzler, H.R. Association of an Asn40Asp (A118G) polymorphism in the mu-opioid receptor gene with substance dependence: a meta-analysis. *Drug Alcohol Depend.*, 83, 2006, pp. 262-268.

[2] Blum, K., Noble, E.P., Sheridan, P.J., Montgomery, A., Ritchie, T., Jagadeeswaran, P., Nogami, H., Briggs, A.H., Cohn, J.B. Allelic association of human dopamine D2 receptor gene in alcoholism. *JAMA*, 263, 1990, pp. 2055-60.

[3] Eugen-Olsen, J., Iversen, A.K., Garred, P., Koppelhus, U., Pedersen, C., Benfield, T.L., Sorensen, A.M., Katzenstein, T., Dickmeiss, E., Gerstoft, J., Skinhøj, P., Svejgaard, A., Nielsen, J.O., Hofmann, B. Heterozygosity for a deletion in the CKR-5 gene leads to prolonged AIDS-free survival and slower CD4 T-cell decline in a cohort of HIV-seropositive individuals. *AIDS*, 11, 1997, pp. 305-10.

[4] Foley, P.F., Loh, E.W., Innes, D.J., Williams, S.M., Tannenberg, A.E., Harper, C.G., Dodd, P.R. Association studies of neurotransmitter gene polymorphisms in alcoholic Caucasians. *Ann. N Y Acad. Sci.*,1025, 2004, pp. 39-46.

[5] Franke, P., Schwab, S.G., Knapp, M., Gänsicke, M., Delmo, C., Zill, P., Trixler, M., Lichtermann, D., Hallmayer, J., Wildenauer, D.B., Maier, W. DAT1 gene polymorphism in alcoholism: a family-based association study. *Biol. Psychiatry*, 45, 1999, pp. 652-654.

[6] Garpenstrand, H., Ekblom, J., Forslund, K., Rylander, G., Oreland, L. Platelet monoamine oxidase activity is related to MAOB intron 13 genotype. *J. Neural. Transm.*, 107, 2000, pp. 523-30.

[7] Grandy, D.K., Zhang, Y., Civelli, O. PCR detection of the TaqA RFLP at the DRD2 locus. *Hum. Mol. Genet.*, 2, 1993, p. 2197.

[8] Hoffmann, S.C., Stanley, E.M., Darrin Cox, E., Craighead, N., DiMercurio, B.S., Koziol, D.E., Harlan, D.M., Kirk, A.D., Blair, P.J. Association of cytokine polymorphic inheritance and in vitro cytokine production in anti-CD3/CD28-stimulated peripheral blood lymphocytes. *Transplantation*, 72, 2001, pp. 1444-1450.

[9] Chiu, Y.F., Liu, S.Y., Tsai, Y.Y. A comparison in association and linkage genome-wide scans for alcoholism susceptibility genes using single-nucleotide polymorphisms. *BMC Genetics*, 6, 2005, p. S89.

[10] Jönsson, E.G., Goldman, D., Spurlock, G., Gustavsson, J.P., Nielsen, D.A., Linnoila, M., Owen, M.J., Sedvall, G.C. Tryptophan hydroxylase and catechol-O-methyltransferase gene polymorphisms: relationships to monoamine metabolite concentrations in CSF of healthy volunteers. *Eur. Arch. Psychiatry Clin. Neurosci.*, 247, 1997, pp. 297-302.

[11] Kašparovská, J., Hříbková, H., Hloušková, R., Novotný, M., Gláslová, K., Šimek, V., Mikeš, V., Zvolský, P., Šerý, O. TaqI A polymorphism of the DRD2 gene and alcoholism in the Czech Republic. *Czech and Slovak Psychiatry*, 99, 2003, pp. 5-9.

[12] Köhnke, M.D., Batra, A., Kolb, W., Köhnke, A.M., Lutz, U., Schick, S., Gaertner, I. Association of the dopamine transporter gene with alcoholism. *Alcohol Alcohol.*, 40, 2005, pp. 339-342.

[13] Lu, R.B., Lee, J.F., Ko, H.C., Lin, W.W., Chen, K., Shih, J.C. No association of the MAOA gene with alcoholism among Han Chinese males in Taiwan. Prog. Neuropsychopharmacol. *Biol. Psychiatry*, 26, 2002, pp. 457-61.

[14] Marcos, M., Pastor, I., González-Sarmiento, R., Laso, F.J. A new genetic variant involved in genetic susceptibility to alcoholic liver cirrhosis: -330T>G polymorphism of the interleukin-2 gene. *Eur. J. Gastroenterol. Hepatol.*, 20, 2008, pp. 855-859.

[15] Parsian, A., Zhang, Z.H. Human dopamine transporter gene polymorphism (VNTR) and alcoholism. *Am. J. Med. Genet.*, 74, 1997, pp. 480-482.

[16] Raber, J., Sorg, O., Horn, T.F., Yu, N., Koob, G.F., Campbell, I.L., Bloom, F.E. Inflammatory cytokines: putative regulators of neuronal and neuro-endocrine function. *Brain Res. Brain Res. Rev.,* 26, 1998, pp. 320-326.

[17] Rigat, B., Hubert, C., Corvol, P., Soubrier, F. PCR detection of the insertion/deletion polymorphism of the human angiotensin converting enzyme gene (DCP1) (dipeptidyl carboxypeptidase 1). *Nucleic Acids Res.*, 20, 1992, p. 1433.

[18] Russ, A.P., Maerz, W., Ruzicka, V., Stein, U., Gross, W. Rapid detection of the hypertension-associated Met235-->Thr allele of the human angiotensinogen gene. *Hum. Mol. Genet.,* 2, 1993, pp. 609-10.

[19] Shinohara, M., Mizushima, H., Hirano, M., Shioe, K., Nakazawa, M., Hiejima, Y., Ono, Y., Kanba, S. Eating disorders with binge-eating behaviors are associated with the s allele of the 3'-UTR VNTR polymorphism of the dopamine transporter gene. *J. Psychiatry Neurosci.*, 29, 2004, pp. 134-137.

[20] Šerý, O., Hladilová, R., Novotný, M., Znojil, V., Zvolský, P. Polymorphism of the IL-6 Gene is in the Relationship with the Disposition to the Alcohol Dependence. *Czech and Slovak Psychiatry,* 99, 2003, pp. 185-188.

[21] Šerý, O., Lochman, J., Častulík, L., Šťastný, F., Přikryl, R., Češková, E. OPRM1 polymorphism is in the relationship with schizophrenia: a new candidate gene. *Czech and Slovak Psychiatry*, 105, 2009 (in press).

[22] Šerý, O., Lochman, J., Zvolský, P., Hlinomazová, Z., Novotný, M. Color vision deficiency in alcoholics and its relationship with the BDNF polymorphism. *Czech and Slovak Psychiatry*, 104, 2008, pp. 115-119.

[23] Šerý, O., Mikes, V., Pitelová, R., Znojil, V., Zvolský, P. The association between high-activity COMT allele and alcoholism. *Neuro Endocrinol Lett.,* 27, 2006, pp. 231-235.

[24] Šerý, O., Theirner, P., Hladilová, R., Štaif, R., Balaštiková, B., Drtílková, I. IL-6 and DRD2 genes are associated with ADHD. *Czech and Slovak Psychiatry,* 99, 2003, pp. 404-409.

[25] Tsai, S.J., Liao, D.L., Yu, Y.W., Chen, T.J., Wu, H.C., Lin, C.H., Cheng, C.Y., Hong, C.J. A study of the association of (Val66Met) polymorphism in the brain-derived neurotrophic factor gene with alcohol dependence and extreme violence in Chinese males. *Neurosci. Lett.*, 381, 2005, pp. 340-343.

[26] Wernicke, C., Smolka, M., Gallinat, J., Winterer, G., Schmidt, L.G., Rommelspacher, H. Evidence for the importance of the human dopamine transporter gene for withdrawal symptomatology of alcoholics in a German population. *Neurosci. Lett.*,333, 2002, pp. 45-48.

In: The International Psychiatry and Behavioral ...
Editor: Nash Boutros
ISBN: 978-1-62257-566-4

Chapter 16

A Double-Blind, Placebo-Controlled, Randomized Clinical Trial of Escitalopram for the Treatment of Affective Disorders in Alcohol Dependent Patients in Early Remission*

E. M. Krupitsky#, S. M. Yerish, A. S. Kiselev, V. A. Berntsev, N. A. Alexandrovsky, M. N. Torban, S. P. Eroshin and O. F. Eryshev

St. Petersburg V.M. Bekhterev Research Psychoneurological Institute, St. Petersburg, Russia

Abstract

Introduction: Results from clinical trials of antidepressants for alcohol dependence are controversial, possibly due to the inclusion of patients with and without co-morbid affective disorders.

Aim: To study the efficacy of one of the most selective SSRIs, escitalopram, for the treatment of alcoholics with co-morbid affective disorders (mild to moderate depression).

Methods: Sixty patients with mild to moderate depression (7-23 on the Hamilton depression scale) were randomized into one of two treatment groups. Patients of the first group were treated with escitalopram (10 mg/day) for 3 months while patients of the 2nd group received an identically looking placebo. All the study subjects were scheduled to come to the clinic on a weekly basis for psychiatric evaluations (severity of depression and anxiety, and craving for alcohol), and to monitor their control of alcohol use and compliance with the study medication (by a riboflavin marker in their urine). Hamilton scales, the Montgomery-Ashberg scale, Spielberger state-trait inventory and Zung scale

---

* Original Publication: Voprosy Narcologii (Problems of addictions), 2009, Number 6, p. 17-34.

Corresponding author: Prof. Evgeny Krupitksy, MD, PhD, Head, Department of Addictions, St. Petersburg Bekhterev Research Psychoneurological Institute, Bekhtereva Street, 3, St. Petersburg 192019, Russia. E-mail: kruenator@gmail.com

were used to assess depression and anxiety. Alcohol cravings were assessed with the Obsessive-Compulsive Drinking scale, Penn Alcohol Craving scale, and Visual Analog Scale of Craving for Alcohol. Alcohol use was evaluated with the Time Line Follow Back technique and by monitoring gamma-glutamiltransferase activity in the blood. Overall treatment effects were assessed with the Clinical Global Impression scale. The study design was double blind.

Results: Escitalopram was significantly superior to the placebo in treating depression, anxiety, alcohol cravings and preventing a relapse to heavy drinking. The number of those who completed treatment was significantly higher in the escitalopram group, with the number of drinking days being significantly lower. Overall treatment effects were significantly better in the escitalopram group.

Conclusion: Escitalopram is an effective medication for alcohol dependence with co-morbid affective disorders.

Keywords: Alcoholism treatment, Escitalopram, Depression, Anxiety

INTRODUCTION

Alcohol dependence is an important medical and social problem which has particular importance due to its wide prevalence and negative social effects [21].

Affective disorders, prevailing among alcohol dependent patients, are closely associated with one of the main symptoms of alcoholism - craving for alcohol (CA). Affective disorders can provoke cravings. Furthermore, cravings are often followed by affective disorders. In the early period of remission, a relapse may often be caused by depression [5, 10].

It should be noted that depression of various severities are a widespread psychopathological phenomena among alcohol dependent patients [8, 24, 40]. A number of population surveys have shown that about 30 percent of alcohol dependent patients have co-morbid depressive disorders of different severities [15, 37]. Besides a depressed mood, alcohol dependent patients manifest other signs of affective disorders: anxiety, dysphoria, irritability, emotional instability and less often – apathy [5]. Timely and adequate treatment of affective disorders in the period of remission is one of the principal ways of remission stabilization and relapse prevention in alcohol-dependent patients.

Some researchers believe that the most promising group of drugs for treating affective disorders in alcohol-dependent patients during remission (abstinence) is the group of selective serotonin reuptake inhibitors – SSRI antidepressants [1, 11, 19, 23]. The effect of craving reduction caused by SSRIs and the fact that they may be considered as an effective component of pharmacological strategies for relapse prevention were already described in the early 1990s [12, 29, 31]. At the same time, it was shown that some SSRIs (citalopram, fluoxetineee) can positively influence alcohol consumption, lowering cravings for alcohol, resulting in a reduced relapse rate [38, 45]. In addition to their anti-depressive effect, SSRIs are able to reduce alcohol-associated aggressive behavior and impulsivity in animal experiments [7]. One of the highly selective SSRIs, citalopram, demonstrated a certain efficacy in maintaining abstincne in alcoholics, according to a recent open randomized clinical trial [44]. A new, highly selective inhibitor of serotonin reuptake, escitalopram, proved effective for treating alcoholism associated with a major depressive disorder [28]. On the other hand, a number of studies showed a limited influence of some SSRIs, sertralinee in particular, on the level of alcohol use in alcohol-dependent patients [26, 35].

As demonstrated by Kranzler et al. in a rigorous clinical trial, fluoxetine was proved to not cause any therapeutic effect on alcohol dependence [22]. The trial of nefazadon carried out by Hautzinger et al. [18] also revealed no significant difference between the active drug and placebo regarding its efficacy in preventing relapse in alcohol-dependent patients. Nevertheless, it should be taken into consideration that neither sertralinee nor nefazadon are characterized by high selectivity in inhibiting serotonin reuptake. It is also important to mention that the negative results were obtained in trials performed on alcohol-dependent individuals recruited from general population, without taking into account presence of co-morbid affective disorders. To explain potential mechanisms of SSRIs' influence on craving for alcohol, a hypothesis for the central serotonin deficiency in alcohol-dependent patients was proposed [12]. A certain ambiguity and lack of integrity of the findings mentioned above concerning the administration of anti-depressants in alcoholism may be due to employing SSRIs of various selectivities. This can also be brought about by using them in the total population of alcohol-dependent individuals, including an essential number of regular alcohol-dependent patients without any co-morbid affective disorders.

Based on these ideas, we hypothesized that highly selective serotonin reuptake inhibitors may be effective to stabilize remission and prevent a relapse in the subpopulation of alcohol dependent individuals, quite common in the initial stage of remission of alcoholism, associated with depressive disorders of mild to moderate severity. In particular, escitalopram, being one of the SSRIs with the highest selectivity, can prove effective in treating alcohol-dependent patients with affective disorders at the early remission stage.

To check this hypothesis, we conducted a double-blind, randomized, placebo-controlled clinical trial of escitalopram efficacy in treating affective disorders and preventing relapse in alcohol-dependent patients at the initial stage of remission (abstinence).

METHODS

The Research Design

Sixty alcohol-dependent patients with co-morbid affective disorders were randomly divided into two groups entering a double-blind placebo controlled clinical trial. The experimental group (29 patients) received escitalopram (10 mg once a day, in the morning); the control group (31 patients) received an identically looking placebo. The patients had been administered medication for three months (13 weeks). During the study period, they were to attend the research center weekly to have their psychiatric symptoms, alcohol use, and medication compliance assessed (the latter- by the fluorescent riboflavin marker in their urine).

SUBJECTS

Men and women aged 18-50 were included into the trial if they had been diagnosed with alcohol dependence according to the criteria of ICD-10, associated with affective disorders (a depression episode, a moderate depression episode, or a recurrent depression disorder); if their test of the expired air proved alcohol to be negative; and they had abstained from taking alcohol for at least 7 days (no alcohol withdrawal symptoms). Only mild or moderate cases of depression (scored 7-23 by the Hamilton scale) were taken. The women were not to be pregnant and they were to agree to use adequate contraception for the trial period. Every patient was to give her or his phone number for follow-up purposes (to follow their weekly visits to the clinic).

Patients were not included into the trial if they were taking another psychotropic drug. They were also not included if they had a marked organic brain lesion, a marked somatic pathology (like a severe disease of the liver, kidneys, or cardio-vascular or nervous systems); a psychotic state or a severe psychiatric disease in their history (schizophrenia, epilepsy, manic-depressive psychosis); any other chemical dependence except alcohol and tobacco; or were receiving another pharmacological treatment or psychotherapy for their alcohol dependence. Every patient entering the trial signed informed consent prior to inclusion into the study.

SELECTION OF PARTICIPANTS AND THE CLINICAL BASIS

The trial was performed in the Department of Narcology (Addiction Psychiatry) of the St. Petersburg Bekhterev Psycho-Neurological Research Institute. The investigators studied medical records of patients admitted to the Narcology department for in-patient treatment to select those meeting the enrollment criteria.

Finally, the idea of the study was explained to the chosen patients, and their informed consent was given. Every patient was enrolled only after his or her signed the informed consent.

MEDICATION

Pharmacists of the Bekhterev Institute, along with the Scientific Production Enterprise "Bios" (St.Petersburg), dispersed escitalopram tablets and produced escitalopram capsules (10 mg) and identically looking placebo capsules (starch). 50 mg of riboflavin were added to both the placebos and the escitalopram capsules as a fluorescent marker of the medication being taken (riboflavin is excreted with urine and it causes fluorescence when irradiated by ultraviolet light of 444 nm wave length, which makes it easy to check the patient's compliance by the fluorescence in his urine being present or absent).

ASSESSMENT TECHNIQUES

To assess the patients' state of health before entering the trial, we employed the total blood count, the blood biochemistry panel and the routine urine test. On the day of enrollment into the trial, the baseline assessment included: a physical examination of the patient; an alcohol breath test; a retrospective analysis of alcohol use for the previous three months according to the technique "Time Line Follow Back" (TLFB) [41], estimating the number of drinking days and the amount of alcohol consumed; a confirmation the ICD-X diagnoses of alcohol dependence and associated affective disorders (a depression episode, a moderate depression episode or recurrent depression disorder) according to ICD-10 criteria; an especially developed clinically structured interview for obtaining the case history; ; and psychometric measurements by a battery of psychometric instruments. The battery of psychometrics contained: the Addiction Severity Index (ASI) [25], a General Assessment of Functioning scale (GAF) (additional scale DSM-IV) [9], the Scale of Clinical Global Impression (CGI) [6], Brief Psychiatric Rating Scale (BPRS) [33], Hamilton Anxiety [17] and Depression [16] Scales, the Montgomeri-Ashberg Depression Rating Scale (MADRS) [27], Zung Self-Assessment Depression scale [39, 48] and Spielberg State Trait Anxiety scale [20, 42], as well as the Pennsylvania Scale [13], Obsessive-Compulsive Drinking Scale [2] and Visual Analog Scale assessing craving for alcohol (Table 1). All the above-mentioned measurements were repeated during the three-month trial period, with the intervals given in Table 1.

In addition to those, to confirm the information provided by the patient on his or her alcohol intake, each patient's blood was taken to measure for gamma-glutamiltransferase activity (GGT) at every weekly visit. This enzyme is a marker for excessive alcohol consumption [46]. Every patient filled in a special form at each visit to determine any present side effects from the therapy.

Table 1.

General study flow chart					
Measures	Baseline	Weekly	Monthly	In the middle of the trial	The final point
Criteria of ICD-10	X				
Inclusion/Exclusion criteria	X				
Breath alcohol test	X	X			X
Case history and physical examination	X				
Addiction severity index	X				X
Clinical Global Impression scale	X			X	X
Time Line Follow Back	X	X			X
Brief Psychiatric Rating Scale	X		X		X
General Assessment of Functioning scale	X			X	X
Pennsylvania Alcohol Craving scale	X	X			X
Obsessive - Compulsive Drinking Scale	X	X			X
Visual Analog Scale of Craving	X	X			X

Table 1. (Continued)

General study flow chart					
Measures	Baseline	Weekly	Monthly	In the middle of the trial	The final point
GGT	X	X			X
Compliance with medication and psychotherapy		X			X
Depression scale (MADRS)	X	X			X
Hamilton anxiety scale	X	X			X
Hamilton depression scale	X	X			X
Zung depression scale	X	X			X
Spielberger State Trait Anxiety scale	X	X			X
Psychotherapy		X			
Adverse events		X			X
Remission log		X			X
Drop out log					X

Compliance with escitalopram was estimated in two ways: by counting the capsules not taken by the patient at each of his/her visits and by determining the riboflavin in the patient's urine by fluorescence under the ultra-violet light with the wave length 444 nm.

Irrespective of the therapy kind (whether escitalopram or the placebo was administered), all the patients involved were given a standardized course of medical management which included elements of cognitive behavioral psychotherapy, according to the guidelines for the addiction patients' counseling [36] at every weekly visit. Thus, each patient without exception was given psychotherapy, including those getting the placebo. A general study flow chart is presented in Table 1.

Randomizing and Blinding

Randomization was performed by means of generating random numbers in Excel. The drugs (escitalopram and placebo) were placed into numbered containers. They were given to the patients at each weekly visit over the three months, according to the double blinding principle. The patients had a three-week store of the drug each time, so that their chance missing of 1 – 2 visits could be covered. The investigators, doctors, patients, and any other staff members taking part in the experiment were unaware which of the groups any particular patient belonged to. The randomization code was kept at the Bekhterev Institute and could be unsealed at any moment in emergency.

Excluding from the Trial

A patient was excluded from the study in case of a relapse to heavy drinking. The renewal of heavy drinking for three or more days in a row without a break, as well as missing three or more visits in a row, was considered a relapse (according to the international standards, “heavy drinking” is understood as taking 5 or more standard drinks a day for a male, 4 or more for a female).

STATISTICAL ANALYSIS

The statistical package SPSS was used to manage the data base and to analyze the data.

In order to preserve confidentiality, all the information in the data base was coded, the patients’ names were mentioned nowhere. The difference was considered statistically significant with $p<0.05$.

The statistical analysis can be divided into three parts: a case history analysis, an analysis of the variables changed over the course of treatment and an analysis of side effects. Analyzing the patients’ case histories is necessary to prove the two groups are quite homogeneous, as any effect of the drug can be discovered only when dealing with homogenous groups. The patients’ characteristics included 91 variables: sex, age, biography data, social status and clinical findings. The analysis of the groups’ homogeneity relied on Fisher’s exact test; Kholmogorov-Smirnov’s tests; the Mann-Whitney test; and a T-test for each individual characteristic, depending on its kind, with the measuring scale corresponding to the normal distribution. The conventional significance level of 0.05 was applied. The analyses showed the groups should be considered homogeneous concerning all the measured characteristics. To evaluate the treatment’s effects, a wide range of methods was used. The significanc associated with the differences of psychometric characteristics were assessed by Friedman and Wilcoxon tests (the changes compared to the baseline), the Mann-Whitney test (between group differences), and the ANCOVA with Bonferroni’s test for *post-hoc* comparisons.

While conducting the ANCOVA, the kind of therapy (escitalopram or placebo) and the time (the week of treatment) were used as independent variables, whereas the psychometric measures and alcohol consumption were considered as dependent variables.

To compare the groups as to such characteristics as the reason for completing the project, the amount of heavy drinking days, the quantity of the alcohol consumed, the number of missing visits or giving up the trial, a correspondence table was made and the Fisher exact test was employed. To compare the groups according to the remission (total abstinence – time to first drink) duration within the trial and according to the length of time before renewal drinking, Mann-Whitney and Kholmogorov-Smirnov tests were applied. The trial’s survival analysis was performed by Kaplan-Meier (an inter-group comparison by means of the chi-square test of Mantel-Kox) depending on the event of dropping out of the study for various reasons.

To estimate the side effects, incidence tables were made that included the presence of any side effects and their number, the number of days with the side effects present, and the number of subjects having the side effects, with Fisher’s exact test being used to appraise the significance of the inter-group difference.

Ethical Aspects

The trial has been approved by the ethical committee of the Bekhterev Institute. Every patient had signed his or her informed consent before entering the study. The patients getting the placebo were not left without any treatment because each patient, with no exception, underwent standard medical management (addiction counseling). The confidentiality of any information concerning the patients participating in the trial was provided by the computers and the data bases protecting codes, as well as by the absence of any patient's names on any document, except the informed consent.

Results

Demographic and Clinical Characteristics

The anamnestic data (both demographic and clinical) are given in Table 2.

As it can be seen from the table, the two patients groups did not have any significant differences in any of the characteristic studies (e.g., their age, sex, duration of their alcohol dependence, etc.) (Table 2). No significant differences in their clinical features, including Addiction Severity Index and Brief Psychiatric Rating Scale scores, have been found.

Table 2. Demographics and Clinical Characteristics

Variables		Means by Groups of patients	
		Escitalopram	Placebo
Number of patients		29	31
Age in years		43.9±1.1	40.9±1.3
Sex	male	22 (75.9%)	25 (80,7%)
	female	7 (24.1%)	6 (19,4%)
Employment (%)	works	55.2±0.1	72,0±0,1
	does not work	44.8±0.1	29,0±0,1
AWS duration (years)		11.6±1.4	9.9±1.3
Duration of the loss of control to stop drinking once started to drink (years)		11.5±1.5	9.5±1.4
Duration of the loss of control on the own behavior under the influence of alcohol (years)		9.8±1.3	10.6±1.7

Note:

1. The mean values are given as M+SE;
2. Any significant difference between the groups is absent;
3. AWS is Alcohol Withdrawal Syndrome.

COMPLIANCE DATA

The indicators of the patients' compliance to taking the drugs were measured by the presence of riboflavin in their urine ranged between 65-100% in both groups, showing over 80% at most visits. No difference between the groups has been found.

Anxiety and Depression

Montgomery-Ashberg Scale (MADRS). The initially elevated level of anxiety and depression, rated by a medical doctor (with Hamilton and Montgomery-Ashberg scales), gradually and considerably decreased in both groups of patients over the course of the study (Table 3). Thus, according to MANOVA, a significant decrease of depression by the Montgomery-Ashberg scale took place by the fourth week of the study in the experimental (escitalopram) group, whereas this happened only by the seventh week in the control (placebo) group.

Measured with the MADRS, the level of depression remained significantly lower than the baseline values from the fourth till the thirteenth week of the study in the escitalopram group, whereas this was only the case during the 7th, 9th, 12th and 13th weeks for the placebo group (Table 3).

The depression value (by MADRS) was much lower in the escitalopram group than in the placebo group. Significant differences between the two groups were noticed on the 6th, 8th, 11th and 12th weeks of the study, and on the 5th and 13th week this difference was close to the statistically significant ones (Table 3).

Hamilton Depression Scale (HDS). A significant reduction of depression, according to this scale, occurred in the patients of the escitalopram group by approximately the 4th week of the study; afterwards the depression level remained significantly lower throughout the trial (Table 3). As for the placebo group, the depression values measured with the HDS decreased significantly by the 5th week, but later they differed from the basal ones only on the 8th and 10th-13th weeks. According to this scale, a significantly lower depression level was recorded in the escitalopram group as compared to the placebo group on the 6th week of the trial, whereas on the 9th and 10th weeks the difference between the two groups was close to being statistically significant (Table 3).

Hamilton Anxiety Scale (HAS). According to this scale, the anxiety level associated with the escitalopram group of patients significantly differed from the baseline on the 4th through 13th weeks of the study, whereas this was the case only on the 12th-13th weeks for the placebo group. The anxiety level measured by the HAS was significantly lower in the escitalopram group than in the placebo group on the 5th-11th weeks of the trial (Table 3).

Zung Depression Scale (ZDS). According to the self-assessment Zung Depression Scale, the depression level was significantly different from the baseline on the 4th-13th weeks in the escitalopram group, and on the 6th-11th and the 13th weeks in the placebo group. We have not revealed any significant difference between the two groups concerning this variable (Table 3).

Spielberger State Trait Anxiety Scale (SAS). According to this questionnaire, a significant reduction occurred for state and trait anxieties in the escitalopram group by the 5th-6th weeks of the therapy, remaining significantly lower than the basal ones afterwards.

Table 3. Dynamics of Psychometric Characteristics over the Course of Treatment

Scales	Medication	Psychometric characteristics according to the week of the study (M±SE)												
		1	2	3	4	5	6	7	8	9	10	11	12	13
MADRS	escitalopram	14.9 ±0.6	13.2 ±0.6	12.2 ±0.6	10.9^{+} ±0.7	9.6^{+} ±0.7	8.1^{+} ±0.8	9.4^{+} ±0.8	7.6^{+} ±0.9	6.0^{+} ±0.8	7.4^{+} ±1.0	5.7^{+} ±1.04	5.5^{+} ±1.0	4.4^{+} ±1.0
	placebo	14.7 ±0.5	14.1 ±0.5	13.1 ±0.6	11.9 ±0.7	11.5 ±0.8	11.9* ±0.9	10.8^{+} ±1.0	10.5* ±1.1	8.7^{+} ±1.5	10.4 ±1.3	9.7* ±1.5	8.7$^{+,*}$ ±1.2	7.5^{+} ±1.5
HDS	escitalopram	14.4 ±0.5	12.5 ±0.5	12.1 ±0.6	10.8^{+} ±0.7	9.4^{+} ±0.7	8.6^{+} ±0.8	9.3^{+} ±0.8	8.19^{+} ±0.9	6.3^{+} ±0.8	6.4^{+} ±1.0	5.5^{+} ±1.0	6.4^{+} ±1.0	4.8^{+} ±1.0
	placebo	14.4 ±0.5	13.6 ±0.5	11.7 ±0.6	11.7 ±0.7	10.7^{+} ±0.8	11.2* ±0.9	10.7 ±1.0	9.4^{+} ±1.1	9.4 ±1.4	9.0^{+} ±1.3	7.4^{+} ±1.4	7.7^{+} ±1.2	6.0^{+} ±1.4
HAS	escitalopram	12.0 ±0.5	11.1 ±0.5	10.3 ±0.6	8.8^{+} ±0.7	7.1^{+} ±0.7	6.1^{+} ±0.8	7.3^{+} ±0.9	6.3^{+} ±0.9	5.0^{+} ±0.9	5.0^{+} ±1.0	3.3^{+} ±1.0	5.1^{+} ±1.0	3.3^{+} ±1.0
	placebo	12.0 ±0.5	11.6 ±0.5	10.9 ±0.6	10.3 ±0.7	10.2* ±0.8	10.7* ±0.9	10.0* ±1.0	9.9* ±1.1	9.0* ±1.4	9.0* ±1.3	7.5* ±1.4	7.6^{+} ±1.2	5.7^{+} ±1.4
ZDS	escitalopram	42.5 ±1.1	40.2 ±1.1	37.5 ±1.3	34.1^{+} ±1.4	32.7^{+} ±1.4	29.7^{+} ±1.6	32.2^{+} ±1.7	31.2^{+} ±1.8	30.7^{+} ±1.7	30.5^{+} ±1.9	29.4^{+} ±2.1	27.3^{+} ±2.0	27.1^{+} ±2.0
	placebo	41.5 ±1.8	38.8 ±1.1	37.1 ±1.2	36.8 ±1.4	35.4 ±1.6	33.2^{+} ±1.9	33.1^{+} ±2.0	31.9^{+} ±2.3	27.3^{+} ±3.0	29.3^{+} ±2.7	28.8^{+} ±3.0	33.4 ±2.4	27.6^{+} ±3.0
SAS State	escitalopram	46.4 ±1.3	46.6 ±1.3	45.7 ±1.5	45.8 ±1.6	41.9 ±1.7	38.8^{+} ±1.8	40.7 ±1.9	37.9^{+} ±2.1	39.8 ±1.9	35.8^{+} ±2.2	35.8^{+} ±2.4	34.4^{+} ±2.3	33.5^{+} ±2.8
	placebo	45.9 ±1.2	44.7 ±1.3	41.9 ±1.4	43.8 ±1.6	42.1 ±1.8	39.9 ±2.2	40.7 ±2.3	41.0 ±2.6	38.4 ±3.4	40.0 ±3.1	38.4 ±3.4	41.4 ±2.8	39.0 ±3.4
SAS Trait	escitalopram	48.5 ±1.3	48.2 ±1.3	46.4 ±1.5	44.7 ±1.7	40.4^{+} ±1.7	38.4^{+} ±1.9	39.7^{+} ±2.0	37.1^{+} ±2.1	38.7^{+} ±2.0	35.7^{+} ±2.3	34.5^{+} ±2.5	35.9^{+} ±2.4	34.3^{+} ±2.4
	placebo	47.0 ±1.3	46.5 ±1.3	44.0 ±1.5	44.2 ±1.7	42.1 ±1.9	41.3 ±2.3	39.2 ±2.4	41.8 ±2.7	38.1 ±3.6	40.4 ±3.2	35.1 ±3.6	39.5 ±2.9	37.4 ±3.6
PACS	escitalopram	7.2 ±0.7	6.5 ±0.7	5.8 ±0.8	4.9 ±0.8	2.5^{+} ±0.9	2.1^{+} ±0.9	2.0^{+} ±1.1	2.0^{+} ±1.1	2.7^{+} ±1.1	3.2 ±1.1	2.2^{+} ±1.3	2.2^{+} ±1.2	2.1^{+} ±1.2
	placebo	6.8 ±0.6	5.4 ±0.7	4.6 ±0.7	4.6 ±0.8	3.4 ±0.9	5.8* ±1.1	2.8 ±1.2	3.8 ±1.3	3.1 ±1.8	3.5 ±1.6	3.6 ±1.8	2.8 ±1.4	2.8 ±1.8

Scales	Medication	Psychometric characteristics according to the week of the study (M±SE)												
		1	2	3	4	5	6	7	8	9	10	11	12	13
PACS	placebo	6.8 ±0.6	5.4 ±0.7	4.6 ±0.7	4.6 ±0.8	3.4 ±0.9	5.8* ±1.1	2.8 ±1.2	3.8 ±1.3	3.1 ±1.8	3.5 ±1.6	3.6 ±1.8	2.8 ±1.4	2.8 ±1.8
OCDS	escitalopram	16.2 ±1.1	12.9 ±1.1	11.8 ±1.3	9.7$^+$ ±1.4	5.5$^+$ ±1.4	4.3$^+$ ±1.6	3.5$^+$ ±1.7	3.6$^+$ ±1.8	3.4$^+$ ±1.7	4.0$^+$ ±1.9	3.3$^+$ ±2.1	3.8$^+$ ±2.0	2.3$^+$ ±2.0
	placebo	14.8 ±1.1	10.3 ±1.1	8.8$^+$ ±1.2	9.2 ±1.4	6.9$^+$ ±1.6	10.0* ±1.8	6.1$^+$ ±2.0	8.2 ±2.3	7.0 ±3.0	7.2 ±2.7	8.2 ±3.0	4.4$^+$ ±2.4	3.8$^+$ ±3.0
VASC	escitalopram	2.2 ±0.3	2.0 ±0.3	1.7 ±0.3	1.5 ±0.3	0.8 ±0.3	0.5$^+$ ±0.4	0.7 ±0.4	0.8 ±0.4	0.5$^+$ ±0.4	0.6 ±0.4	0.9 ±0.5	0.8 ±0.5	0.6 ±0.5
	placebo	2.1 ±0.2	1.5 ±0.3	1.5 ±0.3	1.5 ±0.3	1.3 ±0.4	1.6* ±0.4	1.7 ±0.5	1.3 ±0.5	1.3 ±0.7	1.0 ±0.6	1.3 ±0.7	1.2 ±0.6	0.5 ±0.7

Note: **1**. Significance of difference between the placebo group and the escitalopram group (ANCOVA, T-test with Bonferroni correction for a *post hoc* comparison): * is $p<0.05$. **2**. Significance of difference compared to the basal ones at various stages of treatment (ANCOVA, T-test with Bonferroni correction for a *post hoc* comparison): + is $p<0.05$.

Table 4. Gamma-Glutamiltransferase Activity (GGT)

Medication	GGT activity according to the week of study (M±SE)												
	1	2	3	4	5	6	7	8	9	10	11	12	13
Escitalopram	105.7 ±5.5	93.4 ±8.4	82.1 ±8.8	71.0 ±9.2	69.3 ±9.7	53.6$^+$ ±9.2	59.3$^+$ ±11.0	59.8$^+$ ±11.9	65.9 ±10.3	55.9$^+$ ±11.9	55.5$^+$ ±11.0	60.8 ±11.9	60.0$^+$ ±11.0
Placebo	114.8 ±5.7	81.4 ±8.9	82.3 ±9.9	84.6 ±9.7	60.1$^+$ ±9.7	81.2 ±13.0	78.0 ±13.0	57.2 ±16.8	85.6 ±16.8	75.8 ±14.6	73.7 ±16.8	54.2 ±16.8	58.0 ±20.6

Note: **1**. Significance of difference between the placebo group and the escitalopram group (ANCOVA, T-test with Bonferroni correction for a *post hoc* comparison): * is $p<0.05$. **2.** Significance of the difference compared to the basal ones at various stages of treatment (ANCOVA, T-test with Bonferroni correction for a *post hoc* comparison): + is $p<0.05$.

In the placebo group, both of these variables also decreased; however, due to high inter-individual variability, this decrease did not reach a statistically significant level (Table 3). No significant differences concerning these characteristics have been revealed between the two groups (Table 3).

Scales of Craving for Alcohol. Three scales measuring craving for alcohol were used in this study: the Pennsylvania Alcohol Craving Scale (PACS), Obsessive-Compulsive Drinking Scale (OCDS) and Visual Analog Scale of Craving for alcohol (VASC).

According to the PACS, the intensity of craving was significantly different from the baseline in the escitalopram group on the 5th-13th weeks of the study. Although craving for alcohol gradually decreased in the control group, too, the change was not statistically significant. A significant difference in the intensity of craving between the escitalopram and the placebo group were found in the 6th week of the study (Table 3).

Similar changes of craving were noted according to the OCDS, with the values in later weeks being markedly more significantly different from the baseline ones in the escitalopram group, as well as with insignificant changes between group differences observed in the 6th week (Table 3).

According to the VASC, the craving for alcohol was significantly different from the baseline in the escitalopram group in only the 6th and 9th weeks of the study. In the plcebo group, any change, by the given scale, was absent. There were no differences between the groups either (Table 3).

Biochemical Marker of Drinking

Gamma-glutamiltransferase (GGT). The GGT activity in the escitalopream group was statistically significantly lower than the baseline level in the 6th-8th, 10th-11th and 13th weeks of the study, whereas it was as such only on the 5th week in the placebo group (Table 4). Any significant difference in enzyme activity between groups is absent.

Alcohol Consumption and Dropping out

Drop Out

Ten patients completed treatment in remission in the escitalopram group; another ten patients had a relapse; and nine more patients dropped from the study due to other circumstances, unrelated to drinking. In the placebo group, only five people completed the study in remission, 20 patients dropped out due to a relapse, and 6 patients dropped because of other circumstances. The difference between the groups in the number of patients who relapsed and completed treatment was statistically significant ($p<0.05$; Fisher exact test).

The findings of the Kaplan-Meier survival analysis also essentially demonstrated ahigher level of staying in treatment in the group of patients taking escitalopram (Figure 1). The difference between the escitalopram group and the placebo group was statistically significant (Mantel-Cox test = 0.029).

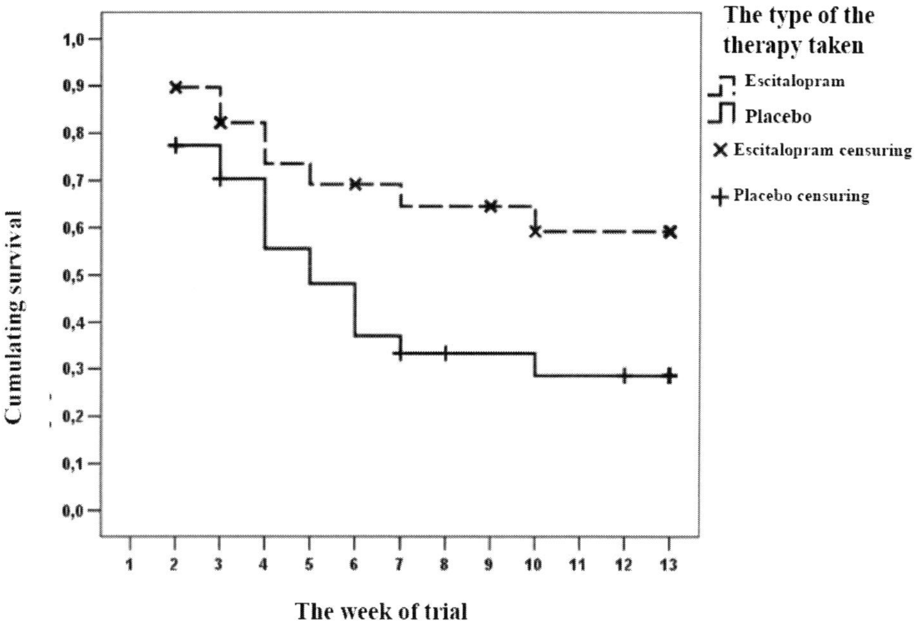

Note:

1. 1 – escitalopram. 2 - placebo.
2. Significance of difference according to the Mantel-Cox chi square method = 0.029.
3. The analysis has been made for the event "relapse".

Figure 1. Kaplan-Meier Survival Analysis.

Alcohol Consumption (Drinking)

The amount of drinking days assessed with the TLFB method was significantly smaller in the escitalopram group (31 days) than in the placebo group (46 days) ($p< 0.05$; Fisher exact test). A relatively small number of alcohol consumption days in the groups is due to the fact that we took into account only slips without relapses to systematic heavy drinking (see above Method section); that is, all patients having a relapse were excluded from the trial on the first day of relapse (see above criteria of exclusion from the trial). The average duration of remission in the escitalopram group (6.6 ± 0.9 weeks) was somewhat higher than in the placebo group (4.9 ± 0.7). However, this difference was not significant. The time to first drink ("break of abstinence") was about the same in both groups: 4.6 ± 3.2 weeks in the escitalopram group vs. 5.0 ± 2.7 weeks in the control group.

General Indicators of the Treatment Effect

Clinical Global Impression Scale (CGI). By the end of the study, "very considerable" or "considerable" improvement was noted in 10 patients of the escitalopram group, and only in 3 patients of the placebo group ($p< 0.05$, Fisher's exact test).

General Assessement of Functioning Scale (GAF). At the baseline, both groups had almost equal estimates by GAF (61.1+1.7 in the escitalopram group; 61.4+ 1.1 in the placebo group). 1.5 months later (the middle of the trial) the GAF scores in the escitalopram group were significantly higher than those of the placebo group (74.3 ± 2.7 vs 62.2 ± 4.3; $p < 0.05$ by the Mann-Whitney test). By the end of the study, approximately the same difference between the groups was maintained (82.0 ± 2.9 in the escitalopram group; 71.7 ± 6.5 in the placebo group; $p=0.1$); however, it did not reach the level of statistical significance due to the decreasing number of patients in both groups by the end of the study and an increasing statistical error of means.

Treatment Tolerability

Adverse Events. Adverse events were recorded in 15 patients out of 29 in the escitalopram group (51.72%), whereas they were noted in 7 patients out of 31 in the placebo group (22.58%) ($p<0.05$, Fisher's exact test). In the excitalopram group, the most frequent adverse events were: irritability, nausea, restlessness, dry mouth, and weight gain. Two patients of the escitalopram group and one person of the placebo group dropped off the study because of the adverse events.

Discussion

The study findings clearly testify that escitalopram is an effective treatment for affective disorders (depression and anxiety) in the initial period of remission in patients ill with alcohol dependence. Even though spontaneous positive dynamics are typical for mild to moderate affective disorders in the initial remission of alcoholism, the severity of depression, according to physician-rated scales (Montgomery-Ashberg and Hamilton scales), reduced much earlier in the patients receiving escitalopram and remained significantly lower than in the placebo group throughout several weeks of the trial. The difference in the anti-anxiety effect between escitalopram and the placebo measured with the Hamilton anxiety scale turned out to be even more pronounced. The anxiety level of the escitalopram group of patients was significantly lower than that of the placebo group throughout most of the study period. According to the patients' rated scales (Spielberger and Zung), changes in anxiety and depression have also demonstrated some advantages associated with escitalopram with a faster reduction of the disorders in patients of the experimantal group. However, there was no significant difference between the two groups according to Spielberger and Zung scales, which appears to be due to a larger inter-individual variability in the subjective assessment of the symptoms. Thus, the findings of the present study quite coincide with those published earlier regarding numerous investigations of marked anti-depressive [3, 14] and anti-anxiety [43, 47] effects of escitalopram.

A faster and more essential reduction of anxiety and depression in patients taking escitalopram was accompanied by a significantly reduced intensity of craving for alcohol, assessed with each of the three scales used for its evaluation in the study. No significant change of craving for alcohol was found in the placebo group. Thus, escitalopram manifested its evident anti-craving effect in alcoholics.

The data on abstinence and alcohol use of the escitalopram group correspond well to those of the escitalopram influence on craving. The patients of the escitalopram group were significantly better in terms of retention in treatment. The number of patients who have completed the project was significantly higher, and the number of days of alcohol use was significantly lower in the escitalopram group of patients. These results are also indirectly confirmed by a more markedly reduced GGT activity (a marker for excessive alcohol use) in the patients taking escitalopram. Thus, the current study demonstrated that escitalopram contributed to remission stabilization and relapse prevention in patients with alcohol dependence. Previously some authors observed the positive effects of citalopram on remission in alcoholism [32], while others - its absence [4, 30]. Escitalopram's effect on remission stabilization and relapse prevention in alcoholism and its marked anti-craving activity, clearly demonstrated in the present study, may have been caused by the inclusion of only those patients with co-morbid affective disorders (mild or moderate depression) into the study. A larger effectiveness of antidepressants for alcoholism treatment in patients with co-morbid depression had been demonstrated earlier in a review by H. Pettinati [34]. This could be due to the intimate interconnection of affective disorders and alcohol dependence. Another possible reason for the higher effectiveness of escitalopram demonstrated in the present study, as compared to the previous contradictive results of administering its predecessor citalopram to treat alcoholism, may be due to higher escitalopram selectivity and strength in inhibiting serotonin reuptake, which results in its superiority over citalopram in the treatment of affective disorders [3, 14].

It should be noted that the physician's general evaluations of the treatment efficacy and social functioning (by CGI and GAF) have also clearly demonstrated that escitalopram has advantages over the placebo. Although the incidence of side effects was significantly higher in the escitalopram group, they were not severe, none of them requiring any special therapy. Only two patients dropped out of the study because of adverse events in the escitalopram group, with one person dropping out of the treatment for the same reason in the placebo group. Thus, this double-blind, randomized placebo-controlled clinical trial showed that escitalopram is effective in treating depression and anxiety of moderate and mild severity in alcohol dependent patients in early remission, it has anti-craving effects and it prevents a relapse to heavy drinking in alcoholics with co-morbid affective disorders.

REFERENCES

[1] Aisberg O.R., Alexandrov A.A. Diagnostic and treatment of alcohol dependence. Minsk, 2007. – p. 22 (in Russian).

[2] Anton R.F., Moak D.H., Latham P.K. The obsessive compulsive drinking scale. *Arch. Gen. Psych.* – 1996. – V. 53. – N. 3. – pp. 225-231.

[3] Aquier P., Robtail S., Lorca P.M., Rive B. Comparison of escitalopram and citalopram efficacy: A meta-analysis. *Int. J. of Psychiatry and Clin. Prac.* 2003. –V.7. – pp. 259-268.

[4] Balldin J., Berggren U., Engel J., Eriksson M., Hard E., Söderpalm B. Effect of citalopram on alcohol intake in heavy drinkers. *Alcoholism: Clinical and Experimental Research.* - 1994. - V. 18. - pp. 1133 – 1136.

[5] Bokiy I.V. Affective disorders in patients with alcohol deprndence and their treatment. *Affective disorders in alcoholism* (edit. Bokiy I.V.). – Leningrad, 1983. – pp. 5-9. (in Russian).

[6] Busner J., Targum S.D., Miller D.S. The Clinical Global Impressions Scale: Errors in Understanding and Use. *Compr Psychiatry.* – 2009. – V. 50. – N. 3. – pp. 257-262.

[7] Caldwell E.E., Miczek K.A. Long-term citalopram maintenance in mice: selective reduction of alcohol-heightened aggression. *Psychopharmacology* (Berl). – 2008. – V. 196. – N. 3. – pp. 407-416.

[8] Crocq M.A. Depression and alcohol. Depression and addiction. *WPA Bulletin on Depression.* – 2001. – V. 5, N. 23. – pp. 1-4.

[9] Diagnostic and Statistical Manual of Mental Disorders: Fourth Edition (DSM-IV) Frances A., Pincus H.A., First M.B. (eds) *Substance Related Disorders.* – 1994. – pp. 325-346.

[10] Eryshev O.F. Nosological comorbidity in substance abuse. Korsakov *Journal of Neurology and Psychiatry.* – 2007. - V. 107 - № 1. - pp. 21-25. (in Russian).

[11] Eryshev O.F., Arkadiev V.V., Ebong K. Modern trends in pharmacotherpy of patients with alcohol dependence. *Psychiatry and psychopharmatherapy.* – 2003. – V. 5. - № 6. – pp. 248-250. (in Russian).

[12] Farren C.K. Serotonin and alcoholism: Clinical and experimental research. *J. Serotonin Res.* – 1995. – V. 2. – N. 1. – pp. 9-26.

[13] Flannery B.A., Volpicelli J.R., Pettinati H.M. Psychometric properties of the Penn alcohol craving scale. *Alc. Clin. Exp. Res.* – 1999. – V. 23. – N. 8. – pp. 1289-1295.

[14] Gorman J.M., Korotzer A., Su G. Efficacy comparison of escitalopram and citalopram in the treatment of major depressive disorders: Pooled analysis of placebo controlled studie. *CNS Spectrums.*- 2002.-V. 7.- pp. 40-44.

[15] Grant B.F., Harford T.C. Comorbidity between DSM-IV alcohol use disorders and major depression: results of a national survey. *Drug Alcohol Depend.* – 1995. – V. 39. – pp. 197-206.

[16] Hamilton M. A rating scale for depression. *J. Neurol. Neurosurg. Psychiatry.* – 1960. – V. 23. – P. 56-62.

[17] Hamilton M. Development of a rating scale for primary depressive illness. *Br. J. Soc. Clin. Psychol.* 1967. – V. 6. – pp. 278-296.

[18] Hautzinger M., Wetzel H., Szegedi A., Scheurich A., Lörch B., Singer P., Schläfke D., Sittinger H., Wobrock T., Müller M.J., Anghelescu I. Combination treatment with SSRI and cognitive behavior therapy for relapse prevention of alcohol-dependent men. Results of a randomized, controlled multicenter therapeutic study. Nervenarzt. – 2005. – V. 76. – N. 3. – pp. 295-307.

[19] Ivanetz N.N., Anokhina I.P. Alcohol dependence. Medical Doctor. – 2004. – № 6. – pp.11-14. (in Russian).

[20] Khanin Y.M. Quick Guide to the scales of reactive and personal anxiety Charles D. Spielberger. LSRIFC. Leningrad., 1976, p. 18 (in Russian).

[21] Koshkina E.A., Spector S.I., Sentsov V.G., Bogdanov S.I. *Medical, social and economic consequences of drug addiction and alcoholism.* – M.: PER SE. – 2008. – p. 288 (in Russian).

[22] Kranzler H.R., Burleson J.A., Korner P., Del Boca F. K., Bohn M.J., Brown J., Liebowitz N. Placebo-controlled trial of fluoxetine as an adjunct to relapse prevention in alcoholics. *American Journal of Psychiatry.* – 1995. – V. 152. – pp. 391–397.

[23] Krupitsky E.M., Iliyk R.D., Eryshev O.F., Tzoy-Podosenin M.V. Modern pharmacotherapy for stabilization of remission and relapse prevention in addiction psychiatry. Bekhterev Review of Psychiatry and Medical Psychology. – 2009. – № 1 (Narcology). – pp. 12–27. (in Russian).

[24] Malin D.I., Yankin E.V., Medvedev V.M., Kovalev A.V. Depression in alcohol dependent patients. Psychiatry and Psychopharmatherapy. – 2004. – V. 6, № 5. – pp. 243-245. (in Russian).

[25] McLellan A.T., Luborsky L., Woody G.E., O'Brien C.P. An improved diagnostic evaluation instrument for substance abuse patients. The Addiction Severity Index. *J. Nerv. Ment. Dis.* – 1980. – V. 168. – N. 1. – pp. 26-33.

[26] Moak D.H., Anton R.F., Latham P.K., Voronin K.E., Waid R.L., Durazo-Arvizu R. Sertraline and cognitive behavioral therapy for depressed alcoholics: results of a placebo-controlled trial. *J. Clin. Psychopharmacol.* – 2003. – V. 23. – N. 6. – pp. 553-562.

[27] Montgomery S.A., Asberg M. A new depression scale designed to be sensitive to change. Br J Psychiatry. – 1979. – V. 134. – pp. 382-389.

[28] Muhonen L.H., Lahti J., Sinclair D., Lönnqvist J., Alho H. Treatment of alcohol dependence in patients with co-morbid major depressive disorder - predictors for the outcomes with memantine and escitalopram medication. *J. Subst. Abuse Treat.* – 2008. – V. 3. – pp. 20-22.

[29] Naranjo C.A., Bremner K.E. Clinical pharmacology of serotonin-altering medications for decreasing alcohol consumption. *Alcohol. Alcohol. Suppl.* – 1993. – V. 2. – pp. 221-229.

[30] Naranjo C.A., Bremner K.E., Lanctot, K.L. Effects of citalopram and a brief psycho-social intervention on alcohol intake, dependence, and problems. *Addiction.* -1995. - V.90. - pp. 87–99.

[31] Naranjo C.A., Kadlec K.E., Sanhueza P., Woodley-Remus D., Sellers E.M. Fluoxetine differentially alters alcohol intake and other consummatory behaviors in problem drinkers. *Clinical Pharmacology and Therapeutics.* – 1990. – V. 47. – pp. 490–498.

[32] Naranjo C.A., Poulos C. X., Bremner K. E., Lanctot, K. L. Citalopram decreases desirability, liking, and consumption of alcohol in alcohol-dependent drinkers. *Clinical Pharmacology and Therapeutics.* – 1992. – V. 51. – pp. 729–739.

[33] Overall J.E., Gorham D.R. The brief psychiatric rating scale. *Psychological Reports.* – 1962. – V. 10. – pp. 799-812.

[34] Pettinati H.M. Antidepressant treatment of co-occurring depression and alcohol dependence. *Biol. Psychiatry.* – 2004. – V.56. – pp. 785–792.

[35] Pettinati H.M., Volpicelli J.R., Kranzler H.R., Luck G., Rukstalis M.R., Cnaan A. Sertraline treatment for alcohol dependence: interactive effects of medication and alcoholic subtype. Alcoholism: *Clinical and Experimental Research.* – 2000. – V. 24. – p. 1041–1049.

[36] Pettinati H.M., Weiss R.D., Miller W.R., Dundon W. Medical Management Treatment Manual: A Clinical Research Guide for Medically Trained Clinicians Providing Pharmacotherapy as Part of the Treatment for Alcohol Dependence. Bethesda, MD: US Department of Health and Human Services: 2004. NIAAA COMBINE Monograph Series, V. 2.

[37] Ross H.E. DSM-III alcohol abuse and dependence and psychiatric comorbidity in Ontario. *Drug Alcohol Depend.* – 1995. – V. 39. – N. 2. – pp. 111-128.

[38] Rossinfosse C., Wauthy J., Bertrand J. SSRI antidepressants and alcoholism. Rev. Med. Liege. – 2000. – V. 55. – N. 11. – pp. 1003-1010.

[39] Rybakova T.G., Balashova T.N. Clinical and psychological characteristics and diagnosis of affective disorders in alcohol dependence. Leningrad., 1988, 27 p. (in Russian).

[40] Salloum I.M., Daiey D.C., Thase M.E. Male depression, alcoholism and violence. UK: Martin Dunitz Ltd., 2000, p. 97.

[41] Sobell M.B., Sobell L.C., Klajner F., Pavan D., Basian E. The reliability of a timeline method for assessing normal drinker college students' recent drinking history: utility for alcohol research. *Addict. Behav.* – 1986. – V. 11 – N. 2. – pp. 149-61.

[42] Spielberger C.D., Gorsuch R.L., Lushene R.E. Manual for the state-trait anxiety inventory. Palo Alto, CA: *Consulting Press*, 1970.

[43] Stahl S., Gergel I., Li D. Escitalopram in the treatment of panic disorder: A randomized, double blind, placebo controlled trial. *J. Clin. Psychiatry.* – 2003. – V. 64. – pp. 1322-1327.

[44] Stella L., Addolorato G., Rinaldi B., Capuano A., Berrino L., Rossi F., Maione S. An open randomized study of the treatment of escitalopram alone and combined with gamma-hydroxybutyric acid and naltrexone in alcoholic patients. *Pharmacol. Res.* – 2008. – V. 57 – N. 4. – pp. 312-317.

[45] Tiihonen J., Ryynanen O.P., Kauhanen J., Hakola H.P., Salaspuro M. Citalopram in the treatment of alcoholism: A double-blind placebo-controlled study. *J. Pharmacopsychiatry.* – 1996. – V. 29. – pp. 27–29.

[46] Vinnitskaya E.V. Alcohol liver disease: clinical course and therapy. *Gastroenterology* – 2007. – № 13. – pp. 53-58. (in Russian).

[47] Waugh J., Goa K. Escitalopram: Review of its use in the management of major depressive and anxiety disorders. *CNS Drugs.* – 2003. – V. 17. – N. 5. – pp. 343-362.

[48] Zung W.W.K. A self-rating depression scale. *Arch. Gen. Psych.* – 1965. – V. 12. – pp. 63-70.

In: The International Psychiatry and Behavioral ...
Editor: Nash Boutros

ISBN: 978-1-62257-566-4

Chapter 17

COMPARATIVE STUDY OF BEER AND HARD LIQUOR USE – RELATED ALCOHOL DEPENDENCY IN SAINT PETERSBURG, RUSSIA*

R. D. Ilyuk*#*, K. V. Rybakova, A. S Kiselev and E. M. Krupitsky
Department of Addictions,
St. Petersburg Psychoneurological Research Institute
named after V.M. Bekhterev, Saint Petersburg, Russia

ABSTRACT

Despite the dramatic increase in beer consumption in the Russian Federation between 1999 and 2009, the incidence and prevalence of alcohol addiction and alcohol psychoses have decreased.

Our study demonstrated that alcohol dependence caused by consuming beer alone is extremely rare (1.2%). 90.3% of study participants consumed different types of alcohol at the same time. Our study of case histories and survey results of alcohol-dependent outpatients with various patterns of hard liquor/beer use demonstrated that alcohol dependence predominantly associated with beer use will correspond with less severe medical and social problems; hard liquor abuse correlates with a higher prevalence of social, legal, somatopsychological problems.

Keywords: alcohol dependence, alcohol abuse, drinks preferences, beer, hard liquor, severity

---

* Original Publication: Ilyuk R.D., Rybakova K.V., Kiselev A.S., Krupitsky E.M. Comparative study of beer and strong alcoholic dependence in Saint Petersburg. Korsakov Journal of Psychiatry and Neurology, 2011, Vol. 211, No. 12.

Mailing address: Department of Addictions, St. Petersburg Psychoneurological Research Institute named after V.M. Bekhterev, 3 Bekhterev St., 192019 Saint Petersburg, Russia, ruslan.iluk@mail.ru

Background

Sociodemographic characteristics of the Russian population are strongly influenced by levels of alcohol consumption [9, 10, 11]: this influence can be direct (such as alcohol poisoning and alcohol-related trauma) and indirect (somatic and psychiatric disorders). The higher the alcohol consumption is, the lower the health indicators are. One of the important impact factors is the alcohol consumption pattern, such as the so-called "northern" and "southern" types of alcohol consumption and abuse [9, 2]. The former is consistent with frequently consuming wine in relatively small doses, and the latter with the less frequent consumption of hard liquor, usually followed by heavy intoxication and aggressive behavior. A correlation exists between the proportion of hard liquor in a country's overall alcohol consumption and life expectancy: countries having a high proportion of hard liquor in their overall alcohol consumption have the men's life expectancy at 10 years less than the women's. In Russia, this gap is 14 years [4, 6]. Those numbers suggest that the change in the structure of alcohol consumption towards a prevalence of soft liquor positively correlated with life expectancy and other health indicators [1, 5]. Considering the prevalence of heavy drinking problems in the Russian Federation, it is important to conduct a comparative study of the severity, characteristics, and socioeconomic impacts of hard and soft liquor dependency.

Study Aims

The aims of the study were to create a complex assessment of the incidence and prevalence of alcohol dependence in the Russian Federation, examine drinking patterns and preferences in alcohol dependent patients, and identify medical and social sequelae of different types of alcohol use in former and current patients of addiction treatment clinics of Saint Petersburg, Russia.

Study Materials

To access the morbidity and prevalence of alcohol dependence and alcohol delirium, we used an open-access nationwide database, local databases of 6 Russian regions and a district database for the Saint Petersburg and Leningrad regions for last 11 years; we also analyzed 200 case histories of alcohol-dependent patients who received inpatient treatment at the addiction treatment department of Bekhterev Institute to study the life and medical histories of patients with different patterns of alcohol use. In addition, we have surveyed 102 random alcohol-dependent patients to access their preferences in alcohol use and interviewed them; we also interviewed 106 patients receiving drug treatment in Saint Petersburg clinics and analyzed the interview data with respect to the type of alcohol predominantly abused by the participants.

Interview subjects had to be men or women between the ages of 18 and 60, diagnosed with alcohol dependence (F-10.2x) as according to the DSM-4, and currently in outpatient treatment at state-run alcohol treatment clinics in Saint Petersburg. The case histories used belonged to men and women between 18 and 70 years of age who were diagnosed with alcohol dependence (F-10.2x).

We had excluded participants with cognitive impairment (as judged by researchers), acute psychosis, and dependence on other drugs (excluding nicotine) from participating in our study.

Study Methods and Instruments

Specifically developed for this study, the study instrument included a set of questions about preferred types of alcohol, the Symptom checklist-90-revised [3], the Drinker Inventory of Consequences–Drinc-2R [7], the SF-36 short-form health survey [12], a visual scale of medical and social functioning (VSMSF), and the Timeline FollowBack (TLFB) [8] scale (as a tool for measuring alcohol use in the last 28 days). SCL-90-R is a multidimensional, self-reporting measure frequently used in clinical and research settings to evaluate and monitor potential problems salient to mental health and substance abuse treatment. The Drinker Inventory of Consequences (DrInc 2-L) (50 items) evaluates lifetime drink-related problems; it has been developed for the Michigan Assistive Technology Clearing House project (MATCH).

The Short-Form Health Survey (SF-36) is used to investigate quality of life through a general evaluation of health. The scale has 36 items which evaluate: physical functioning, role limitation due to physical and emotional problems, bodily pain, general health perceptions, vitality, social functioning, and general mental health.

The TLFB is a method to assess recent alcohol, cigarette, marijuana, and other drug use. It involves asking clients to retrospectively estimate their alcohol, drug, marijuana or cigarette use for a specific time period prior to the interview date. For alcohol, clients are asked to estimate amounts and types of alcohol consumed. For cigarettes and marijuana, individuals are asked to estimate the number of cigarettes or joints smoked per day. (Analyzing the TLFB data, we have used results from the last 28 days of alcohol use. The standard serving of alcohol equals 14 grams of alcohol. A heavy drinking day is a day when the normal daily amount of alcohol was exceeded – 5 or more standard drinks for men, 4 or more standard drinks for women.)

Data Analysis

Data was entered into a Microsoft Access database and exported to SPSS version 12.0 for analysis. To compare the data from the case histories of groups of beer and hard liquor drinkers we used ANOVA and the Mann–Whitney U test. For the evaluation of drinking preferences we used descriptive statistics.

Data collected from 106 current patients of alcohol treatment clinics has been tested using the Kolmogorov–Smirnov test (K–S test) and then (depending on the results) by using ANOVA with the *post hoc* Bonferroni test and Games-Howell test (with Levene's test). Cross tabulation tests and Fisher's exact test have been used for qualitative indicators and variables with a small number of values. Also, Kendall's tau coefficient has been used to measure the associations within each of the groups.

Results of Incidence and Prevalence Analyses

Results from the analysis of the official data from the Russian Ministry of Health suggest that the number of individuals registered with the diagnosis of alcohol dependence was nearly constant during the last 11 years; these numbers even demonstrate a slight (7%) decrease by 2009 (1,524.37 per 100,000 pop.) in comparison with 1,999 results (1,632.51 per 100,000 pop.). The latter is a national trend, but it is specifically visible in Saint Petersburg where the prevalence has dropped 36% (720.06 per 100,000 pop. in 2009 vs. 1,632.51 per 100,000 pop. in 1999). The number of individuals hospitalized with alcohol-related psychoses increased almost 60% by 2003 (96.16 per 100,000 pop.) if compared with 1999 (60.63 per 100,000 pop.). However, starting in 2003, this indicator was decreasing and reached 73.96 per 100,000 pop. in 2009. Some regions (i.e., Saint Petersburg) had a lower prevalence rate in 2009 than in 1999 (25% lower in Saint Petersburg). The dynamic of incidence associated with alcohol dependence is similar to that of the prevalence of alcohol-related psychoses: by 2003, the alcohol addiction incidence increased by 48% to the 1999 level (159.10 per 100,000 pop. vs. 107.96 100,000 pop.) and then decreased to 112.52 per 100,000 pop. in 2009. In some regions (i.e., Saint Petersburg and Leningrad Region), the incidence in 2009 was 48.84 per 100,000 pop., showing an almost 30% decrease in comparison to 1999 (109.32 per 100,000 pop.).

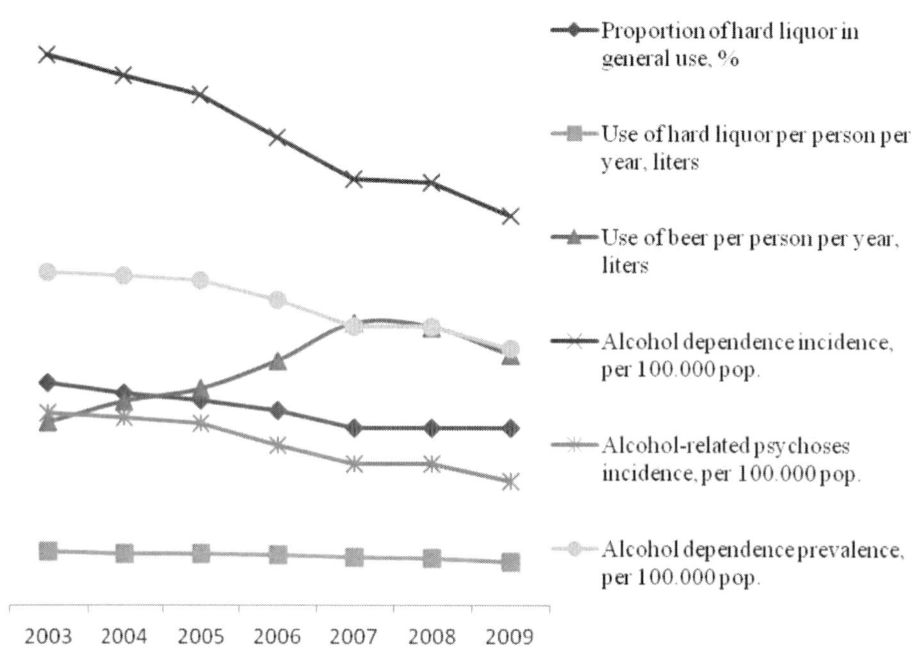

Figure 1.

An almost two-fold increase of incidence associated with alcohol-related psychoses in the Russian Federation and in most of the other regions during the period between 1999-2003 (31.16 per 100,000 pop. to 55.52 per 100,000 pop.) was followed by a decrease in 2004-2009 (54.01 per 100,000 pop. to 35.67 per 100,000 pop.). An analysis of regional differences reveals that the highest rates of incidence and prevalence associated with alcohol dependence and psychoses are typical for regions where the proportion of hard liquor in its overall consumption is higher (e.g., central and northern regions of Russia). These rates are much lower in the South.

Another trend we have found is that the proportions of hard liquor use and hard liquor consumption per person per year have decreased since 1999. This has been accompanied by a simultaneous increase of beer and long drink consumption (Figure 1).

Preferences of Alcohol Use in Alcohol Addiction Treatment Patients

One hundred and two participants have been recruited for this part of the study. Sixteen participants' questionnaires have been excluded from the analysis because of not being completely filled out; 86 questionnaires have been used for analysis. Based on the drinking preferences, we have divided the subjects into 5 groups.

Beer Drinkers – 1.2% of overall number of participants (1 female, 28 years old). The only type of alcohol this respondent consumed during her lifetime was beer.

Hard Liquor Drinkers – 8.1% of participants. The mean age in this group was 47.17 (SD = 6.37) years. These subjects did not consume beer and other types of long drinks during their lifetimes. Within last month, 28.6% of this group used wine and liquors and 71.4% used hard liquor. The largest group of participants was compiled of individuals who used both hard and soft liquors – 78 (90.7%). We have divided them into following groups:

Predominantly Beer Drinkers – 16.3% of participants (14 individuals). The mean age in this group was 41.75 (SD = 12.88). In this group, the proportion of hard liquor used in their lifetimes was lower than 10%. 35.7% of the subjects preferred beer, 21.4% - long drinks, 14.3% - wine and liquors, 28.6% - hard liquor. During the last month, 78.6% of patients preferred beer, 7.1% - soft drinks, 7.1% - hard liquor.

Predominantly Hard Liquor Drinkers – 62.8% of all participants (54 individuals). The mean age in this group was 46.43 (SD = 10.10). In this group, the proportion of hard liquor used in their lifetimes was over 80%; the lifetime preferred drink for 11.3% of patients was beer, for 5.7% - long drinks, 28.3% - wine and liquors, and 54.7% – hard liquor. The preferred drink of the last month for 14.8% of patients was beer, 3.8% - long drinks, 16.7% - wine and liquor and 64,8% - hard liquor.

No Preference Group – 11.6% of all participants. The mean age of this group was 41.6 (SD = 10.57). In this group, the proportion of hard liquor used during their lifetimes was 21–79%. The preferred lifetime liquor for 40% of patients was beer, 10% - long drinks, 20% - wine and liquors, for 30% - hard liquor. During the last month, 60% of patients preferred to drink beer, 40% - hard liquor.

MEDICAL AND SOCIAL CONSEQUENCES OF ALCOHOL DEPENDENCE IN SUBJECTS WITH DIFFERENT PATTERNS OF ALCOHOL DEPENDENCE

The case history analysis (Table 1) revealed that 157 (78.5%) subjects had a diagnosis of alcohol dependency with a predominant use of hard liquor. The other 43subjects (21.5%) diagnosed predominantly drink of beer. Twelve participants preferred strong (over 5% alcohol content) beer and 31 preferred usual beer. The mean age of the predominantly beer drinkers was 39 ± 11, and the age was significantly (p = 0.009) lower than in the hard liquor drinkers' group at 46 ± 10.6. Social and demographical characteristics and somatic health statuses had no statistically significant differences across the groups. Predominantly beer drinkers had significantly (p = 0.01) lower scores on the family adaptation scale of VSMSF: 4.2 ± 2.2 vs. 6.15 ± 2.0 in the predominantly hard liquor drinking group. The age of regular drinking was almost identical for the both groups: 26.8 ± 7.4 and 25.5 ± 7.9 respectively. Regular beer drinking appeared to be associated with a faster onset of the withdrawal syndrome at: 5.1 ± 3.5 years vs. 6.0 ± 2.7 for predominantly hard liquor drinkers. The mean age of developing a withdrawal syndrome was lower than in the hard liquor group – 30.2 ± 9.1 years vs. 32.6 ± 8.1 years (p = 0.04). The severity of the withdrawal syndrome on the VSMSF scale was 5.7 ± 1.0 for hard liquor drinkers and 4.9 ± 1.0 for the beer drinking group (p = 0.01).

Table 1. Medical and social characteristics of alcohol dependent patients

	Predominantly hard liquor drinkers		Predominantly beer drinkers		
	Mean	SD	Mean	SD	P
Age	45.96	10.58	39.04	11.02	0.01*
Social adaptation (family)	4.22	2.18	6.15	2.03	0.01*
Years since first use of alcohol	28.15	10.21	22.47	9.86	0.01*
Years before first episode of withdrawal	6.03	2.68	5.07	3.47	0.04*
Age of first withdrawal episode	32.61	8.13	30.23	9.12	0.04*
Withdrawal severity	5.69	1.00	4.91	1.11	0.01*
Duration of withdrawal	4.74	0.92	4.23	1.07	0.03*
Standard drinks/ last month	280.00	124.45	249.00	111.37	0.02*
Maximal daily alcohol tolerance	353.13	146.88	318.02	133.42	0.02*
Duration of binge	10.75	8.82	6.40	4.22	0.06
Somatic health problems	6.41	1.11	5.60	1.03	0.04*
Mental health problems	7.10	1.59	6.48	1.61	0.02*
Asocial behavior	2.37	1.21	1.91	1.21	0.03*
Number of hospitalizations	3.29	2.86	2.58	2.20	0.19
Number of detoxifications	3.27	2.79	2.79	2.13	0.55

*significant difference ($p \leq 0.05$) in Mann–Whitney U test.

The mean duration of withdrawal in the beer drinkers was 4.8 ± 0.9 days vs. 4.2 ± 1.0 days for hard liquor group (p = 0.03). Twenty one participants had seizures during their withdrawal syndrome; of them, 17 (81%) had a hard liquor dependency and 4 (19%) had a beer dependency. Thirteen patients had alcohol-related psychoses in their medical histories; of them, only 1 has been a beer drinker. Alcohol addiction with the predominant use of hard liquor was characterized by a higher ($p = 0.02$) daily alcohol tolerance at 353 ± 146.9 grams of alcohol vs. 318 ± 132.4 grams for the beer drinkers. Significant differences were also found for alcohol-related mental and physical problem scales of the VSMSF: physical harm from the alcohol use in the hard liquor drinking group was 6.4 ± 1.1 vs. 5.6 ± 1.0 ($p < 0.05$); the mental health scale differences were 7.1 ± 1.6 и 6.48 ± 1.6 ($p = 0.02$) respectively.

Medical and Social Characteristics of Alcohol Dependent Patients in Treatment

Using the "Alcohol Consumption in the Last 28 Days" graph data, 106 study participants hava been divided into five groups:

The hard liquor drinking group consisted of 17 (16.04%) alcohol dependent patients: 12 men (70.59%) and 5 women (29.41%), only drinking hard liquor (vodka, brandy, whiskey, wine). According to the TLFB results, the mean number of hard drinking days was 18.89 (SD = 8.52). In this group, strong beer (over 5% alcohol content) had been used in the past by 3 people (17.65%), beer with less than 5% alcohol content – 1 person (5.88%), hard liquor – 100% respondents. The mean quantity of alcohol used in a day was 129.61 ml (SD = 98.22). The mean age of participants was 43.06 years (SD = 8.36). An attractive motivation for alcohol abuse was found in 9 participants (52.94%), hedonistic – in 8 (47.06%), activational – in 2 (11.76%), submissive – in 1 (5.88%), pseudocultura l– in 2 (11.76%), caused by withdrawal symptoms – in 4 (23.53%). Twelve participants used alcohol alone (70.59%). Sixteen participants (94.12%) received medical treatment for alcohol problems.

The beer drinking group consisted of 30 (28.3%) alcohol dependent patients: 23 men (76.67%) and 7 women (23.33%), only drinking beer. The number of participants in the beer drinking group is larger because we deliberately recruited beer drinkers for our study. According to the TLFB results, the mean number of hard drinking days was 14.57 (SD = 10.87). In this group, hard liquor had previously been used by 14 participants (46.67%), strong beer (over 5% alcohol content) have previously been used by 20 people (66.67%), beer with less than 5% alcohol content – 23 people (76.67%), hard liquor – 14 (46.67%) respondents. The mean quantity of alcohol used in a day was 81.28 ml (SD = 62.40). The mean age of participants was 39.93 years (SD = 10.94). The slow development of a withdrawal syndrome was reported by 4 participants (13.33%), mid-pace development – by 10 (33.33%), and fast – by 16 (53.33). An attractive motivation for alcohol abuse was found for 10 participants (33.33%), hedonistic – for 16 (53.33%), activational – for 3 (10.00%), pseudocultural– for 7 (23.33%), caused by withdrawal symptoms – for 3 (10.00%). Nineteen participants used alcohol alone (63.33%). Twenty-nine participants (96.67) received medical treatment for alcohol problems.

The predominantly hard liquor drinking group consisted of 19 (17.92%) alcohol dependent patients: 13 men (68.42%) and 6 women (31.58%) who were predominantly using hard liquor (over 80% on the heavy drinking days) and much smaller amounts of beer. According to the TLFB results, the mean number of hard drinking days was 12.57 (SD = 6.98) – of them, "hard liquor" days were 12.07 (SD = 7.40) and "beer" days – 0.51 (SD=1.54). For this group, hard liquor had previously been used in 100% of the participants, strong beer (over 5% alcohol content) had previously been used by 8 people (42.11%), beer with less than 5% alcohol content – 14 people (73.68%). The mean quantity of alcohol used in a day was 89.20 ml (SD = 54.07). The mean age of participants was 46.58 years (SD = 10.94).

An attractive motivation for alcohol abuse was found in 14 participants (73.68%), hedonistic – in 10 (52.63%), activational – in 1 (5.26%), pseudocultural – in 2 (10.53%), caused by withdrawal symptoms – in 5 (26.32%). Fourteen participants used alcohol alone (73.68%). 16 participants (84.21%) received medical treatment for alcohol problems.

The predominantly beer drinking group consisted of 21 (19.81%) participants, 19 men (90.48%) and 2 women (9.52%) who predominantly (over 80%) used beer on their hard drinking days and had significantly smaller hard liquor use. According to TLFB results, the number of hard drinking days was 15.96 (SD = 7.10), heavy drinking days with predominant use of beer – 14.48 (SD = 6.66), and hard liquor – 1.49 (SD = 1.06). The lifetime use of beer stronger than 5% was registered in 17 participants (80.95%) and beer with alcohol content less than 5% – 15 participants (71.43%), hard liquor – 100% of the participants. The mean amount of alcohol consumed in a heavy drinking day was 87.08 ml (SD = 44.25). The mean age of participants was 35.57 yers (SD = 8.02). An attractive motivation for alcohol abuse was reported by 10 participants (47.62%), hedonistic– by 14 (66.67%), activational – by 2 (9.52%), submissive – by 1 (4.76%), pseudo cultural – by 10 (47.62%), caused by withdrawal syndrome – by 5 (23.81%). Ten participants (47.62%) used alcohol alone. Seventeen patients (80.95%) received medical help for alcohol dependence.

The no preference group consisted of 19 (17.92%) subjects – 14 men (73.68%) and 5 women (26.32%) without any preferences in alcohol use. The number of heavy drinking days in the TLFB for the patients of this group was 17.73 (SD = 9.46), of them using hard liquor – 7.03 (SD = 4.52) and beer – 10.70 (SD = 6.62). Over their lifetimes, strong beer had been used by 15 participants (78.95%), beer with an alcohol content of less than 5% – 15 participants (78.95%), hard liquor - all 100% participants. The mean daily alcohol consumption was 110.22 ml (SD = 71.63). The mean age was 44.05 years (SD = 8.51). An attractive motivation was found in 5 respondents (26.32%), hedonistic – in 12 (63.16%), activational – in 6 (31.58%), pseudocultural – in 4 (21.05%), and withdrawal-syndrome related – in 9 (47.37%). Fourteen participants used alcohol alone (73.68%). 18 patients (94.74%) received medical help for alcohol abuse.

Statistically significant differences between groups were discovered (Table 2):

The mean age in the hard liquor drinking group was 43.06 years (SD = 8.36), and it was significantly ($p \leq 0.05$) higher than in the predominantly beer drinking group – 35.57 years (SD = 8.02). In the predominantly hard liquor drinking group, the mean age was 46.58 years (SD = 9.06), and it was higher ($p \leq 0.05$) than in the beer drinking group – 39.93 years (SD = 10.94) and the predominantly beer drinking group – 35.57 years (SD = 8.02); in the no preference group, the mean age was 44.05 years (SD = 8.51), and it was significantly higher ($p \leq 0.05$) than in the predominantly beer drinking group – 35.57 years (SD = 8.02).

Using the VSMSF questionnaire, the study on dysfunctional social behavior reveled differences between groups: in the hard liquor drinking group, the rating of dysfunctional social functioning of 5.18 (SD = 3.73) was higher ($p \leq 0.05$), than in the beer drinking group – 2.93 (SD = 2.48) and in the no preference group – 2.47 (SD = 2.22). Similar results were registered in the predominantly hard liquor drinking group, in which group the dysfunctional behavior was more common ($p \leq 0.05$) – 5.16 (SD = 2.61) than in the beer drinking group – 2.93 (SD = 2.48), and no preference group – 2.47 (SD = 2.22).

Table 2. Sociodemographic and clinical characteristics of alcohol dependent patients/ patterns of alcohol use

	Hard Liquor Drinkers		Beer Drinkers		Predominantly Hard Liquor Drinkers		Predominantly Beer Drinkers		No Preference Group	
	Mean	SD	Mean	SD	Mean	SD	Mean	SD	Mean	SD
Age	43.06^{3}	8.36	39.93^{5}	10.94	$46.58^{5,8}$	9.06	$35.57^{3,8,10}$	8.02	44.05^{10}	8.51
Years since first use of alcohol	23.41	8.21	20.03	12.38	26.32	12.97	17.05	7.28	23.63	9.49
Age of first use of alcohol	18.18	5.16	17.70	4.69	18.89	6.15	17.71	3.59	18.84	4.75
Age of heavy drinking	28.12	7.62	26.40	8.36	27.21	6.64	22.19	5.15	26.47	6.99
Dysfunctional social behavior (from 1 to 10 VSMSF)	$5.18^{1.4}$	3.73	$2.93^{1.5}$	2.48	$5.16^{5.9}$	2.61	4.48	3.87	$2.47^{4.9}$	2.22
Problems with law	$7.41^{1.4}$	3.81	$3.57^{1.5}$	4.43	6.79^{5}	4.37	6.24	4.55	4.47^{4}	4.87
Withdrawal syndrome (от 1 до 10 VSMSF)	7.00	2.29	6.07	1.84	6.26	2.05	6.35	2.30	7.37	1.54
Age of amount control loss	30.29	7.99	30.56	10.46	29.47	7.89	26.45	5.67	29.77	8.06
Age of situational control loss	30.07	7.91	31.54	9.56	31.13	8.75	26.95	5.85	29.67	7.53
Maximal daily alcohol tolerance (in lifetime)	19.00	10.31	14.05	8.09	20.58	9.39	17.99	7.79	21.99	12.00
Number of hospitalizations for somatic problems	2.71	3.75	1.73	2.46	1.26	1.10	2.14	1.80	2.16	1.57
Number of remissions after treatment	1.59	2.15	1.90	2.09	1.63	2.31	1.76	3.28	1.58	1.57
Alcohol-related personality changes	1.94	0.66	1.87	0.68	2.11	0.66	1.90	0.62	2.05	0.52
Seizures during withdrawal	1.35	0.49	1.11	0.38	1.11	0.32	1.33	0.48	1.32	0.48

*Significant difference ($p \leq 0.05$) in Mann–Whitney U test: [1] – hard liquor drinkers and beer drinkers, [2] – hard liquor drinkers and predominantly hard liquor drinkers, [3] – hard liquor drinkers and predominantly beer drinkers, [4] – hard liquor drinkers and no preference group, [5] – beer drinkers and predominantly hard liquor drinkers, [6] – beer drinkers and predominantly beer drinkers, [7] – beer drinkers and no preference group, [8] – predominantly hard liquor drinkers and predominantly beer drinkers, [9] – predominantly hard liquor drinkers and no preference group, [10] – predominantly beer drinkers and no preference group.

The scales associated with problems with the law were higher ($p \leq 0.05$) in the hard liquor drinking group – 7.41 (SD = 3.81) than in the beer drinking group – 3.57 (SD = 4.43); in the patients who preferred beer – 6.79 (SD = 4.37), it was higher than in the beer drinkers group – 3.57 (SD = 4.43); in the hard liquor drinking group – 7.41 (SD = 3.81) higher than in the no preference group – 4.47 (SD = 4.87).

The age of the first withdrawal syndrome in the group of predominantly hard liquor drinkers was 35.63 years (SD = 6.97), and it was significantly higher ($p \leq 0.05$) than in beer drinking group – 31.40 years (SD = 9.39). The time before the withdrawal syndrome's first episode was 8.42 years (SD = 3.91) in the hard liquor preference group, and it was higher ($p \leq 0.05$) than in the beer drinking group – 5.0 years (SD = 3.43) and in the no preference group – 5.0 years (SD = 3.07). The same indicator in the hard liquor drinking group was 6.47 years (SD = 3.39), and it was 5.90 years (SD = 3.70) in the predominantly beer drinking group.

Compared with the beer drinkers, psychiatric problems during the withdrawal syndrome were more often (70.59% vs. 30.0%, $p \leq 0.05$) registered by the hard liquor drinking group . Using the VSMSF scale, the study associated with craving intensity demonstrated that the highest level of craving were with the participants from the no preference group – 5.63 (SD = 4.11); that is significantly ($p \leq 0.05$) higher than in the hard liquor drinking group – 1.94 (SD = 2.97), predominantly hard liquor drinking group – 2.84 (SD=3.30) and beer drinking group – 3.97 (SD = 3.38). This indicator was significantly higher in the predominantly beer drinking group – 4.43 (SD = 3.89) in comparison to the hard liquor drinking group – 1.94 (SD = 2.97). In the hard liquor drinkers, craving episodes 1-2 times a week were found more often (58.82% vs. 15.79%, $p \leq 0.05$) than in the no preference group. In comparison to the beer drinking group, we found more patients in the predominantly hard liquor drinking group (63.16% vs. 36.67%, $p \leq 0.05$) that had craving episodes once or twice a week. Furthermore, the difference wassignificantly more (63.16% and 15.79%, $p \leq 0.05$) when compared to the no preference group.

Subjects from the predominantly hard liquor drinking group reported coronary artery disease more often than patients from the beer drinking group (15.79% and 0%, $p \leq 0.05$) and predominantly beer drinkers (15.79% vs 0%, $p \leq 0.05$). Patients from the hard liquor drinking group reported having hypertension stage I more often than patients from the beer drinking group (29.41% vs. 3.33%, $p \leq 0.05$) and predominantly beer drinkers (29.41% vs. 4.76%, $p \leq 0.05$). Hypertension stage II was reported most often by the no preference group (21.05% vs. 0%, $p \leq 0.05$) in comparison with beer drinkers. In the beer drinking group, somatic disorders during the withdrawal syndrome were the most rare when compared with hard liquor drinkers (40.0% vs. 5.88%, $p \leq 0.05$), the no preference group (40.0% vs. 10.53%, $p \leq 0.05$), and predominantly beer drinkers (40.0% vs. 9.52%, $p \leq 0.05$). The mean number of seizure episodes as a complication of the withdrawal syndrome in the hard liquor drinking group, 1.35 (SD = 0.49) was higher than in the predominantly beer drinking group – 1.33 (SD = 0.48). This indicator was even lower in the no preference group 1.32 (SD = 048) and in predominantly hard liquor drinkers – 1.11 (SD = 0.32) and the beer drinkers – 1,11 (SD = 0.38). Alcohol-related personality changes were most often reported by predominantly hard liquor drinkers 2.11 (SD = 0.66), with lower frequencies in the no preference group - 2.05 (SD = 0.52), hard liquor drinkers group - 1.94 (SD = 0.66), predominantly beer drinkers – 1.90 (SD = 0.62) and beer drinkers – 1.87 (SD = 0.68). An attractive motivation for drinking was most frequent at the predominantly hard liquor drinkers (73.68% vs. 26.32%, $p \leq 0.05$) if compared with the no preference group.

SCL-90-R test results (table 3) demonstrated that hard liquor drinkers have a higher rating on the scale of “depression” than in both the beer drinking groups. Predominantly hard liquor drinkers showed a similar trend. The “Phobic symptoms” scale results are higher in hard liquor drinkers than compared with the beer drinkers and predominantly beer drinkers; predominantly hard liquor drinkers demonstrated similar results. The “psychosis” scale results were higher in the hard liquor drinking groups than in the beer drinkers. General severity index results were lower in the beer drinking group than in the hard liquor drinking groups and in the no preference group. The overall sum of the SCL-90-R results across all scales was lower in the beer drinkers than in the hard liquor drinking groups.

SF-34 questionnaire results (table 4) demonstrated statistically significant differences in the “BP” scale – in the beer drinkers, this index was higher than in hard liquor drinkers, predominantly hard liquor drinkers and the no preference group. Statistically significant correlations are presented in Table 5. More details on results of the DrInC-2 instrument are available online: http://bekhterev.spb.ru/content/43/res_alco_report_tables.pdf

Thus, the study of medical and social characteristics of 106 patients with alcohol dependence who were receiving outpatient drug treatment in Saint Petersburg revealed some differences in the characteristics of alcohol dependence depending on the predominant type of alcohol abused. At the time of the study, the youngest participants belonged to the beer-preferring groups of beer drinkers and predominantly beer drinkers; older respondents demonstrated predominantly hard liquor consumption (hard liquor drinkers, predominantly hard liquor drinkers and no preference group subjects).

Social consequences: The most pronounced social and legal consequences of alcohol use are typical for hard liquor drinkers and predominantly hard liquor drinkers. The burden of these problems is caused by early onset of abuse, consumption of higher doses of alcohol and the predominant use of hard liquor on the heavy drinking days. Dysfunctional social behavior, such as absenteeism from work or school, having a blue-collar job or being unemployed, financial problems, and administrative and criminal offenses are more typical for the subjects belonging to the groups of heavy liquor drinkers. In the beer drinking groups these consequences are not as usual.

Medical consequences: Hard liquor drinkers demonstrated a higher frequency of craving, used higher volumes of alcohol, had more acute withdrawal symptoms, and demonstrated a tendency to drink alone rather than in group. Medical interventions for the subjects from this group often are limited to detoxification alone; alcohol-related somatic disorders contribute to the increased severity of withdrawal. Subjects from the no preference group demonstrated the highest craving figures.

Weekly and bi-weekly craving episodes are the most often reported by the beer-preferring participants. Beer use at a young age leads to a more rapid and earlier developing alcohol dependency. A high tolerance and preference for stronger types of beer are associated with more acute episodes of craving. Medical treatment received by the beer drinkers was usually more effective and leaded to a higher proportion of remissions (table 5).

Table 3. SCL-90-R results of alcohol dependent patients/ patterns of alcohol use

Показатель	Hard Liquor Drinkers		Beer Drinkers		Predominantly Hard Liquor Drinkers		Predominantly Beer Drinkers		No Preference group	
	Mean	SD	Mean	SD	Mean	SD	Mean	SD	Mean	SD.
SCL-90 Somatization (SOM)	0.89	0.56	0.59	0.39	0.95	0.57	0.68	0.64	0.80	0.70
SCL-90 Obsessive-compulsive disorders (O-C)	0.91	0.57	0.61	0.45	0.79	0.46	0.53	0.41	0.70	0.66
SCL-90 Interpersonal sensitivity (INT)	0.73	0.61	0.46	0.42	0.78	0.55	0.52	0.60	0.71	0.64
SCL-90 Depression (DEP)	$1.04^{1,3}$	0.61	$0.60^{1,5}$	0.55	$1.02^{5,8}$	0.66	$0.63^{3,8}$	0.54	0.80	0.73
SCL-90 Anxiety (ANX)	0.91	0.70	0.57	0.41	0.78	0.44	0.75	0.66	0.76	0.70
SCL-90 Hostility (HOS)	0.79	0.69	0.41	0.32	0.68	0.58	0.70	0.67	0.47	0.40
SCL-90 Phobic Anxiety (PHOB)	$0.46^{1,3}$	0.55	$0.17^{1,5}$	0.27	$0.36^{5,8}$	0.36	$0.20^{3,8}$	0.36	0.29	0.51
SCL-90 Paranoid Symptoms (PAR)	0.77	0.40	0.44	0.44	0.54	0.61	0.65	0.62	0.68	0.64
SCL-90 Psychosis (PSY)	0.35^{1}	0.41	$0.19^{1,5}$	0.32	0.36^{5}	0.28	0.33	0.48	0.34	0.59
SCL-90 Sum	71.29^{1}	38.43	$45.13^{1,5}$	30.63	68.74^{5}	35.31	52.62	43.77	60.68	54.69
SCL-90 General Severity Index GSI	0.79^{1}	0.43	$0.50^{1,5,7}$	0.34	0.76^{5}	0.39	0.58	0.49	0.67^{7}	0.61
SCL-90 Present Symptomatic Distress Index PSDI	1.66	0.45	1.38	0.34	1.50	0.39	1.39	0.37	1.51	0.55
SCL-90 Positive Symptom Total PST	41.47	16.01	31.30	16.08	44.16	16.91	33.57	20.25	36.68	21.79

Significant differences between groups ($p \leq 0.05$) in Mann–Whitney U test: [1] –hard liquor drinkers and beer drinkers, [3] – hard liquor drinkers and predominantly beer drinkers, [5] – beer drinkers and predominantly hard liquor drinkers, [7] – beer drinkers and no preference group, [8] – predominantly hard liquor drinkers and predominantly beer drinkers.

Table 4. SF-36 results of alcohol dependent patients/ patterns of alcohol use

Показатель	Hard Liquor Drinkers		Beer Drinkers		Predominantly Hard liquor Drinkers		Predominantly Beer Drinkers		No Preference group	
	Mean	SD.	Mean	SD	Mean	SD	Mean	SD	Mean	SD
SF-36 Physical functioning (PF)	91.18	13.75	88.50	19.35	81.32	22.41	87.14	15.94	87.89	13.16
SF-36 Role physical functioning (RP)	45.59	42.61	69.17	42.39	44.74	40.47	64.29	43.71	61.84	40.28
SF-36 Pain (BP)	71.59[1]	22.98	88.23 [1,5,7]	17.41	67.58[5]	21.93	80.00	27.14	72.11[7]	24.53
SF-36 General health (GH)	52.88	19.67	56.87	18.86	55.68	20.32	54.38	17.57	56.37	17.49
SF-36 Vitality (VT)	55.29	15.56	54.50	18.82	50.00	20.68	55.95	15.94	49.21	27.60
SF-36 Social functioning (SF)	63.24	22.74	71.25	24.38	60.53	24.39	67.86	21.50	65.79	20.35
SF-36 Role emotional functioning (RE)	56.86	46.79	67.78	44.19	35.09	39.24	68.25	41.47	66.67	44.44
SF-36 Mental helath (MH)	58.82	14.41	59.73	16.20	50.53	17.95	57.52	15.20	50.53	23.26
SF-36 Physical health (PHc)	47.99	7.73	51.89	8.57	48.10	8.07	49.99	7.07	49.92	7.08
SF-36 Mental health (MHc)	40.32	10.08	41.56	10.17	35.46	12.02	41.46	9.47	38.68	11.33

Significant differences between groups ($p \leq 0.05$) in Mann–Whitney U test : [1] – hard liquor drinkers and beer drinkers, [5] – beer drinkers and predominantly hard liquor drinkers, [7] – beer drinkers and no preference group.

Table 5. Statistically significant correlations between alcohol use/alcohol use consequences indicators

Hard liquor drinkers ($p \leq 0.05$)	Withdrawal severity (VSMSF)	Mean daily alcohol intake (0.39)
	Duration of withdrawal	Mean daily alcohol intake (0.40)
	Number of treatment episodes	Number of treatment episodes limited with detox only (0.51)
	Ago of situation control loss	Family relationships (–0.44)
	Age of first alcohol use	Alcohol-related mental health problems (VSMSF) (–0.39)
	ANX (SCL-90)	Age of first episode of regular drinking (–0.37) and age of first episode of withdrawal (–0.38)
	GSI (SCL-90)	Age of first episode of regular drinking (–0.40) and age of first episode of withdrawal (–0.40)
	Interpersonal relationships problem (DrInC-2)	Age of first use of alcohol (–0.36), Mean daily alcohol intake (–.047), number of remissions (–0.41)
Predominantly hard liquor drinkers ($p \leq 0.05$)	PHOB (SCL-90)	Years of alcohol use (0.35)
	Duration of withdrawal	Number of hospitalizations for somatic disorders (0.39)
	Severity of withdrawal (по VSMSF)	O-C (SCL-90) (0.46), VT (–0.34), MH (SF-36) (–0.35)
	Dysfunctional social behavior (VSMSF)	Hard liquor heavy drinking days/ heavy drinking days (0.42), beer drinking days/ heavy drinking days(–0.42)
	Years of drinking alcohol	PF (–0.42), PHc (SF-36) (–0.35)
	Age of starting of regular drinking	Maximal day alcohol tolerance (–0.38), O-C (SCL-90) (–0.37), INT (SCL-90) (–0.36), PAR (SCL-90) (–0.58)
	PAR (SCL-90)	Age of the first episode of withdrawal syndrome (–0.37)
Beer drinkers ($p \leq 0.05$)	Number of treatment episodes	Number of remissions (0.37)
	Spontaneous remissions	Number of hospitalizations with somatic disorders (0.43), mean day dose of alcohol (TLFB) (–0.45),number of days of heavy drinking (TLFB) (–0.43); use of strong beer during last year (–0.48)
	Craving level (VSMSF)	Proportion of strong beer in overall alcohol used (0.33)
	Years since the first alcohol use	Mental health problems related to alcohol use (VSMSF) (0.27)
	Somatic problems (VSMSF)	Mean daily dose of alcohol (0.38)
Predominantly beer drinkers ($p \leq 0.05$)	Withdrawal severity (VSMSF)	Maximal daily tolerance (0.38), number of treatment episodes (0,.35)
	Age of situation control lost	Maximal daily alcohol tolerance (0.39)
	Withdrawal syndrome duration of development (years)	Mean daily alcohol intake (–0.46)
	Usual binge duration	RE (SF-36) (–0.42), MHc (SF-36) (–0.34)
	Number of spontaneous remissions	Dysfunctional social behavior (DrinC-2) (–0.49)
	RE (SF-36)	Age of loss of amount control (–0.39)

No Preference Group ($p \leq 0.05$)	Craving level(VSMSF)	Mean weekly dose of alcohol (0.67)
	Somatic health problems (VSMSF)	Mean weekly dose of alcohol (0.67)
	HOS (SCL-90)	Problems with law (0.56)
	Currently working	Mean weekly dose of alcohol (–0.73)
	Dysfunctional social behavior (VSMSF)	Age of regular alcohol use (–0.43), age of amount control loss (–0.69) and situation control loss (–0.63)
	Age of regular alcohol use	O-C (SCL-90) (–0.52), DEP (SCL-90) (–0.51), ANX (SCL-90) (–0.47), FOB (SCL-90) (–0.43)
	Age of the first withdrawal episode	O-C (SCL-90) (–0.43), DEP (SCL-90) (–0.46), ANX (SCL-90) (–0.40), FOB (SCL-90) (–0.41)
	Age of amount contol loss / situation control loss	O-C (SCL-90) (–0.64/–0.63), DEP (SCL-90) (–0.57/–0.55), ANX (SCL-90) (–0.59/–0.64), FOB (SCL-90) (0/–0.46)
	Remissions as a result of treatment	DEP (SCL-90) (–0.45), FOB (SCL-90) (–0.52)
	Intrapersonal problems (DrinC-2)	Age of first use (–0.42), withdrawal duration (–0.36)

Beer drinkers consumed less alcohol per day and were generally more responsive to the treatment, but their withdrawal syndromes might be more severe in cases of high tolerance to alcohol. In these groups, patients with an early onset of addiction problems had higher alcohol tolerance and heavier drinking days within the last month. Regarding medical problems, subjects from the hard liquor drinking group are more likely to have seizures during the withdrawal syndrome (possibly caused by the toxic effectassociated with high doses of ethanol on the CNS).

Patients from these groups have higher proportions of coronary heart diseases and hypertension. Also, subjects from hard liquor groups are more likely to report other medical problems. Beer drinkers have less medical problems and pains that can interfere with active living.

Psychiatric problems: Alcohol-related personality disorders are more typical for subjects from hard liquor drinking groups: in our study, they demonstrated the highest rates on depression, phobic anxiety and psychosis scales of the SCL-90.

In the case of hard liquor drinkers, the early onset of alcohol problems is accompanied by psychiatric symptoms including anxiety and hostile behavior. A heavy withdrawal syndrome in this group of patients is correlated with high rates on the obsessive-compulsive scale and has a negative impact on a daily life.

In the No Preference group, the early onset of alcohol problems as associated with high rates on depression, anxiety, phobic anxiety, paranoid, and obsessive-compulsive scales of the SCL-90. For patients of this group, the severity of personality disorders is proportional to the significance of addiction problems.

In beer drinkers, the consumption of massive amounts of alcohol provokes more severe psychiatric complications. Patients with the early onset of alcohol problems demonstrate more emotional problems. Prolonged periods of beer use are associated with impulsivity and decreased levels of behavioral control.

LIMITATIONS

The study had a relatively small sample size; results of the study are partly based on data provided by the subjects that might have caused a recall of memory bias, attention bias, and bias related to researchers' interpretation of subjects' interviews.

CONCLUSION

Our analysis of the alcohol dependence incidence/prevalence official data from the Ministry of Health suggests that between 1999 and 2009 the incidence/prevalence figures did not increase significantly; the last 7 years of this period demonstrated a downward trend for these indicators.

The above changes have occurred despite an increase in consumption of beer and long drinks in Russia during that period and may be associated with a decrease in their share in the total consumption of alcohol. The distribution analyses of drinking preferences demonstrated that alcohol-dependent patients mostly drink both hard liquor and beer. The sole use of beer is rare – only 1.2% of participants reported it; 8.1% of alcohol- dependent patients in the study would only drink hard liquor or wine. In the group of patients drinking hard liquor, long drinks and beer, 90.7% prefer hard liquor.

An analysis of case histories of alcohol-dependent patients demonstrated that, despite its relatively rapid formation, beer dependence shows a slower progression than in the case of hard liquor. Alcohol dependence with the predominant use of beer is associated with consuming less alcohol, a milder withdrawal syndrome with fewer complications. An evaluation of alcohol-dependent patients in drug treatment demonstrated that hard liquor drinkers used more pure alcohol, had more hard drinking days and more medical and social problems during the last month than beer drinkers.

Higher proportions of hard liquor in the consumption are associated with a more severe dependence, and physical and mental disorders. The mixed drinking pattern and use of beer with higher alcohol content is associated with a higher craving. Beer drinkers have better chances to receive effective treatment. The beer drinkers are likely to have less medical and social problems than beer/hard liquor or only hard liquor users.

REFERENCES

[1] Alcohol in postwar Europe: A discussion of indicators on alcohol consumption and alcohol-related harm. ECAS II / Ed. by. H. Leifman, E. Osterberg, M. Ramstedt. – Stockholm: *National Institute of Public Health, European* Commission, 2002. P.237.

[2] Alcohol in postwar Europe: Consumption, drinking patterns, consequences and policy responses in 15 European countries. ECAS I // Ed. by T. Norstrom. – Stockholm: *National Institute of Public Health, European Commission,* 2001, pp.213-19.

[3] DeRogatis L.R. SCL-90-R administration, scoring and procedures manual // Baltimore, 1977. — P. 4–8.

[4] European Health for All database, 2008: http://www.human-resources-health.com/content/6/ 1/8.

[5] Global Status Report on Alcohol –World Health Organization, *Department of Mental Health and Substance Abuse*. – Geneva. – 2004, P.94.

[6] International Profile. Alcohol and Other Drugs. – WHO. – Toronto, Ontario. – 1994. – p.175.

[7] Miller, W.R., Tonigan, J.S. and Longabaugh, R. (1995). The Drinker Inventory of Consequences (DrInC): An Instrument for Assessing Adverse Consequences of Alcohol Abuse. Project MATCH Monograph Series, Vol. 4. DHHS Publication No. 95-3911. Rockville, MD: *National Institute on Alcohol Abuse and Alcoholism.*

[8] Sobell, L.C, Agrawal, S., Sobell, M.B., Leo, G.I., Young, L.J., Cunningham, J.A., Simco, E.R. Comparison of a quick drinking screen with the timeline followback for individuals with alcohol problems. J. *Stud. Alcohol* 64: 858-861, 2003.

[9] Vrublevsky A.G. Varianty alcogolisma: zakonomernosti techeniya i principy prognosirovaniya. – Moscow, Medicina, 1989. – 49 p.10. Nemtsov A.V. Alcogolnaya istoria Rossii: Noveyshiy period. – Moscow.: MNIIP, «Librocom», 2009. – 320 p. 11. Politika po kontrolu krisisnoy smertnosti v perehodny period. / Editors Shkolnikov V.M., Chervyakov V.V. – Moscow.: *PROON*, 2000. – 191 p.

[10] Ware J.E., Kosinski M. Interpreting SF-36 summary health measures: a response // *Qual. Life Res.* — 2001. — Vol. 10, № 5. — P. 405–413.

In: The International Psychiatry and Behavioral ...
Editor: Nash Boutros

ISBN: 978-1-62257-566-4

Chapter 18

TREATMENT OF FAMILY CODEPENDENCY AS A FACTOR PROMOTING REMISSION IN OPIATE ADDICTS

Natalia Baranok[*]
The State Health Care Center,
Murmansk Regional Narcological Center Murmansk, Russia

ABSTRACT

During their participation in a12-month outpatient rehabilitation program,142 opiate addicts (age 26.3±2.1 years, 96 males, 46 females)were randomly assigned to one of two groups: relatives of patients from thefirst group participated in the 12-month program consisting ofindividual and group behavioral interventions aimed to treat co-dependence,whereas therelatives of patients fromsecond group received only a few sessions of routine counseling for relatives of drug addicts. Patients of both groups were treated alike with an opiate antagonist (naltrexone) and cognitive behavioral intervention. Patients of the first group demonstrated significantly better rehabilitation outcomes: better retention in their rehabilitation program, a higher rate of abstinence, improved social functioning and a stronger motivation to stay clean.

Keywords: Opiate dependence, rehabilitation, codependence

INTRODUCTION

Studies in the areas of remission and relapse associated withopiate dependence are important due to theirhigh prevalence rate, constantly growing incidence rate, and a relatively low response rate. Among top-priority tasks of modern addiction psychiatry is to develop

[*] Natalia Baranok, Chief of the social rehabilitation department of the state health care institution "Murmansk Regional Narcological Center". Business phone number: 8(8152) 45-69-42, Mobile phone number: 8-921-2722511, E-mail: drbaranok@mail.ru

effective methods of treatment and rehabilitation. Together with pharmacotherapy, psychosocial methods are very important in drug abuse treatment (e.g., psychotherapeutic treatment, therapeutic community, Narcotics Anonymous, etc.). Considering that pharmacological methods of remission stabilization in opiate dependence treatment are limited by compliance, lack of readiness to change, and some other factors, it is extremely important to develop effective psychosocial interventions to improve compliance with pharmacotherapy and to prevent a relapse.

According to M.V.Demina et al. [5], among opiate addicts who seek treatment, over 70% come from so-called "intact families", enablingfamily members of drug addicts to participate in the rehabilitation process. The importance associated withthe role of family members in the treatment and rehabilitation processesof drug addicts is obvious. It is quite common that a family develops a state of codependency if one of their members is an addict. There is no consistent definition of that term; furthermore, if relationships in families with a drug addict wereinitially called "codependent", now the term is considered to be wider in psychological publications and refers to any close relations where an inadequate obsession with some other person's life leads to an adjustment disorder [6, 7].

Researchers give different interpretations to codependency in families of drug addicts. Some suggest that codependency is a kind of addictive behavior; others try to find in it some features of an endogenetic process (protracted atypical endogenous depression with a prevailing anxiety depersonalized symptomatology and paranoiac reactions) [5]. According to V.D. Moskalenko [2], codependence is a way of pathologic personality development. Distinctive psychopathologic abnormalities of codependents, revealing features of their peculiar lifestyle and attitude toward themselves and others, come within the ICD 10 (International Classification of Diseases) as "Disorders of adult personality and behavior".

The behavior of codependent relatives is not only a factor that maintains drug use, but quite often it even complicates the process of treatment and rehabilitation, as the inadequate behavior of the codependent person, either directly or by implication, leads to the patient's refusal of further treatment and involvement in rehabilitation programs, and, inturn, to the relapse.

Research Aim

The aim of this study was to study how treatingthe codependence in relatives (who participate in a special psychotherapeutic program) of patients with opiate dependence influences the effectiveness of the opiate dependence treatment.

Materials and Methods

The study inclusion criteria included: an initially low potential for rehabilitation (less than 45 on Potential Rehabilitation Scale), lack of permanent job, living together with relatives, and diagnosis of codependence symptoms in the latter. During the 45-day program of in-patient rehabilitation,142 opiate addicts (average age [M±SD]26.3±2.1 years; 96 men, 46 women) were randomly divided into 2 groups: the relatives of the first group participated in a special codependence rehabilitation program, whereasthe relatives of the other group received only brief routine drug counseling. The first group included 70 patients (49 men, average age – 26.5±3.6 years, average duration of drug use – 6.5±3.5 years); the second group was composed of 72 patients (47 men, average age – 26.5±2,. years, average duration of drug use – 7.2±3.4 years). Amajor fractionof the patients had a college education (80% in the first group, 76% in the second). There was no significant difference between the groups in terms of clinical and demographic characteristics.

All patients completed a full course (45 days) of in-patient rehabilitation (a psychotherapeutic program based on a cognitive behavioral approach) and were transferred to an outpatient rehabilitation program. All patients at the outpatient treatment stage (6 months) were administered either an oral opiate receptor blocking agent, naltrexone (50 mg/day, 67 people in the first group and 68 people in the second one), or an injectable, long acting, sustained release naltrexone (Vivitrol, 380 mg monthly, 3 patients in the first group and 4 in the second). Within the first two months, patients weekly visited an addiction psychiatrist for a counseling session and urine drug tests. Then, during the period from 3 to 6 months, patients attended a clinic every other week, andthen monthly during the following 6 months. All patients were administered a urine drug test monthly (immunoassay method). The psychometric test battery included a Scale of a Rehabilitation Potential (RP) [3] administered during the period of in-patient rehabilitationat6 months and oneyear after starting the rehabilitation program, as well as a study of the patient's motivational attitudes with the "Motivation for Drug Consumption and Quitting" (MDCQ) [1],administereda week before finishing the in-patient rehabilitation course, and then again 3 and 6 months after participatingin the rehabilitation program.

The relatives of patients in both groups were examined at the very beginning of the study during the period of in-patient rehabilitation in order to measure the severity of codependence with the Structured Clinical Interview based on criteria outlined in the paper of B.Weinhold and J.Weinhold [4]. All relatives participated in the study were diagnosed as codependent according to criteria of a rating scale for codependence [4], and then randomized into either a special program of psychotherapy for codependent persons which included group sessions twice a month and individual counseling (initially – weekly, then – twice a month) throughout the period of treatment (12 months) (1 group), or attended only several routine sessions of brief, individual counseling for relatives of drug addicts (2 group). Relatives of patients in both groups had a high level of codependece (56±4.5 on the scale of B.Weinhold and J.Weinhold in the first group, 60.5±3.8 – in the second one). 80% of the relatives of patients in the first group attended 82% of appointed sessions during the treatment regimen's participation period.

Theproportion of patients in remission was the primary outcome variable demonstrating the effectiveness associated withthe treatment of drug dependence. Changes of rehabilitation potential and motives for quitting drugs were secondary indicators.

RESULTS

According to the results, the numbers of patients in remission in the first group after 3, 6 and 9 months of treatment weresignificantly higher than in the second group (Table 1). The difference between the groups at 12 months was close to the level of significance.

Table 1. Proportion of patients in remission during treatment

Groups	Percentage of patients in remission during treatment [number of patients (%)]				
	1 month	3 months	6 months	9 months	12 months
1 group	56 (80)	45 (64)	26 (37)	22 (31)	19 (27)
2 group	51 (71)	34 (47)*	15 (21)*	12 (17)*	10 (14)+

Note: Statistical significance of differences between the groups (Fisher's exact test):
* - $p<0.05$; + - $p=0.062$

Table 2. Total intensity of the motivational factor for drug use during treatment (Motivation for Drug Use Scale)

Groups	Intensity of the motivational factor for drug use at different stages of treatment (M±SD)		
	1 month	3 months	6 months
1 group	54.7±13.9	35.8±5.9	20.6±4,4
2 group	55.2±8.9	45.1±9.1*	23.8±4,1*

Note: Statistical significance of differences between the groups (Student t-test): * - $p<0.05$.

Initially, the groups did not differ significantly on the Motivation for Drug Use Scale in terms of the rate of motivation for drug use (Table 2). The structure of motivation did not differ either: low levels of conformativemotives and high levels of euphoric motives prevailed in both groups.After 3 months, a large decline associated with thegeneral intensity of the motivational factor for drug use in both groups occurred; however, in the first group,those motives were less intenseat both 3 and 6 months than in the second (Table 2).

At the beginning of the study,motivations for quitting the drugs and the structure of motives on the Motivation for Drug Use Scale did not differ significantly between the groups.Furthermore, the average intensity of the factor was 63.4±7.2 in the first group and 62.6±9.3 in the second group;the motive associated withavoiding family problems was the strongest in both groups; and motives associated withpoor living conditions, fear of stigma, problems at work and concerns about their health were less important.

A significant increase of the total intensity associated with the subjects'motives for quitting had failed to occur in both groups during the period of treatment: after a 3-month period, the total intensity of motives for quitting was 70.2±9.4 in the first group and 67.5±7.2 in the second one, after a 6-months interval – 73.2±4.1 and 72.1±5.2 respectively. However, at the three-month time point, the motive for avoiding family problems became significantly higher in the first group compared to the second one: 10.0±1.7 vs. 8.1±2.0 ($p<0.05$).The rehabilitation potential of the patients in both groups was growing in direct correspondence with the duration of remission in the groups (Table 3), mainly owing to Block III (social status) and Block II (clinical symptoms) of this instrument. The rehabilitation potential in the first group of patients after 6 months of treatment increased and reached the normative level, whereasthe level of rehabilitation potential forthe the second group ofpatients remained at a relatively low level (Table 3). The differences in the rehabilitation potential between two groups were significant at6 months of treatment, basically owing to more pronounced positive changes of the social status of the patients in the first group.

DISCUSSION

The results of this study demonstrated that, throughthe process of codependency management,the involvement of relatives of the patients suffering from opiate dependence makes it possible to increase the rate of abstinence, and duration and remission. In addition, in the hierarchy of motives to quit opiates, treating the codependence of relatives contributes to a decreasedgeneral level of motivation for drug use and an increasedmotivation for avoiding family problems.

When in the rehabilitation process,changing forms of relatives' codependent behaviorsfor more constructive ones, leads to a faster increase of rehabilitation potential forthose patients with an opiate addiction . The increase of RP occurs mainly dueto a faster re-socialization of the patients motivated to improve their family and work status, possibly because of more adequate behaviorson the part oftheir relatives, affording the patients an opportunity to be autonomous (i.e., self-sufficient, owing to a considerable decrease of hyper-protection by relatives – up to its total lack thereof).

A study associated withthe psychological features of mothers of drug addicts with an opiate dependence demonstrated thatthose relatives who did not participate in a correction program for their codependent behavior showed a tendency to restrict the patient's self-sufficiency [7].

Table 3. Changes of Rehabilitation Potential over the course of remission

Groups	Changes of Rehabilitation Potential over the course of remission (M±SD)					
	1 month		6 months		12 months	
	Overall RP index	Block III of RP	Overall rehabilitation potential index	Block III of RP	Overall RP index	Block III of RP
Group 1	40.5±5.6	7.5±2.8	64.3±3.8	24±4.2	73.3±2.8	31±2.2
Group 2	37.4±7.1	6±2.8	50.2±4.2*	17±3.4*	71.5±2.2	29.5±2.6

Note: Statistical significance of differences between the groups(Student t-test): * - $p<0.05$.

CONCLUSION

1. Involving opiate addicts' relatives in a psychotherapeutic codependence treatment program increases the effectiveness of the opiate dependence treatment.
2. The social adaptation proceeds faster for those opiate addicts whose relatives participate in the codependence treatment program, resulting in a positive impact witha significantly faster growth rate of rehabilitation potential.

3. Involving opiate addicts' relatives in a psychotherapeutic program for managing codependence contributes to a faster and pronounced decrease in the intensity of motivation for drug use.
4. Avoidance of family problems is a leading motive for quitting opiates in the hierarchy of motives to quit drugs, and its intensity depends on the successful management of codependent behavior patterns of patients' relatives.

REFERENCES

[1] Baranok N.V. A study of motivation of opiate addicts for drug use and to quit drugs. *Medical Academic Journal,* 2010. Vol. 10. No. 5. – p. 199. (in Russian).

[2] Moscalenko V.D. Codependency: a family disease – M.: *PER SE*, 2004. – 26 p. (in Russian).

[3] Protocol "Rehabilitation of drug addicts (Z50.3)". Ministry of Health of the Russian Federation as of 22.10.2003 № 500 «Patient management protocol 'Rehabilitation of drug addicts (Z50.3)». URL: http://rudoctor.net/medicine2009/bz-jw/med-kmzag/index.htm (access date 18.03.2011). (in Russian).

[4] Weinhold B., Weinhold J., *Breaking Free of the Codependency Trap*. Published in Russian: Moscow: Class, 2003, p.224.

[5] Chirko V.V., Demina M.V. Parents of Drug addicts: Psychopathology of codependency. *Problems of Addiction Psychiatry* (VoprosyNarcologii), 2005, No. 2, p.19–29 (in Russian).

[6] Shapoval I.A. *Living a life of codependence*. – Moscow: University book, 2009, p. 40.

[7] Shishkova A.M. Psychological aid to mothers of drug addicts. *Bulletin of the Russian State Pedagogical University named afer A.I. Gertsen*., 2008, V.29 (65), p. 470-475 (in Russian).

VIOLENCE

In: The International Psychiatry and Behavioral ...
Editor: Nash Boutros

ISBN: 978-1-62257-566-4

Chapter 19

The Psychosocial Impact of Political Violence on Palestinian and Jewish Adolescents*

Alean Al-Krenawi#
Memorial University, St. John's Newfoundland, Canada

Abstract

A sample of school-attending adolescents, both girls and boys, aged 14-18 (453 Jewish and 508 Palestinian) participated in this study. The research instruments included a traumatic events survey (TEV), Brief Symptoms Inventory (BSI), PTSD questionnaire, Peer Relations questionnaire (PRQ), Aggression questionnaire (AQ), and Family Assessment Device (FAD). Exposure to political violence was shown to have negative effects on mental health. Findings revealed that Jewish participants reported more exposure to political violence, and Palestinian participants reported more symptoms of somatization, phobic anxiety, psychoticism, PTSD, family functioning problems, and aggression (specifically physical aggression and anger). Parental education, socio-economic status (SES) and family stresses are discussed in relation to these findings. The Palestinians since 1948 have experienced a double trauma of exposure to political violence and negative social and psychological response to the discrimination and racism against them in Israel. The conclusion considers implications for policy and practice.

Keywords: Political violence, PTSD, Palestinians, Israeli, adolescents

---

* Original Publication: Alean Al-Krenawi. The Psychosocial Impact of Political Violence on Palestinian and Jewish Adolescents. The Arab Journal of Psychiatry (2010) Vol.21 No.2Page (112- 136).
# Corresponding author: Alean Al-Krenawi, PhD. Professor and Dean, School of Social Work. aalkrenawi@mun.ca, alean@bgu.ac.il

Introduction

Exposure to political violence is related to post-traumatic stress disorder (PTSD), depression, anxiety, and behavioral problems [3, 24, 35, 73]. But it may also be associated with such positive outcomes as pro-social behaviour and positive self-esteem [46]. The present paper is among the first to compare Jewish and Palestinian adolescent respondents to political violence within Israel. Results show high levels of problems in both populations. In contrast to previous scholarship[21], the paper finds that Palestinians reported less exposure to political violence but experienced higher impacts. One of the major factors explaining this differential experience was socioeconomic status (SES). By focusing on both populations living in Israel, greater insight can be obtained into similar and divergent subjective experiences of political violence. Consequently the nature of the required medical and allied disciplinary responses to political violence can be tailored to suit these needs.

Political Violence in the Israeli Context

War was part of the Middle East prior to the 1948 creation of Israel and continues since that date [48]. Since September 2000, many people have been killed and injured as a result of the ongoing political violence, with numbers much higher in the West Bank and Gaza Strip [8, 21]. People from throughout the region are directly vulnerable to political violence, and experience it daily and vicariously through the experiences of those with whom they are close [48].

Today, Israel is home to approximately 7.6 million people. Of these, about 1.5 million or 19.4% are Palestinian. Eighty-two percent of the Palestinians in Israel are Muslim, 9% are Christian, and 9% are Druze [51]. Prior to 1948, Palestinians made up the majority of inhabitants of Palestine, but subsequent to the establishment of the state of Israel, 84% of the Palestinian population was exiled and became refugees [41]. Those who were left became a minority. About a quarter of those who remained were displaced from their homes to other locations, thus becoming internal refugees [13, 74].

The Palestinian minority is considered to be a society in transition, caught between Eastern and Western cultures due to the process of Westernization within Israel [2, 1]. The Palestinian minority has significantly higher rates of poverty, unemployment, infant mortality and school attrition than the Jewish majority [58]. Many Palestinian Arabs in Israel live under a military regime and experience social exclusion, leaving them in a conflict of dual identity as both Israeli and Palestinian. Although they live in the state of Israel, their selfidentification has been shown to be more emotionally connected with being Palestinian and with the Palestinians in the Occupied Territories [32]. Furthermore, it has been postulated that the Israeli component of the Arabs' collective identity does not include a sense of belonging to the state, identifying with it, and developing a sense of attachment because the national superstructure excludes their identity [59].

Since its inception, the very definition of Israel as a Jewish state has cast Arab national identity and social status into ambiguity [59]. Social identity is thought to be the means through which individuals understand themselves in their social context. Moreover, understanding the processes of identity formation in the context of intergroup conflict is particularly important, since social identity is critical to understanding how people act. When groups are in conflict, their members are placed under great pressure to conform to the values and practices of the favoured group [23]. Furthermore, the period of adolescence is a critical time where individuals are searching to secure a stable and consistent identity [71]. Palestinian adolescents' identity is a combination of identity formation during adolescence, the reality of belonging to a traditional culture in a Western nation, and the unique manifestations of the Israeli context, in which Muslim adolescents are viewed as part of a "hostile" non-assimilating minority. Relating to the Jewish-Israeli perspective, Kelman states that inherent to Jewish-Israeli identity is the negation of the Palestinian "other" and the portrayal of this other as "the enemy" [42]. Palestinians experience a double trauma of exposure to political violence, and negative social and psychological responses. As such, this study raises questions about the identity of Arab youth in Israel. A previous study on Palestinian communities in Israel reveals strong identity towards Palestinian national heritage and negative attitudes towards Israeli policies towards Palestinian citizens. Authors have categorized the Arab minority in Israel as significant, non-assimilating (differing from the majority in language, religion, nation, culture and ethnic descent), dissident (rejecting the State's official ideology of Zionism), and hostile (viewed by the Jewish majority as untrustworthy) [61]. Nonetheless, Smooha asserts that a hybrid identity is emerging that may be referred to as "Palestinians in Israel" and that "conveys the primacy of Palestinian affiliation and orientation, without renouncing Israeli connections" 62. In addition, Amara & Schnell's empirical study found that Arabs in Israel feel strongly attached to at least three identities [12]. The identity of Muslim adolescents in Israel reflects the components of identity of the adult Muslim population in Israel outlined here. Furthermore, the identity of Muslim adolescents in Israel is an amalgamation of identity formation during adolescence, the reality of belonging to a traditional culture in a Western nation, and the unique manifestations of the Israeli context, in which Muslim adolescents are viewed as part of a "hostile" non-assimilating minority. In fact, Hujierat (2005) [38] pointed out that the identity of Muslim adolescents in Israel may change with the political situation evident in a specific moment in time.

The same study asked Muslim adolescents in Israel to categorize themselves as Muslim, Arab, or Palestinian and found that those whose major identity was Muslim had relatively low collective self-esteem. [38]. Furthermore, the group that chose to characterize themselves as Muslimexpressed little interest in acculturation into Israeli society. Thus, the findings of the study pointed out that the Arab youth in the Israeli context are living in a multi-traumatic environment; they are exposed to political events, and living in the margins of Israeli society compare to their Jewish peers but having identity problems from living in two different worlds simultaneously.

The Jewish population in Israel is highly diverse. A country of immigrants, the majority remain Sephardim (European origins), with the remainder Ashkenazi (from other parts of the world). Most places on the globe are represented. Recent places of migration include Russia, the former Eastern Bloc countries, and Ethiopia. The post-1967 context has seen a considerable number of Jewish settlements constructed in the West Bank and Gaza Strip, although now only those in the West Bank remain. Recent estimates hold that upwards of 300,000 settlers are in the West Bank [44]. There are tremendous variances in SES and most other well-being indicators throughout the Jewish sector of Israel. It is vital to emphasize the heterogeneity of this population. Palestinians in Israel and Jewish-Israelis often live in separate cities, although there are major centers that mix the two backgrounds, including: Jaffa, Tel Aviv, Haifa, Akko, Lod, and Ramlah.

Methodology

The sample consisted of school-attending adolescents, both girls and boys, aged 14-18 from Israel (453 Jewish and 508 Palestinian). The sample was recruited from three urban centers: Tel-Aviv, Jaffa and Haifa. These three centers are district cities with heterogeneous populations in culture, religion and class. Additionally, the sample was recruited from Ariel, s a West Bank settlement that is more homogeneous. All three cities were subject to suicide bombings and other politically violent events since the outbreak of the Intifada in September 2000. To ensure comparable internal diversity, the Palestinian sample was recruited from Palestinian-villages, cities and mixed cities where Palestinian and Jewish peoples live. We randomly selected schools and then randomly selected co-educational classes (grades 8-12) within the schools. Graduate and undergraduate students were trained to distribute and administer the the data collection, including answering any respondent queries. Research assistants were both gender and ethnically matched with the students. Thus Jewish-Israeli schoolgirls were interviewed by Jewish-Israeli female research assistants, etc.

The Following Research Instruments Were Used

1) *Background Socio-demographic Questionnaire* – Thirteen items covered the socioeconomic status of participants' family, their parent's education, gender, ethnicity, age, family structure and dwellings.

2) *Political Violence* – To assess level of exposure to political violence, the researcher created an 18-item Traumatic Event Questionnaire[7] tailored to each community's primary language (Hebrew or Arabic), and to modes of exposure to political violence (for example, questionnaire asked about bomb to Palestinian-Israeli adolescents or missile attacks to Jewish-Israeli adolescents). The responses had nominal scales on self-reported individual and friend/relative exposure. The total score was computed by summing all positive answers (range of scale 0–18) with a higher score indicated more exposure to political violence. The internal reliability of the questionnaire was adequate among both the Jewish adolescents (Cronbach's alpha = 0.71) and among Palestinian-Israeli adolescents (Cronbach's alpha = 0.85).

3) *Mental Health* – Mental health was assessed by clinically relevant psychological symptoms in adolescents. For this aim the Brief Symptom Inventory (BSI) was used [19, 23]. This measure consists of 53 self-reported items covering nine symptom dimensions: somatization, obsession-compulsion, interpersonal sensitivity, depression, anxiety, hostility, phobic anxiety, paranoid ideation, psychoticism; and a composite measure of General Severity Index (GSI). A mean score was computed for each sub-scale and it ranged from 0-4 with a higher score indicating more mental health problems (scores of 2.52 and above indicate Positive clinical diagnosis). The internal reliability of the nine odd-scales is adequate (Cronbach's alpha = 0.71-0.81) and the test-retest reliability is satisfactory (r= 0.60-0.90). The measure also has a moderate level of validity, which was measured by comparison to the

MMPI. Norms and scores among youth populations in Israel and the United States are available for comparison. The internal reliability of the current measure, in general, and of its sub-scales was measured in a Jewish research population [60] with reasonable results (Cronbach's alphas range from 0.62 to 0.90). In the current study the reliability of the sub-scales among the Jewish-Israeli adolescents was Cronbach's alpha 0.66–0.85 and 0.95 for the GSI, and among the Palestinian-Israeli adolescents 0.64–0.86 for the sub-scales and 0.96 for the GSI.

4) *PTSD – Post-traumatic stress disorder* was measured by the PTSD Symptom Scale: The PSS-I [31]. This measure is a 17-item instrument in which each symptom is rated on a 4-point scale. Sub-scale scores are calculated by summing items in each of the PTSD symptom clusters: re-experiencing, avoidance and arousal. A mean score was computed for each sub-scale and total scale with results ranging from 1–4, with a higher score indicating more PTSD. The scale has high internalconsistency (Cronbach's alpha = 0.85) and moderate to high correlations with other measures of psychopathology. The PSS-I has high test-retest reliability (r = 0.80) and inter-rater reliability (k = 0.91). In the current study the reliability of the total score was Cronbach's alpha 0.88 and sub-scales ranged from 0.76–0.79 among the Jewish-Israeli adolescents and 0.89 for total score and 0.74–0.79 for the sub-scales among the Palestinian-Israeli participants.

5) *Social Functioning* – To assess the social functioning of the adolescent participants we used the Peer Relations questionnaire, which is a standard measure for assessing peer group relationships [37]. The questionnaire, consisting of 25 questions, is suitable for respondents aged 12 and older. The sum score of the instrument was computed (ranging from 0-100), with a higher score indicating more problems in relationships with friends. The measure has a cut-off point at 35 points: individuals who score below 35 are categorized as being within the norm and those who score above 35 are categorized as having problems. The measure has high internal reliability (Cronbach's alpha = 0.94) and a low standard measure error (4.44). The peer group measure also has high validity and is able to discriminate between clinical and normal populations. Based on prior research the internal reliability of the measure has been found to be high in an Israeli study of Jewish adolescents 60 (Cronbach's alpha = 0.93, N=146), and in studies among Bedouin-Arab adolescents (Cronbach's alpha = 0.89, N=256) [11]. The reliability of the scales among the Jewish-Israeli adolescents in the current study was Cronbach's alpha 0.93 and 0.92 among the Palestinian-Israeli adolescents.

6) *Aggression* –To assess adolescents' aggressive responses and their ability to channel those responses in a safe, constructive manner, the Aggression Questionnaire (AQ) was used. This 34-item instrument 17 assesses adolescents' aggression on four sub-scales: physical aggression, verbal aggression, anger and hostility. A mean score was computed for each sub-scale and total scale. Each scale ranges from 1-5 with a higher score indicating more aggressive behaviors. The internal consistency of the AQ is relatively high (Cronbach's alpha = 0.89). The AQ is a stable instrument with good test-retest correlations of 0.80. Scores on the AQ sub scales were moderately correlated with each other. However, when the variance in the correlations due to the anger score was partialed out, correlations were not significant. This supports the theoretical validity of the AQ in that the associations between physical aggression, verbal aggression, and hostility are due to their connection with anger. Scores also had good concurrent validity [22]. In the current study the reliability among the Jewish-Israeli participants was Cronbach's alpha 0.89 for the total scale and 0.72–0.85 for the sub-scales,

and among the Palestinian-Israeli participants 0.90 for the total scale and 0.67–0.85 for the sub-scales.

7) *Family Functioning*– In order to assess the overall health and pathology of participants' family functioning The McMaster Family Assessment Device (FAD) was used [26, 40]. The FAD describes structural and organizational properties of the family group and the patterns of transactions among family members which have been found to distinguish between healthy and unhealthy families. This instrument includes 60 items on six dimensions of family functioning and one general functioning scale. All sub-scales range from 1-4, with a higher score indicating more problems in a family's functioning. Cut-off points discriminating between "clinical" and "normal" families in American populations are available, though there are none for Israeli families. The scale has satisfactory reliability (Cronbach's alpha = 0.72-0.92), good test-retest reliability (r = 0.66) and high validity, as indicated by comparing the scale's scores to other measures of the same matters [26, 50]. Due to the lack of relevant cut-off points, we used only the 12 items that assess the family's general functioning. A recent study [55] found that these 12 items give a satisfactory picture of the family's general functioning. In the current study the reliability among was adequate (Cronbach's alpha 0.84 among Jewish-Israeli adolesencents and 0.72 among the Palestinian-Israeli adolescents).

Data analysis proceeded in four parts. First we examined differences between the two ethnicities using T test and Chi square analysis s. Second we examined the associations between ethnicity and participant exposure to traumatic events, psychosocial, family functioning, PTSD and aggression using xx. Third, we examined the association between political violence and dependent variables using Pearson correlations. Finally, we conducted multiple regressions to assess how political violence and ethnicity are associated with the dependent variables.

RESULTS

Table 1 shows the results of Chi-square tests and independent sample t-tests. Jewish-Israeli parents had higher education, higher SES, and lower unemployment than their Palestinian-Israeli counterparts.

Table 2 shows that Jewish-Israeli adolescents reported more exposure to political violence than Palestinian-Israeli adolescents. No consistent results were found regarding mental health symptoms, using the general severity index. Palestinian-Israeli participants reported more phobic anxiety, psychoticism, PTSD, family and social problems, and aggression (physical), while Jewish-Israeli participants reported more paranoid ideation and aggression (verbal). Table 3's shows that political violence had a positive significant correlation for Jewish-Israeli participants on the general severity index and the PTSD index and aggression, but not on family or social functioning. For Palestinian-Israeli participants, political violence was found to correlate with mental health symptoms, aggression, family and social functioning. These associations with political violence remained significant af controlling for economic status, parents' education, gender, and religiosity. As summarized in table 4, respondents exposed to greater political violence reported higher levels of various mental health symptoms (somatization, obsession-compulsion, depression, anxiety, hostility, phobic anxiety, paranoid ideation, psychoticism, GSI), and more PTSD symptoms.

Table 1. Socio-demographic variables by ethnicity

	Jewish-Israeli (n=453)	Palestinian-Israeli (n=508)	Significant test
Gender, %			
Male	44.9	37.9	$\chi 2 = 4.59$*
Female	55.1	62.1	
Age, mean (sd)	15.35 (0.66)	15.53 (1.02)	t=3.03**
Religiosity, %			
Very religious	4.8	4.5	$\chi 2 = 23.65$***
Religious	34.2	36.3	
Traditional	51.4	40.6	
Not religious	9.6	18.6	
No. of siblings, mean (sd)	2.00 (1.14)	3.66 (1.83)	t=16.31***
Father's education			
Less than 8 years	2.4	10.5	$\chi 2 = 47.09$***
8-9 years	8.1	15.5	
10-11years	14.0	12.0	
12 years	39.2	24.9	
13 years or more	36.3	37.1	
Mother's education			
Less than 8 years	1.6	8.6	$\chi 2 = 60.85$***
8-9 years	4.0	14.2	
10-11 years	8.4	10.3	
12 years	45.9	30.5	
13 years or more	40.0	36.5	
Father's employment status			
Works	87.7	75.8	$\chi 2 = 21.24$***
Does not work	12.3	24.2	

Table 1. (Continued)

	Jewish-Israeli (n=453)	Palestinian-Israeli (n=508)	Significant test
Mother's employment status			
Works	80.4	61.9	$\chi 2$ =166.91***
Does not work	19.6	38.1	
Parents' marital status			
Married	83.8	90.4	$\chi 2$ =8.95**
Unmarried	16.2	9.6	
Family' economic status			
Low	4.1	5.5	$\chi 2$ =30.74***
Average	55.4	37.0	
High	40.5	57.4	

* $p<0.05$; ** $p<0.01$; *** $p<0.001$.

Table 2. Political violence and psychological functioning by ethnicity

	Jewish-Israeli (n = 453)		Palestinian-Israeli (n = 508)		t value
	Mean	SD	Mean	SD	
Political Violence					
Traumatic Events Questionnaire	3.11	2.61)	2.21	(2.78)	5.05***
Mental Health Symptoms (BSI)					
Somatization	0.81	(0.71)	0.84	(.66)	0.85
Obsession-Compulsion	1.16	(0.80)	1.19	(.64)	0.53
Interpersonal Sensitivity	1.01	(0.90)	0.99	(.79)	0.21
Depression	0.96	(0.76)	0.95	(.77)	0.25
Anxiety	1.13	(0.77)	1.06	(065)	1.52
Hostility	1.11	(0.93)	1.12	(.77)	0.09
Phobic Anxiety	0.56	(0.60)	0.82	(067)	6.11***
Paranoid Ideation	1.36	(0.87)	1.14	(.75)	4.04***
Psychoticism	0.77	(0.75)	0.85	(.67)	1.74*
General Severity Index	0.99	(0.64)	1.00	(.56)	0.30
Post-traumatic stress disorder (PTSD)					
PTSD Symptom Scale	1.29	(0.39)	1.25	(.48)	7.97***
Re-Experiencing	1.28	(0.44)	1.53	(.56)	7.44****
Avoidance	1.24	(0.39)	1.47	(.53)	7.38***
Arousal	1.37	(0.52)	1.59	(.58)	6.00***
Family Functioning					
Family Assessment Device	1.81	(0.51)	1.91	(0.46)	3.07**
Social Functioning					
Index of Peer Relations	17.79	(14.49)	19.24	(15.58)	1.45
Aggression					
Buss-Perry Aggression Questionnaire	1.99	(0.58)	2.21	(.60)	3.40***
Physical Aggression	1.83	(0.78)	2.08	(085)	4.72***
Verbal Aggression	2.57	(0.82)	2.46	(.78)	2.01*
Anger	1.79	(0.67)	2.11	(.70)	7.05**
Hostility	1.97	(0.67)	1.96	(.69)	0.14

PTSD – Post traumatic stress disorder; BSI – Brief symptom inventory.

* p <.05; ** p<.01; *** p<.001.

Table 3. Pearson product moment correlation coefficients between measures: Jewish-Israeli participants above the diagonal, andPalestinian-Israeli participants below the diagonal

	1	2	3	4	5	6
1. Political violence	.20***	.27***	.07	.06	.17***	
2. General Severity Index (GSI)	.20***		.47***	.47***	.39***	.54***
3. Post-traumatic stress disorder (PTSD)	.31***	.58***		.25***	.23***	.25***
4. Family Assessment Device (FAD)	.18***	.40***	.36***		.42***	2.9***
5. Index of Peer Relations (IPR)	.17***	.42***	.37***	.38***		.25***
6. Aggression	.21***	.39***	.40***	.14***	.24***	

Table 4. Political violence, nationality, and socio-demographic variables as predictors of Psycho-social functioning: Standardized coefficients (β), unstandardized coefficients (b) and 95% confidence intervals of multiple regression

	Political violence	Nationality	Economic status	Parents education	Gender	Religion	R^2	F value
Mental health symptoms (BSI)								
Somatization								
Β	.16***	.07*	-.18***	.04	.19***	-.03	.10	15.21***
B	.04	.10	-.12	.02	.26	-.03		
95% CI	.02 to .05	.01 to .19	-.16 to -.08	-.02 to .07	.17 to .35	-.09 to .03		
Obsession-compulsion								
Β	.15***	.04	-.20***	-.01	.13***	.02	.09	13.76***
B	.04	.06	-.14	-.01	.19	.02		
95% CI	.02 to .06	-.03 to .16	-.18 to -.09	-.06 to .04	.09 to .28	-.04 to .08		
Interpersonal sensitivity								
β	.13***	.04	-.25***	.03	.20***	.04	.13	20.69***
b	.04	.07	-.20	.02	.44	.05		
95% CI	.02 to .06	-.04 to .18	-.25 to -.15	-.03 to .07	.23 to .45	-.02 to .12		
Depression								
β	.13***	.04	-.25***	.03	.20***	.04	.13	20.69***
b	.04	.07	-.20	.02	.44	.05		
95% CI	.02 to .06	-.04 to .18	-.25 to -.15	-.03 to .07	.23 to .45	-.02 to .12		

	Political violence	Nationality	Economic status	Parents education	Gender	Religion	R^2	F value
Depression								
β	.18***	.04	-.25***	-.01	.14***	-.03	.12	20.08***
b	.05	.07	-.18	-.01	.22	-.03		
95% CI	.03 to .07	-.04 to .17	-.23 to -.13	-.05 to .04	.13 to .32	-.10 to .03		
Anxiety								
β	.15***	-.02	-.17***	-.01	.20***	.06	.11	17.37***
b	.04	-.03	-.11	-.01	.29	.05		
95% CI	.02 to.06	-.13 to .06	-.16 to -.07	-.05 to .03	.20 to .39	-.01 to .11		
Hostility								
β	.17***	.05	-.12***	.01	-.01	.02	.05	7.13***
b	.05	.08	-.10	.01	-.01	-.01	.03	
95% CI	.03 to .07	-.03 to .20	-.185 to -.05	-.05 to .06	-.13 to .10	-.05 to .10		
Phobic anxiety								
β	.11**	.22***	-.19***	.05	.19***	.02	.14	22.56***
b	.03	.28	-.12	-.03	.25	.02		
95% CI	.01 to .04	.19 to .36	-.16 to -.08	-.07 to .01	.17 to .33	-.04 to .07		
Paranoid ideation								
β	.17***	-.10**	-.16***	.02	.12***	.03	.09	14.07***
b	.05	-.16	-.12	.01	.19	.03		
95% CI	.03 to .07	-.27 to -.05	-.17 to -.07	-.04 to .07	.09 to .30	-.04 to .10		
Psychoticism								
β	.18***	.10**	-.24***	-.03	.12****	-.02	.12	19.03
b	.05	.15	-.16	-.02	.18	-.02		
95% CI	.03 to .06	-.01 to .15	-.17 to -.10	-.04 to .04	.14 to .29	-.04 to .06		
General Severity Index								
β	.20***	.06	-.24***	-.01	.18***	.01	.14	22.80***
b	.04	.07	-.14	-.01	.22	.01		
95% CI	.03 to .06	-.01 to .15	-.17 to -.10	-.04 to .04	.14 to .29	-.04 to .06		
Post traumatic stress disorder (PTSD)								
PTSD								
β	.30***	.31***	-.14***	-.02	.10**	-.01	.18	31.63***
b	.05	.27	-.06	-.01	.09	-.01		

Table 4. (Continued)

	Political violence	Nationality	Economic status	Parents education	Gender	Religion	R^2	F value
95% CI	.04 to .06	.21 to .23	-.08 to -.03	-.03 to .02	.03 to .14	-.04 to .04		
Re-experiencing								
β	.26***	.29***	-.13***	-.02	.11**	.02	.16	26.54***
b	.05	.29	-.06	-.01	.11	.02		
95% CI	.04 to .06	.22 to .36	-.09 to -.03	-.04 to .02	.05 to .18	-.03 to .06		
Avoidance								
β	.26***	.28***	-.14***	-.02	.06	.01	.14	23.88***
b	.04	.26	-.06	-.01	.06	.01		
95% CI	.03 to .06	.20 to .32	-.09 to .03	-.04 to .02	-.01 to .12	-.04 to .04		
Arousal								
β	.26***	.24***	-.10***	.01	.10**	-.02	.12	19.54***
b	.05	.27	-.05	.01	.11	-.02		
95% CI	04 to .07	.19 to .34	-.08 to -.02	-.04 to .04	.04 to .18	-.06 to .03		
Family functioning								
Family assessment device								
β	.13***	.14***	-.19***	-.09*	-.06	-.10**	.09	14.01***
b	.02	.14	-.09	-.04	-.06	-.06		
95% CI	.01 to .04	.07 to .20	-.11 to .06	-.07 to -.01	-.13 to .01	-.10 to -.02		
Social functioning								
Index of peer relations								
β	.12***	.05	-.20***	-.01	-.07*	-.04	.06	9.70***
b	.02	.06	-.10	-.01	-.08	-.03		
95% CI	.01 to .04	-.02 to .13	-.14 to -.07	-.04 to .03	-.15 to -.01	-.08 to .02		
Aggression								
Buss-Perry aggression questionnaire								
β	.18***	.14***	-.05	-.03	-.13***	-.01	.06	9.76***
b	.04	.17	-.03	-.02	-.16	.01		
95% CI	.02 to .05	.09 to .25	-.07 to .01	-.05 to .02	-.24 to -.08	-.05 to .06		

	Political violence	Nationality	Economic status	Parents education	Gender	Religion	R^2	F value
Physical aggression								
β	.14***	.19***	-.02	-.05	-.32***	.01	.14	23.77***
b	.04	.31	-.02	-.04	-.53	.01		
95% CI	.02 to .06	.21 to .42	-.07 to 03	-.09 to .02	-.64 to -.43	-.06 to .08		
Verbal aggression								
β	.09*	-.05	-.01	.01	.02	-.02	.01	1.73
b	.03	-.09	.01	.01	.04	-.02		
95% CI	.01 to .05	-.20 to .03	-.05 to .05	-.05 to .05	-.08 to .15	-.09 to .05		
Anger								
β	.17***	.24***	-.03	-.04	-.04	-.02	.08	12.32***
b	.05	.35	-.02	-.03	-.07	-.02		
95% CI	.03 to .06	.25 to .44	-.06 to .02	-.07 to .02	-.16 to .03	-.08 to .04		
Hostility								
β	.15***	.02	-.11**	.01	.01	.04	.04	6.01***
b	.04	.03	-.07	.01	.01	.04		
95% CI	.02 to .06	-.07 to .12	-.11 to .03	-.04 to .05	-.08 to .11	-.02 to .10		

* p <.05; ** p<.01; *** p<.001.

Nationality: 0=Jewish-Israeli, 1=Palestinian-Israelis.

Gender: 0=male, 1=female.

In addition, exposure to political violence was found to be a significant predictor of problems in family functioning, social functioning and aggression.

Ethnicity was also found to be a major predictor. Palestinian-Israelis had more symptoms of somatization, phobic anxiety, psychoticism and less paranoid ideation. Additionally, they had more PTSD symptoms, family functioning problems and aggression, specifically, physical aggression and anger. Regression results did not indicate significant interactions for any of the dependent variables. Findings show that exposure to political violence has a detrimental effect on social and mental health for both Jewish-Israeli and Palestinian-Israeli participants.

Several sociodemographic factors were significant predictors of social and mental functioning. Participants with higher SES had less mental health symptoms, PTSD symptoms, less family and social functioning problems and less anger. Parents' education likewise was associated with family functioning. Girls tended to have more mental health symptoms and PTSD symptoms and boys tended to have more problems with peers and aggression. Religiosity was not associated with any of the dependent variables.

DISCUSSION

Seven points bear emphasis. First, political violence is a major predictor of psychosocial functioning. This was true for both Jewish-Israeli and Palestinian-Israeli respondents. This finding is highly consistent with previous scholarship. Exposure to war can lead to such major problems as PTSD responses, and anxiety attacks [16, 68, 69, 67, 34]. Like exposure to domestic and community violence (among victims and witnesses), war can produce psychological trauma; cognitive, emotional, and behavioral problems; [45] and other maladaptive strategies for coping with violent behavior [29, 30, 54]. Children exposed to violence are more likely to develop violent behavior leading to juvenile delinquency [53, 78] and are more likely to display aggression and to legitimate violence. [15, 28]. Previous research on Palestinians in the West Bank shows well-established connections between political, domestic, community, and school violence. [10] Among Jewish Israeli adolescents exposed to war, there is comparable evidence of self-perceived problems in psychological growth and mild to severe PTSD [47].

Second, there are important differential responses to political violence. Ffemale respondents had more mental health symptoms and PTSD symptoms. Boys had more problems with peers and increased aggression. Religiosity did not predict any of the dependent variables. Jewish-Israeli participants, were more exposed to political violence than their Palestinian-Israeli counterparts. But for both sample groups, and indeed for anyone, exposure to violence can be a major influence on adolescent development [9]. Adolescence itself is already a critical period, characterized by major changes in biological, psychological, and social systems [27, 63] as well as by major social and situational challenges [20]. Moreover, adolescents have reached a stage of cognitive development and awareness [52] wherein consequences of exposure to violence may include PTSD reactions, dropping out of school, behavior problems, delinquency; lack of security and dissolution of social structures, and perceived threats to physical, emotional, and social development [20, 30, 53, 77]. Previous research shows that responses to living in a context of violence and trauma are not universal in nature and can manifest in a range of mild-to-severe psychological disorders [14], or no disorder at all. Indeed, there is no universal response to highly stressful events, and many of those exposed to the excesses of war heal within community, as personal recovery is deeply rooted in social recovery [66].

Third Palestinian-Israeli respondents had more mental health problems, PTSD symptoms, family and social problems and more aggression. The preceding discussion outlines the negative impact on a precarious period of human development – adolescence. But one needs to read these findings in the context of the already existent stresses on the Palestinian-Israeli families because of pressure to survive economically and culturally as a minority. Almost 60% of non-Jewish children in Israel live in poverty; this is 2.5 times higher than the Jewish population poverty rates (Israeli Central Bureau of Statistics, 2009). In the Jewish sector, 15% of children have unemployed parents, compared with 23% of Palestinian-Israeli children [39].

Families are already weakened and therefore people might need to seek outside support services. Yet research confirms lack of services and lower service utilization rates for relevant services, for youth in particular [56, 57]. And funding for social and allied services for the Palestinian-Israeli sector is markedly lower than those for their Jewish-Israeli counterparts. There are long-term implications that bear emphasis. The youth demographics are particularly profound; those who are 15 years old and under constitute about 41% of the Palestinian-Israeli community; those under age 20 are a little under 50% of the Palestinian-Israeli sector [39].There are great issues of risk, given the proportions of youth who are exposed to political violence. Yet the Palestinian-Israelis experience a double trauma: like their Jewish-Israeli counterparts they are exposed to political violence; but their population has higher unemployment, lower SES, and lower funding for educational, health, and social services. [18].

There are likewise implications to family structures. The impact on the family unit – in Palestinian-Israeli and Jewish-Israeli sectors – bears emphasis. Various studies have shown that exposure to political violence leads to a multitude of significant changes in the structure and every day actions of the family unit [40, 75]. The family unit, when subjected to political violence, becomes highly vulnerable to various stress-related factors [9, 43, 64]. Familial relations become overburdened by conflict as traditional normative understandings that define the family unit, structure and hierarchy are challenged; parents may lose employment, and gender and age roles may be challenged [65].

Fourth, this is double trauma. it is expected that the group that was exposed to more political violence (Jewish-Israeli) would show more mental health symptoms, but the reverse was true. Palestinian-Israelis report more symptoms, social, and family problems. What can explain this? In part, it may be because Palestinian-Israeli communities receive less money for counseling and professional services; they are less inclined to seek outside services; and they are the clients of service systems that are already underfunded [4, 5]. Then there is the social significance of death – which needs to be understood in its immediate impact on those who are associated with the dead, as well as a wider community and political symbol of ongoing war-related trauma. Traumatic events such as the death of friends, community members, and relatives require culturally specific, and clinically particular, services [8, 9]. Particularly with high context communities in which community linkages are vital, bereavement responses need to be situated collectively, and such community responses may be an impetus for consciousness development and community learning, as we discuss below.

Fifth, the socio-economic status of Palestinian-Israeli is lower than that of Jewish-Israelis. This has implications for all areas of life, including responses to trauma and health. Economic status and level of education are known to be associated with the psychological well-being of families and individuals. Previous scholarship correlates low levels of education and unemployment with high risk factors for poor mental health [36]. Indeed, chronic poverty has a deleterious impact on many life domains, including basic needs, family and social relations, leisure, and self-esteem [76]. According to Tolman and Wang (2005) [70], domestic violence is associated with various forms of material deprivation, as well as increased welfare dependence and decreased work reliance. Other studies have linked job loss to domestic violence (e.g., Moore and Selkowe, cited in Tolman and Wang, 2005) [70]. Low educational attainment has also been found to be associated with domestic violence [72]. Domestic violence, in turn, has been linked to increased rates of mental health problems, including depression, suicidal ideation and PTSD [70]. Moreover, since the education system is a part of the broader society, there is reason to believe that there is a relationship between an environment of political violence and high rates of school violence [10].

Sixth, this study shows that Palestinian-Israeli adolescents' ability to cope with their complex reality is harder than that of their Jewish-Israeli counterparts due to lower educational levels, unemployment, domestic violence, and social and economic discrimination and deprivation. According to Slone (2003) [59], the adolescent period is a developmental with its predominance of identity-seeking characteristics, the quest for autonomy, and the facility of emotionality in the midst of a volatile external situation. It has been noted that the overall issue of Arab in Israel identity has become even more complex against the background of the Israeli-Palestinian conflict (Slone, 2003). These multiple aspects of the Palestinian-Israeli adolescent's reality raise questions as to their implications on that individual's social and personal identity and trajectory into adulthood. The period of adolescence is a critical time, in which individuals search to secure a stable and consistent identity [71]. Following one study's assertion that under constructivist assumptions, one's identity is not eternally fixed but can be shaped by external events and the attempts of ethnic entrepreneurs to mobilize constituencies 49, there is a need to examine the identity construction of adolescent Palestinians in the context of both their immediate environment and Israeli society as a whole.

Finally, there are myriad implications for human service and teaching professionals, policy makers, and political actors. Psycho-educational and psychotherapeutic models of intervention need to be developed for Palestinian-Israeli and Jewish-Israeli populations that are culturally sensitive and relevant [2, 3]. Services should take into account distinctive characteristics within populations. There are profound diversities in the communities in terms of geographic and other forms of identity. Leverage may be made to encourage Palestinian-Israeli families who might be reluctant to receive services. One such leverage is the well-being of children, a priority around which all community members may rally [6.] Sufficient funding, and sufficient relevance need to occur, and all community stakeholders can be usefully brought together to ensure collaboration and the maximized targeting of needs with services. Likewise, popular psycho-educational campaigns can be aptly deployed in schools and community milieu, in order to bring about awareness and to provide support and access to services. Strategies of poverty reduction and community economic development could likely reduce the double trauma of Palestinian life. And throughout, there are linkages between all aforementioned systems; political actors, policy people, service administrators and providers, as well as the communities they serve, need to work collaboratively and the insights from each constituency need to be reciprocally shared [33].

Conclusion

The present study provides compelling evidence that while political violence and behavioral and emotional problems were high among all respondents, they were particularly high among Palestinian-Israeli youth. Any increase in mental health services directed towards youth and their families would be beneficial to either population but especially to those who are vulnerable to various trauma-related health problems.

The researcher was surprised by the extent of the relationship between low socioeconomic status and problematic responses to trauma, as well as by the impact of the Palestinian-Israeli double trauma. The findings provide evidence that Palestinians, particularly those in poverty, suffer significantly, raising questions about the long-term health of this sector of society, their feelings of social exclusion, and hence the peace process. Investments in jobs, funding for municipal, health, and social services, and other means of increasing social inclusion and raising socioeconomic status are all worthy goals for reducing gaps between Jewish-Israeli and Palestinian-Israeli populations. This double trauma that Palestinian-Israelis face is central to this analysis. Thus for the long term's sake and for the future of the region, investment in the Palestinian-Israeli community is worthwhile. In the end, helping those vulnerable who are exposed to trauma is a viable objective for service providers, scholars, and perhaps most importantly of all, policy makers and political actors.

Declaration of Conflict of Interest

None

References

[1] Al-Haj, M. (1989). Social research on family lifestyles among Arabs in Israel. *Journal of Comparative Family Studies, 20*(2), 175-95.

[2] Al-Krenawi, A., and Graham, J.R. (2000). Culturally sensitive social work practice with Arab clients in mental health settings. *Health and Social Work, 25*(1), 9-22.

[3] Al-Krenawi, A., and Graham, J.R. (2004). Somatization among Bedouin-Arab women: Differentiated by marital status. *Journal of Divorce and Remarriage, 42*(1/2), 131-143.

[4] Al-Krenawi, A., and Graham, J.R. (2006). A comparison of family functioning, life and marital satisfaction, and mental health of women in polygamous and monogamous marriages. *International Journal of Social Psychiatry, 52*(1), 5-17.

[5] Al-Krenawi, A., and Graham, J.R. (2007). The provision and use of social services among the Bedouin-Arab indigenous population in Israel. *Social Development Issues. 29*(1), 100-118.

[6] Al-Krenawi, A., Graham, J.R. and Al-Krenawi, S. (1997). Social work practice with polygamous families. *Child and Adolescent Social Work Journal, 14*(6), 444-458.

[7] Al-Krenawi, A., Graham, J.R., and Kanat-Maymon, Y. (2009). Analysis of trauma exposure, symptomatology and functioning in Jewish Israeli and Palestinian adolescents. *British Journal of Psychiatry*, *195*, 427-432.

[8] Al-Krenawi, A., Graham, J.R., and Sehwail, M. (2002). Bereavement responses among Palestinian widows, daughters, and sons following the Hebron massacre. *Omega: Journal of Death and Dying*, *44*(3), 241-255.

[9] Al-Krenawi, A., Graham, J.R., and Sehwail, M. (2004). Mental health and violence/trauma in Palestine: Implications for helping professional practice. *Journal of Contemporary Family Studies, 35*(2), 185-210.

[10] Al-Krenawi, A., Lev-Wiesel, R., and Sehwail, M. (2007). Psychological symptomatology among Palestinian male and female adolescents living under political violence 2004–2005. *Community Mental Health Journal, 43*(1), 49-56.

[11] Al-Krenawi, A., and Slonim-Nevo, V. (2002). Mental health aspects of Arab-Israeli adolescents from polygamous versus monogamous families. *The Journal of Social Psychology, 142*(4), 446-60.

[12] Amara, M., and Schnell, I. (2003). Identity repertoires among Arabs in Israel. *Journal of Ethnic and Migration Studies*, *3*(1), 175-193.

[13] Arab Association for Human Rights, (15-22 July, 2003). More house demolitions in the Negev. *Weekly Review of the Arab Press in Israel,* 126. Retrieved August 1, 2003, from http://www.arabhra.org.

[14] Baker, A.M. and Shalhoub-Kevorkian, N. (1999). The effects of political and military trauma on children: The Palestinian case. *Clinical Psychology Review, 19,* 935-950.

[15] Bandura, A. (1998). Mechanisms of moral disengagement. In W. Reich (Ed.), *Origins of terrorism: Psychologies, ideologies, theologies and state of mind* (pp. 161-191). Washington DC: Woodrow Wilson Center Press.

[16] Barber, B.K. (1999). Political violence, family relations, and Palestinian youth functioning. *Journal of Adolescent Research, 14*, 206–230.

[17] Buss, A.H., and Perry, M. (2002). The aggression questionnaire. *Journal of Personality and Social Psychology*, *63*(3), 452-59.

[18] Boudreaux, R. (2008, February 26). Israel: Digital gap between Arabs and Jews. *Los Angeles Times.* Retrieved September 14, 2009, from http://latimesblogs.latimes.com/babylonbeyond/2008/02/israel-digital.html

[19] Canetti, L., Shalev, A.Y., and De-Nour-Kaplan, A. (1994). Israeli adolescents' norms of the Brief Symptom Inventory (BSI). *Israel Journal of Psychiatry and Related Sciences, 31*(1), 13-18.

[20] Cicchetti, D., and Rogosch, F. A. (2002). A developmental psychopathology perspective on adolescence. *Journal of Consulting and Clinical Psychology, 70,* 6-20.

[21] Cohen, M., and Eid, J. (2007). The effect of constant threat of terror on Israeli Jewish and Arab adolescents. *Anxiety, Stress, and Coping, 20*(1), 47-60.

[22] Corcoran, K., and Fischer, J. (2000). *Measures for clinical practice.* New York: Free Press.

[23] Derogatis, L., and Spencer, P. (1982). *The brief symptom inventory (BSI): Administration, scoring and procedures, Manual I.* Baltimore: Johns Hopkins.

[24] Durakovic-Belko, E., Kulenovic, A., and Dapic, R. (2003). Determinants of post-traumatic adjustment in adolescents from Sarajevo who experienced war. *Journal of Clinical Psychology, 59*, 27–40.

[25] Elbedour, S., Bastien, D.T., and Center, B.A. (1997). Identity Formation in the Shadow of Conflict: Projective Drawings by Palestinian and Israeli Arab Children from the West Bank and Gaza. *Journal of Peace Research, 34*(2), 217-231.

[26] Epstein, N.B., Baldwin, L.M., and Bishop, D.S. (1983). The McMaster Family Assessment Device: Reliability and validity. *Journal of Marital and Family Therapy, 9*(2), 171-180.

[27] Feldman, S., and Elliott, G. (Eds.). (1990). *At the threshold: The developing adolescent.* Cambridge, MA: Harvard University Press.

[28] Fitzpatrick, K.M. (1997). Fighting among America's youth: A risk and protective factors approach. *Journal of Health and Social Behavior, 38*, 131-148.

[29] Flannery, D., Singer, M., and Wester, K. (2001). Violence exposure, psychological trauma, and suicide risk in a community sample of dangerously violent adolescents. *Journal of the Academy of Child and Adolescent Psychiatry, 40*(4), 435-444.

[30] Flannery, D., Wester, K., and Singer, M. (2004). Impact of violence exposure at school on child mental health and violent behaviour. *Journal of Community Psychology, 32*(5), 559-574.

[31] Foa, E.B., Riggs, D., Dancu, C.V., and Rothbaum, B.O. (1993). Reliability and validity of a brief instrument for assessing posttraumatic stress disorder. *Journal of Traumatic Stress, 6*, 459-73.

[32] Ganim, A., and Smooha, S. (2001). *Attitudes of the Arabs to the State of Israel.* Haviva Institute of Peace Research. Retrieved September 14, 2009, from http://66.155.17.109/peace/ publications.

[33] Graham, J., and Barter, K. (1999). Collaboration: A social work practice method. *Families in Society: The Journal of Contemporary Human Services, 80*(1), 6-13.

[34] Gurwitch, R.H., Kees, M., and Becker, S.M. (2002). In the face of tragedy: Placing children's reactions to trauma in a new context. *Cognitive and Behavioral Practice, 9*(4), 286-295.

[35] Hadi, F.A. (1999). Predicting psychological distress in children. *Journal of the Social Sciences, 27*(1), 73- 87.

[36] Harpham, T., Grant, E., and Rodriguez, C. (2004). Mental health and social capital in Cali, Colombia. *Social Science and Medicine, 58*(11), 2267–2277.

[37] Hudson, W.W. (1982). *The Clinical Measurement Package: A field manual.* Chicago: Dorsey Press.

[38] Hujierat, M. (2005). *The collective identity of Arab-Israeli students: Identity complexity and collective self-esteem.* Ph.D dissertation, Beer-Sheva, Israel: Ben-Gurion University of the Negev.

[39] Israeli Central Bureau of Statistics. (2009). *Statistical Abstract of Israel 2009 No. 60.* Retrieved September 14, 2009, from http://cbs.gov.il/reader/

[40] Joshi, P.T., O'Donnell, D.A., Cullins, L.M., and Lewin, S.M. (2006). Children exposed to war and terrorism. In M.M. Feerick and G.B. Silverman (Eds.), *Children exposed to violence* (pp, 53-84). Baltimore, MD: Paul H. Brookes Publishing.

[41] Kanaana, S. (1992). *Still on vacation! The eviction of the Palestinians in 1948.* Ramallah and Jerusalem Shaml-Palestinian Diaspora and Refugee Centre.
[42] Kelman, H.C. (1987). The Political Psychology of the Israeli-Palestinian Conflict. *Political Psychology*, *8*, 347–63.
[43] Khamis, V. (2005). Posttraumatic stress disorder among school age Palestinian children. *Child Abuse and Neglect, 29*(1), 81-95.
[44] Kraft, D. (2009, July 28). Number of settlers in West Bank has doubled. *The Independent.* Retrieved September 14, 2009, from http://www.independent.ie/world-news/middle-east/number-of-settlers-in-west-bank-has-doubled-1843605.html
[45] Kuther, T. L. (1999). A developmental-contextual perspective on youth co-victimization by violence. *Adolescence, 34*, 669-714.
[46] Laufer, A., Raz-Hamama, Y., Levine, S. Z., and Solomon, Z. (2009). Posttraumatic growth in adolescence: The role of religiosity, distress and forgiveness. *Journal of Social and Clinical Psychology*, *28*, 862-880.
[47] Laufer, A and Solomon, Z. (2006). Posttraumatic Symptoms and Post-traumatic Growth among Israeli Youth Exposed to Terror Incidents. *Journal of Social and Clinical Psychology*, *25*(4), 429-447.
[48] Lavi, T., and Solomon, Z. (2005). Palestinian youth of the Intifada: PTSD and future orientation. *Journal of the American Academy of Child Adolescent Psychiatry*, *44*, 1176–1183.
[49] Lowrance, S. (2005). Being Palestinian in Israel: Identity, protest, and political exclusion. *Comparative Studies of South Asia, Africa and the Middle East, 25*(2), 487-499.
[50] Miller, I.W., Epstein, N.B., Bishop, D.S., and Keitner, G.I. (1985). The McMaster Family Assessment Device: Reliability and validity. *Journal of Marital and Family Therapy, 11*(4), 345-356.
[51] Nir, O. (2003). *Israel's Arab minority, policy brief: Middle East Institute*. Retrieved September 29, 2008, from www.mideasti.org/articles/doc22.html
[52] Osofsky, J.D. (2004). *Young children and trauma: Intervention and treatment.* New York: The Guilford Press.
[53] Osofsky, H.J., and Osofsky, J.D. (2001). Violent and aggressive behaviors in youth: A mental health and prevention perspective. *Psychiatry: Interpersonal and Biological Processes, 64*(4), 285-295.
[54] Overstreet, S., and Braun, S. (2000). Exposure to community violence and post-traumatic stress symptoms: Mediating factors. *American Journal of Orthopsychiatry, 70,* 263-271.
[55] Ridenour, T.A., Daley, J.G., and Reich, W. (1999). Factor analysis of the family assessment device. *Family Process*, *38*(4), 103-129.
[56] Savaya, R. (1995). Attitudes towards family and marital counseling among Israeli Arab women. *Journal of Social Service Research*, *21*(1), 35-51.
[57] Savaya, R. (1998). The under-use of psychological services by Israeli Arabs: An examination of the roles of negative attitudes and the use of alternative sources of help. *International Social Work, 41,* 195-209.
[58] Sikkuy. (2004). *Sikkuy Report 2004.* Retrieved September 14, 2009, from http://www.sikkuy.org.il/english/reports.html

[59] Slone, M. (2003). The Nazareth Riots: Arab and Jewish Israeli Adolescents Pay a Different Psychological Price for Participation. *The Journal of Conflict Resolution, 47*(6), 817-836.

[60] Slonim-Nevo, V., and Shraga, Y. (2000). Psychological and social adjustment of Russian-born and Israeli-born Jewish adolescents. *Child and Social Work Journal, 17*(6), 455-75.

[61] Smooha, S. (1999). The status quo option. In: S. Ozacky-Lazar, A. Ghanem, and I. Pappe (Eds.), *Seven roads: Theoretical options for the status of the Arabs in Israel* (pp. 23-28). Geva'at Haviva, Israel: Peace Research Institute.

[62] Smooha, S. (2004). Arab-Jewish relations in Israel as a deeply divided society. In: A. Shapira (Ed.), *Israeli Identity in Transition*. (pp. 31-67). New York: Praeger.

[63] Spear, L.P. (2000). The adolescent brain and age-related behavioral manifestations. *Neuroscience and Biobehavioral Reviews, 24,* 417-463.

[64] Srour, R.W. (2005). Children living under a multi traumatic environment. *Israel Journal of Psychiatry, 42*(2), 88-95.

[65] Suad, J. (2004). Conceiving family relationships in post-war Lebanon. *Journal of Comparative Family Studies, 35*(2), 271-293.

[66] Summerfield, D. (2000). War and mental health: A brief overview. *British Medical Journal, 321,* 232-235.

[67] Thabet, A.B.M., Abed, A.M., and Vostanis P. (2002). Emotional problems in Palestinian children living in a war zone: A cross-sectional study. *Lancet, 359*(9320), 1801-1805.

[68] Thabet, A.B.M., and Vostanis, P. (2004). Co morbidity of PTSD and depression among refugee children during war conflict. *Journal of Child Psychology and Psychiatry, 45*(3), 533-542.

[69] Thabet, A.B.M., and Vostanis, P. (2005). Child mental health problems in the Gaza strip. *Israel Journal of Psychiatry, 42*(2), 84-87.

[70] Tolman, R.M., and Wang, H.C. (2005). Domestic violence and women's employment: Fixed effects models of three waves of women's employment study data. *American Journal of Community Psychology, 36,* 147-158.

[71] Tsou, A. (2002). *Understanding the influence of ethnic identity and acculturation on psychological adjustment among Chinese American adolescents.* PhD dissertation, Berkley: California School of Professional Psychology.

[72] Vest, J. R., Catlin, T. K., Chen, J. J., and Brownson, R. C. (2002). Multistate analysis of factors associated with intimate partner violence. *American Journal of Preventive Medicine, 22*(3), 156-164.

[73] Vizek-Vidovic, V., Kutervac-Jagodic, G. and Arambasic, L. (2000). Posttraumatic symptomatology in children exposed to war. *Scandinavian Journal of Psychology*, 41, 297- 306.

[74] Wakim, W. (1994). The National Committee for the Defence of the Rights of the Uprooted in Israel, presented at the first *Conference for Human Rights in Arab Society*, held in Nazareth.

[75] Weine, S., Muzurovic, N., Kulauzovic, Y., Besic, S., Lezic, A., Mujagic, A., Muzurovic, J., Spahovic, D., Feetham, S., Ware, N., Knafl, K., and Pavkovic, I. (2004). Family consequences of refugee trauma. *Family Process, 43*(2), 147-60.

[76] Wilton, R. (2004). Putting policy into practice? Poverty and people with serious mental illness. *Social Science and Medicine, 58,* 25-39.

[77] Yurtbay, T., Alyanak, B., Abali, O., Kaynak, N., and Durukan, M. (2003). The psychological effects of forced emigration on Muslim Albanian children and adolescents. *Community Mental Health Journal, 39,* 203-212.

[78] Zingraff, M.T., Leiter, J., Myers, K.A., and Johnson, M.C. (1993). Child maltreatment and youthful problem behavior. *Criminology, 31,* 173-202.

In: The International Psychiatry and Behavioral ...
Editor: Nash Boutros
ISBN: 978-1-62257-566-4

Chapter 20

THE FREQUENCY OF LAW BREAKING AND COMPULSORY HOSPITALIZATION AMONG MENTALLY ILL PEOPLE IN KATOWICE, POLAND

***Eliza Górniak*[1], *Karolina Furczyk*[2] *and Krzysztof Krysta*[3*]**

[1]Department of Psychiatry and Psychotherapy,
Medical University of Silesia, Katowice, Poland
[2]The Clinic of Psychiatry and Psychotherapy,
Rostock University, Rostock, Germany
[3]Department of Psychiatry and Psychotherapy,
Medical University of Silesia, Katowice, Poland

ABSTRACT

Background: It is a common belief that mental disorders are widely associated with dangerous, threat-posing behavior and law-breaking. This paper analyzes the problem of law-breaking by the mentally disordered.

Method: The analysis of cases concerning compulsory psychiatric treatment or confinement in a medical institution on the grounds of mental incompetence to commit an offence or mental unfitness to stand trial obtained from the court and the public prosecutor's office in Silesia from 2007 to 2009.

Results: 14 cases were analyzed. All the offenders were male, mean age was 44.6. All the offenders were diagnosed by psychiatrists, most of them with schizophrenia (n=10 cases). Other diagnoses included paranoic syndrome (n=1), bipolar affective disorder with manic episode (n=1), schizoaffective disorder (n=1), and delusional syndrome (n=1). 9 out of 14 offenders were diagnosed prior to the offence, some of whom were also hospitalized (n=5). 8 of the analyzed cases concerned use of violence, 3 concerned larceny, 2 concerned posing a threat to the life or health of others, and 1 concerned fraud. 2 of the offenders were previously sentenced for other offences. 12 of

* Corresponding Author: Krzysztof Krysta, MD, Department of Psychiatry and Psychotherapy, Medical University of Silesia, Katowice, Poland, krysta@mp.pl

the offenders were compulsorily treated by psychiatrists, 10 of whom are still hospitalized at the time of writing this report.

Conclusion: The small number of the cases analyzed (14 cases in the whole of a few thousand) suggests that mentally disordered persons do not break the law often. There seems to be a higher risk associated with the male gender, though. Also, the frequency of violent acts and offences committed despite previous treatment is disturbing.

Keywords: psychiatric disorders, law-breaking, violence

INTRODUCTION

It is a common belief that mentally ill persons are violent, unpredictable and that they often pose a threat to the health and safety of others. These widely held opinions contribute to creating and reinforcing stigma attached to mental illness (Filipovits and Farkas, 2008; Furczyk et al., 2011).

The fact remains, however, that although mental illnesses are associated with increased risk of violent behavior, the association is not independent of modifying factors such as psychoactive substance abuse, history of family violence or other environmental stressors. Violent behavior may result in law-breaking attitudes (Fazel et al, 2009a; Elbogen Johnson, 2009; Fazel et al, 2009b).

According to Polish law a person who, as a result of psychiatric illness, mental retardation or other disturbance in psychiatric functions, has no ability to control his or her own behavior or to fully recognize its possible outcome, although breaking the law, does not commit a crime (Polski Kodeks Karny, 2009).

In such cases, if the behavior is destructive and socially harmful, and it is probable that this kind of conduct repeats, a person may by the court's decision be detained in an appropriate medical facility (Polski Kodeks Karny, 2009). Therefore, a number of Polish court cases resulting in compulsory psychiatric treatment or confinement in a medical institution on the grounds of mental incompetence to commit a crime reflect the frequency of law breaking among the mentally ill.

The aim of this paper is to present and characterize the cases of law breaking by the mentally disordered in the city of Katowice. The legal qualification of committed offences and the results of legal proceedings with special emphasis on the aspect of violent behavior is described.

METHOD

For the purposes of this research, the records of all the cases from the years 2007 to 2009 were obtained from two Public Prosecutor's Offices and one District Court of Katowice. All of the cases that resulted in withdrawing the case on the grounds of the defendant's mental unfitness to stand trial or in stating their mental incompetence to commit an offence were selected and analyzed.

Results

Only 14 out of a few thousand of all cases were found to fit the research criteria. All the defendants were male. Their mean age was 44.6 years. At the time of the offence, the youngest of the defendants was 21, while the oldest was 72 years old. During the course of the legal proceedings, all of the defendants were examined, observed and diagnosed by forensic psychiatrists. In most cases the final diagnosis was that of schizophrenia (10 cases, 9 of which were diagnosed as paranoid schizophrenia, while the remaining 1 was schizophrenia combined with mental retardation). Other defendants were diagnosed with paranoid syndrome (n=1), psychotic manic episode in the course of the bipolar affective disorder and concomitant alcohol dependence (n=1), schizoaffective disorder (n=1) and persistent delusional syndrome (n=1). 9 out of 14 defendants had been treated and diagnosed by psychiatrists before breaking the law; however, in three cases after examination by sworn experts the diagnoses were changed.

Five out of these 9 defendants had also been hospitalized for psychiatric reasons before they broke the law, while the rest of them had only been treated as outpatients. Eight out of 14 analyzed cases were associated with violence, and in most of them (n=5) the violence was directed against the defendant's family members. As for the legal qualification of the offences the defendants were accused of committing, the analysis revealed 8 cases of assault, 3 cases of larceny, 2 cases of posing a threat to the life or health of others, and 1 fraud. All cases of larceny involved objects of very small value. To give a vivid example, one case involved a gold fish.

Two defendants had been accused of committing other crimes in the past, while for the rest of them the analyzed cases were their first contact with the law. As a result of the legal proceedings, twelve of the defendants were hospitalized and compulsorily treated. Ten of them are still hospitalized at the time of writing this report.

Discussion

According to the information found on the Katowice court's website, an average number of cases taking place each year in the offices which provided the data for this analysis reaches a few thousand. With this taken into consideration, the described 14 cases are found to constitute only a very small portion of the whole number of cases.

This strongly contrasts with a popular image of violent, dangerous 'madmen' known from the media, influencing the way persons with mental illness are seen by society (Cutcliffe and Hanningan, 2001).

Analyses conducted in other parts of Poland, as well as abroad, confirm this conclusion. Between 1997 and 2002 in the Polish city of Szczecin and the surrounding area there were 128 cases in which compulsory psychiatric treatment of the defendant was considered by the court. As a result of the legal proceedings, the court decided that institutionalization in a medical facility was necessary in 85 of these cases (Kolasinski and Korecka, 2004). In 1998, in Baltimore, 14 out of 11497 defendants tried for different crimes pleaded insanity (Janofsky, Vandewalle, and Rappeport, 1989). All of them were male, which seems to confirm differences between men and women with regard to criminal and violent behavior (Vaske et al., 2011)

The hereby presented analysis showed schizophrenia to be the most common disease diagnosed in the researched group of defendants, a fact which confirms that this disease is associated with aggressive and criminal behavior (Fazel et al., 2009a; Ran et al, 2010; Haller, Dittrich, and Kocsis, 2004). In some of the described cases a matter of occasional alcohol abuse by the defendants was also raised. Alcohol abuse is known to increase the risk of aggressive behavior, mostly directed against the subject's own family members (Fazel et al., 2009b; Thompson and Kingree, 2006). This kind of aggression was particularly common in the presented cases, which might be attributed both to the fact that the defendants were mentally disturbed and to the coexisting problem of alcohol abuse.

A large number of mentally ill defendants presented in this paper had been diagnosed and treated by psychiatrists even before they broke the law. In these cases treatment did not prevent the disordered from committing the crime, although, as the related papers show, an early diagnosis, systematic and frequent visits to a psychiatrist, as well as treating concomitant addictions, all result in significant reduction of the risk of criminal behavior (Thompson and Kingree, 2006; Van Dorn et al., 2011).

The presented analysis confirms the results of other similar research. Amongst the mentally disordered it is male patients diagnosed with schizophrenia who are especially inclined to present with criminal behavior. Violence in this group of patients is most often directed against their own family members, which also is related to alcohol abuse. The fact that a lot of crimes were committed in spite of the fact that the defendants were being treated by psychiatrists suggests that the doctor-patient relationship needs continuous improvement and the scale of criminal risk has to be carefully and individually assessed in each and every case. Still, although there clearly is an association between mental disorders and aggressive or criminal behavior, the number of cases against the mentally ill seems minute when compared to the whole number of cases. There is an urgent need to start a public discussion concerning this matter to influence the whole society, and through this prevent stigmatization of the mentally disordered.

References

Cutcliffe Jr, and Hanningan B. (2001) Mass media, 'monsters' and mental health clients: the need for increased lobbying. *Journal of Psychiatric and Mental Health Nursing, 8*, 315-21.

Elbogen EB, and Johnson SC. (2009) The intricate link between violence and mental disorder: results from the National Epidemiologic Survey on Alcohol and Related Conditions. *Archives of General Psychiatry, 66*, 152-61.

Fazel S, Grann M, Carlström E, Lichtenstein P, Långström N. (2009) Risk factors for violent crime in Schizophrenia: a national cohort study of 13,806 patients. *The Journal of Clinical Psychiatry, 70*, 362-9.

Fazel S, Långström N, Hjern A, Grann M, and Lichtenstein P. (2009) Schizophrenia, substance abuse, and violent crime. *JAMA, 301*, 2016-23.

Filipovits D, and Farkas M. (2008) Violent behaviour and stigmatisation among psychiatric patients. Psychiatria Hungarica, *23,* 420-9.

Furczyk K, Gorniak E, Skowronek R, Gajda M, Krysta K, and Krupka-Matuszczyk I. (2011) The way young people see the mentalny ill: a questionnaire study. *Psychiatria Danubina, 23*, 46-49.

Haller R, Dittrich I, and Kocsis E. (2004) How dangerous are patients with mental disorders? *Wiener medizinische Wochenschrift, 154,* 356-65.

Janofsky JS, Vandewalle MB, and Rappeport JR. (1989) Defendants pleading insanity: an analysis of outcome. *The Journal of American Academy of Psychiatry and the Law, 17,* 203-11.

Kolasinski B, and Korecka D. (2004) Internacja psychiatryczna- teoria i praktyka. *Prokuratura i Prawo, 6*, 135-156.

Polski Kodeks karny . Art. 31. § 1. and Art.94 § 1.(Dz. U. z dnia 2 sierpnia 1997 r).

Ran MS, Chen PY, Liao ZG, Chan CL, Chen EY, Tang CP, Mao WJ, Lamberti JS, and Conwell Y. (2010) Criminal behavior among persons with schizophrenia in rural China. *Schizophrenia Research, 122,* 213-8.

Thompson MP, and Kingree JB. (2006) The roles of victim and perpetrator alcohol use in intimate partner violence outcomes. *Journal of interpersonal violence*, *21*, 163-77.

Van Dorn RA, Andel R, Boaz TL, Desmarais SL, Chandler K, Becker MA, and Howe A. (2011) Risk of arrest in persons with schizophrenia and bipolar disorder in a Florida Medicaid program: the role of atypical antipsychotics, conventional neuroleptics, and routine outpatient behavioral health services. *The journal of clinical psychiatry*, *72*, 502-8.

Vaske J, Wright JP, Boisvert D, and Beaver KM. (2011) Gender, genetic risk, and criminal behavior. *Psychiatry research***,** *185*, 376-81.

INDEX

A

abuse, 7, 10, 14, 104, 178, 179, 180, 181, 183, 188, 190, 191, 192, 193, 194, 195, 196, 221, 234, 257, 258, 267, 308
access, 33, 37, 258, 280, 298
acculturation, 285, 303
acid, 256
action potential, 116
action research, 199, 200, 201, 202, 203, 207
acupuncture, 30, 33, 34
acute schizophrenia, 18, 26
ADA, 36, 45, 46
adaptation, 146, 147, 152, 158, 262, 279
Addiction Severity Index (ASI), 7, 243
adenosine, 120
adipose, 38
adipose tissue, 38
adiposity, 38, 50
adjustment, 7, 276, 301, 303
Administration for Children and Families, 195, 197
administrators, 213, 298
adolescent development, 296
adolescent female, 55
adolescents, 55, 60, 61, 62, 63, 164, 169, 180, 194, 201, 283, 285, 286, 287, 288, 296, 298, 300, 301, 303, 304
adulthood, 177, 178, 192, 193, 298
adults, 51, 52, 62, 83, 107, 145, 152, 158, 180
advantage effect, 18
adverse effects, 33, 41
adverse event, 252, 253
advocacy, 127
aerobic exercise, 43
affective disorder, 3, 4, 5, 8, 9, 11, 12, 61, 122, 171, 239, 240, 241, 242, 243, 252, 253, 256, 305, 307
Africa, 302
age, 5, 7, 13, 19, 20, 21, 26, 31, 38, 41, 58, 61, 90, 98, 99, 100, 118, 121, 124, 128, 129, 148, 150, 152, 164, 167, 181, 183, 190, 191, 199, 204, 212, 220, 223, 245, 246, 259, 261, 262, 263, 264, 266, 267, 270, 271, 275, 276, 286, 297, 302, 303, 305, 307
agencies, 178, 179
aggression, 183, 190, 235, 254, 283, 287, 288, 294, 295, 296, 297, 300, 308
aggressive behavior, 240, 258, 287, 302, 308
aggressive personality, 105
AIDS, 236
akathisia, 36
alcohol abuse, 9, 11, 13, 14, 256, 257, 263, 264, 267, 308
alcohol consumption, 7, 8, 10, 240, 243, 245, 251, 255, 258, 264, 273
alcohol dependence, 10, 219, 220, 223, 232, 233, 234, 235, 238, 239, 240, 241, 242, 243, 246, 252, 253, 254, 255, 256, 257, 258, 260, 261, 264, 267, 272, 307
alcohol problems, 263, 264, 272, 273
alcohol research, 256
alcohol use, 8, 11, 13, 239, 241, 243, 253, 254, 258, 259, 263, 264, 265, 267, 268, 269, 270, 271, 309
alcohol withdrawal, 242
alcoholics, 9, 13, 14, 223, 232, 234, 237, 238, 239, 240, 253, 255
alcoholism, 10, 13, 20, 219, 220, 232, 233, 236, 237, 240, 241, 252, 253, 254, 255, 256
algorithm, 37, 45, 47
allele, 223, 224, 225, 226, 227, 228, 229, 230, 231, 237
alters, 123, 255
American Heart Association, 53
American Psychiatric Association, 36, 47, 49, 50, 78, 82, 121, 168

amphetamines, 57
amplitude, 17, 18, 19, 21, 22, 23, 24, 25
analgesic, 10
anatomy, 120
anger, 283, 287, 296
angiotensin converting enzyme, 237
annealing, 222
ANOVA, 22, 23, 117, 259
anticonvulsant, 88, 111
antidepressants, 65, 66, 67, 113, 117, 120, 165, 170, 239, 240, 253, 256
antipsychotic, 25, 27, 30, 40, 41, 42, 47, 48, 50, 51, 52, 53, 54, 67, 69, 72, 88, 111
antipsychotic drugs, 25, 50, 53, 67
antisocial personality, 4, 104, 105
antisocial personality disorder, 4
anxiety, 3, 4, 8, 10, 11, 12, 14, 15, 20, 65, 68, 106, 113, 162, 163, 180, 234, 239, 240, 244, 247, 252, 253, 254, 256, 272, 276, 284, 286, 288, 293, 296
anxiety disorder, 4, 10, 11, 12, 14, 15, 106, 256
APA, 36, 168
apathy, 240
Arab countries, 179
Arab world, 177, 178, 179, 194
aripiprazole, 91, 92, 94, 95, 98, 99, 111, 167, 170
arousal, 287
arrest, 309
arrests, 6
arterial hypertension, 38, 42
arteriovenous malformation, 164
ASI, 7, 8
assault, 11, 193, 235, 307
assessment, 20, 41, 42, 50, 75, 76, 78, 81, 82, 88, 93, 94, 96, 100, 103, 105, 106, 108, 127, 128, 130, 143, 146, 152, 153, 158, 203, 213, 243, 252, 258, 294, 302
assessment techniques, 76
asymmetry, 17, 25, 27
atherosclerosis, 50
ATP, 38
atrial fibrillation, 170
atrophy, 164, 171, 172
attachment, 201, 284
Attention Deficit Hyperactivity Disorder (ADHD), 89, 106, 237
attitudes, 195, 277, 306
attribution, 165
attribution bias, 165
auditory cortex, 17, 19, 20, 24, 25
auditory stimuli, 18, 19, 20
authority, 73
autism, 63, 199, 200, 201, 202, 203, 205, 212, 213, 214, 215
autonomy, 298
avoidance, 287
awareness, 68, 101, 178, 179, 194, 296, 298
axons, 233

B

bacteria, 68
basal ganglia, 165
base, 222, 245
basic needs, 298
batteries, 79
Beck Depression Inventory, 115, 117
beer, 257, 259, 261, 262, 263, 264, 265, 266, 267, 268, 269, 270, 272, 273
behavior modification, 211
behavior therapy, 254
behavioral manifestations, 303
behavioral problems, 202, 284, 296
behaviors, 81, 201, 203, 204, 207, 210, 211, 214, 237, 255
Beijing, 34
Belgium, 161
beneficial effect, 56, 167
benefits, 202, 212
benzodiazepine, 94
bias, 67, 72, 143, 148, 152, 165, 190, 192, 272
bile, 46
bile acid sequestrant, 46
biochemistry, 243
biological activity, 66, 67, 68, 69, 71
biological systems, 67
bipolar disorder, 3, 4, 5, 8, 9, 10, 11, 12, 13, 36, 61, 87, 89, 90, 92, 93, 97, 98, 99, 100, 104, 105, 106, 109, 111, 113, 164, 167, 169, 309
blood, 31, 38, 42, 102, 221, 240, 243
blood pressure, 38, 42
body image, 171
body mass index (BMI), 38, 40, 42, 43, 52, 60, 102
bones, 116, 162
brain, 17, 18, 25, 26, 27, 33, 34, 56, 66, 67, 68, 116, 120, 122, 123, 162, 164, 165, 166, 169, 172, 220, 233, 235, 238, 242, 303
brain abnormalities, 26
brain damage, 166
brain structure, 18
brain tumor, 164
Brazil, 35, 36, 38
Brno, 219, 221

C

CAD, 45
calibration, 21
campaigns, 298
candidates, 146
cannabis, 6, 7, 13, 57
carbamazepine, 88, 91, 92, 98, 99, 111
carbohydrate, 40, 43
cardiovascular disease, 35, 36, 38, 39, 42, 50, 51, 53
cardiovascular disease, 39
cardiovascular disorders, 42
cardiovascular risk, 40
caregivers, 81, 204
case studies, 163, 165, 172
case study, 169, 195, 201, 214
cash, 128
cataplexy, 57
catatonia, 56, 57, 58, 59, 60, 61, 62, 63
catatonic, 55, 56, 57, 59, 60, 61, 62, 63
catatonic schizophrenia, 55, 56, 57, 60, 62, 63
catharsis, 202
Caucasians, 236
causation, 235
CDC, 194, 213
central nervous system, 18, 78, 219, 235
cerebral blood flow, 26
challenges, 191, 215, 296
chemical, 13, 30, 242
chemokine receptor, 221
Chicago, 50, 301
child abuse, 177, 178, 179, 180, 190, 191, 192, 193, 194, 195, 196, 197
child maltreatment, 195, 197
childhood, 56, 63, 178, 191, 192, 193, 194, 196, 197, 201
children, 6, 8, 11, 38, 55, 58, 61, 62, 63, 151, 153, 159, 164, 178, 179, 192, 194, 195, 199, 200, 201, 202, 203, 204, 205, 207, 210, 211, 212, 213, 214, 215, 297, 298, 300, 301, 302, 303, 304
China, 29, 309
cholesterol, 42
chromatography, 222
chronic diseases, 50
citalopram, 167, 240, 253, 254, 255
cities, 286
clarity, 67, 151
classes, 99, 286
classification, 30, 143, 161, 162, 163, 167, 168
clients, 13, 259, 297, 299, 308
clinical application, 75
clinical assessment, 190
clinical depression, 8, 9
clinical diagnosis, 19, 286
clinical examination, 90, 205
clinical presentation, 13
clinical symptoms, 29, 38, 279
clinical trials, 37, 76, 82, 239
clozapine, 29, 30, 31, 32, 33, 34, 40, 43, 47, 48, 53, 62, 91, 92, 98, 99, 111, 167
clusters, 287
CNS, 123, 219, 220, 233, 234, 235, 254, 256, 272
cocaine, 7, 9, 11, 13
cocaine abuse, 13
coffee, 221
cognition, 75, 76, 79, 81, 82, 83, 122, 128, 130, 171
cognitive abilities, 60, 129, 143
cognitive ability, 143, 144
cognitive deficit, 26, 75, 78, 81
cognitive deficits, 26, 75, 78, 81
cognitive development, 296
cognitive domains, 75, 78
cognitive dysfunction, 79
cognitive function, 75, 76, 81, 146, 147
cognitive impairment, 20, 25, 75, 76, 78, 164, 259
cognitive level, 5
cognitive performance, 60, 76, 81
collaboration, 298
college students, 256
colleges, 177, 179, 181, 182, 183, 185, 191
Colombia, 301
coma, 20
combination therapy, 46
commercial, 154
communication, 117, 130, 153, 200, 201, 202, 203, 204, 205, 207, 210, 211, 213, 214
communication skills, 201, 204, 205, 207, 210, 211
communities, ix, 50, 128, 213, 285, 297, 298
community, 14, 129, 180, 197, 286, 296, 297, 298, 299, 301, 302
comorbidity, 11, 13, 14, 15, 104, 106, 254, 256
compensation, 204
complex partial seizure, 171
complexity, 70, 202, 301
compliance, 34, 71, 88, 96, 97, 100, 101, 207, 208, 209, 211, 239, 242, 247, 276
complications, 40, 43, 60, 179, 272, 273
comprehension, 130, 131, 149, 152
compulsion, 286, 288, 292
computer, 21, 57
computer software, 21

concussion, 192
conductance, 166
conference, 36, 50
confidentiality, 245, 246
confinement, 305, 306
conflict, 12, 36, 37, 49, 121, 284, 297, 298, 303
conflict of interest, 12, 36, 37, 49, 121
congruence, 210
connectivity, 25, 116
consciousness, 66, 192, 297
consensus, 12, 35, 36, 37, 40, 43, 46, 48, 76, 96, 103, 105, 106
Consensus, v, vi, 35, 37, 50, 76, 87
consent, 59, 61, 117, 147, 221, 242, 246
constipation, 33, 60
construct validity, 146
construction, 298
consulting, 62, 202
consumers, 10, 76
consumption, 4, 6, 7, 8, 10, 12, 255, 257, 258, 261, 267, 272, 273
containers, 244
control condition, 21
control group, 21, 30, 33, 40, 120, 199, 202, 203, 204, 205, 207, 210, 221, 223, 241, 250, 251
controlled studies, 163
controlled trials, 37
controversial, 239
controversies, 179
conversations, 58, 204
cooling, 143
cooperation, 117, 221
coordination, 37
coronary artery disease, 266
coronary heart disease, 50, 51, 52, 272
correlation, 18, 22, 24, 25, 47, 71, 81, 223, 258, 288, 292
correlation coefficient, 22, 81, 223, 292
correlations, 76, 267, 270, 287
cortex, 17, 18, 25, 26, 28, 116, 124
cost, 36
cough, 68
counseling, 212, 214, 244, 246, 275, 277, 297, 302
covering, 286
cranium, 117
craving, 239, 240, 241, 243, 250, 252, 253, 254, 266, 267, 273
creatinine, 102
crimes, 8, 11, 307, 308
criminal behavior, 308, 309
crises, 178
critical period, 296
criticism, 179, 197
Cross-national, 14
cross-sectional study, 303
CRP, 50
CSF, 236
CSS, 223
CTA, 222
cues, 28, 65, 72, 201
culture, 179, 285, 286
CVD, 36
cycles, 90, 92, 95, 97, 98, 99, 101, 105, 222
cycling, 10, 111
cytokines, 237
Czech Republic, xi, xii, 219, 236, 237

D

data analysis, 32
data collection, 286
database, 41, 258, 259, 273
deaths, 39
defects, 200, 201, 202
defendants, 307, 308
defense mechanisms, 72
defibrillation, 59
deficiencies, 202
deficiency, 58, 201, 237, 241
deficit, 19, 25, 26, 27, 31, 78, 106, 235
dehydration, 58
delinquency, 296
delirium, 258
delusions, 20, 25, 161, 162, 163, 166, 167, 168, 171, 172
dementia, 108, 127, 128, 129, 142, 143, 144, 162, 164
demographic characteristics, 78, 117, 277
demographic data, 148, 181, 182
denaturation, 222
dendritic cell, 234
denial, 61, 163, 168, 181, 183, 191, 192
Department of Health and Human Services, 195, 197
Department of Justice, 197
dependent variable, 205, 245, 288, 296
depressants, 241
depression, 4, 8, 9, 13, 20, 25, 63, 65, 66, 67, 69, 72, 88, 90, 95, 96, 104, 105, 110, 115, 116, 117, 118, 119, 120, 121, 122, 123, 162, 164, 165, 167, 169, 170, 171, 194, 234, 239, 240, 242, 243, 244, 247, 252, 253, 254, 255, 256, 267, 272, 284, 286, 288, 298, 303
depressive symptoms, 10, 113, 117, 163, 180
deprivation, 39, 298

depth, 31
despair, 163, 167
detection, 21, 200, 221, 222, 236, 237
detoxification, 5, 6, 267
developing countries, 40
developmental disorder, 200
developmental psychopathology, 300
deviation, 149
dexamethasone suppression test, 124
diabetes, 35, 36, 37, 38, 39, 40, 41, 42, 43, 44, 46, 47, 50, 51, 52, 54, 102, 106
diabetic patients, 43
Diagnostic and Statistical Manual of Mental Disorders, 82, 254
diagnostic criteria, 129
diet, 39, 42, 43, 46
Dietary Guidelines, 53
dieting, 48
differential diagnosis, 56
diffusion, 59
directors, 70
disability, 11, 192
discrimination, 28, 283, 298
diseases, 39, 42, 61, 66, 164, 168, 212, 219, 234
disorder, ix, 3, 4, 5, 6, 7, 8, 10, 11, 12, 13, 14, 25, 26, 46, 50, 52, 56, 71, 78, 100, 104, 105, 106, 115, 117, 121, 161, 162, 163, 164, 167, 168, 171, 180, 194, 200, 202, 205, 210, 212, 213, 214, 235, 242, 243, 276, 287, 291, 292, 293, 297, 301, 302, 305, 307
disposition, 219, 220, 232, 233, 234, 235
dissociation, 27, 190
distress, ix, 150, 155, 156, 157, 167, 302
distribution, 3, 18, 52, 230, 234, 272
diversity, 286
DNA, 220, 221, 222, 233
doctors, 31, 70, 71, 244
DOI, 72
domestic violence, 298
dominance, 19, 26
dopamine, 67, 69, 72, 120, 123, 165, 170, 220, 221, 235, 236, 237, 238
dopamine agonist, 170
dopaminergic, 67, 72, 234
dorsolateral prefrontal cortex, 18, 115, 116, 120, 121, 165, 166
dosage, 59, 60, 69, 88, 93, 96, 97, 99, 107
drawing, 11, 194, 211
drinking patterns, 258, 273
drug abuse, 14, 20, 196, 276
drug action, 72
drug addict, 255, 275, 276, 277, 279, 280
drug addiction, 255
drug consumption, 7
drug dependence, 234, 235, 277
drug interaction, 103, 108
drug therapy, 17, 25, 43, 46, 99
drug treatment, 19, 36, 43, 46, 88, 104, 105, 108, 258, 267, 273
drugs, 6, 7, 10, 12, 39, 43, 46, 48, 66, 67, 68, 76, 88, 91, 94, 95, 98, 99, 234, 235, 240, 244, 247, 259, 277, 278, 280
DSM, 5, 90, 113, 221
DSM-IV-TR, 117, 129, 161, 162, 168
dyslipidemia, 36, 40, 42, 45, 52
dysphoria, 180, 240
dystonia, 36

E

eating disorders, 190
economic consequences, 255
economic development, 298
economic status, 288, 290, 298
editors, 121, 122
education, 5, 21, 22, 37, 43, 66, 129, 181, 182, 183, 191, 192, 200, 203, 212, 214, 236, 277, 283, 286, 288, 289, 292, 293, 294, 295, 296, 298
educational attainment, 298
educational background, 148
educational programs, 200
educational system, 178
EEG, 21, 58
Egypt, 177, 180, 193
elaboration, 223
elders, 144
electric current, 31, 116
electrical fields, 116
Electroconvulsive Therapy, 61, 63
electrodes, 21
electrolyte, 56
electrolyte imbalance, 56
electrophoresis, 222
elongation, 233
e-mail, 65, 132, 134, 142
emergency, 13, 56, 101, 244
emigration, 304
emission, 170
emotion, 58
emotional information, 66, 68, 72
emotional problems, 259, 272, 299
emotional responses, 68, 71
emotional state, 69, 201
emotional well-being, 146, 157
emotionality, 298

empathy, 201, 202, 214
employees, 37
employment, 6, 70, 146, 191, 289, 290, 297, 303
employment status, 289, 290
encephalitis, 164
encoding, 144
endangered, 70
endocrine, 40, 237
endocrine disorders, 40
endocrinology, 37
endogenous depression, 276
endonuclease, 222
energy, 146, 154, 157
England, 196
enlargement, 164, 172
enrollment, 242, 243
entrepreneurs, 298
environment, 56, 67, 120, 178, 235, 285, 298, 303
environmental aspects, 39
environmental stress, 306
enzyme, 233, 243, 250
enzymes, 220
epidemic, 38, 39, 40, 50
epidemiologic, 14, 15, 38
epidemiologic studies, 38
epidemiology, 161, 168
epilepsy, 27, 33, 145, 146, 148, 152, 153, 154, 155, 156, 157, 158, 159, 164, 173, 242
episodic memory, 128
equipment, 200
ERPs, 17, 18, 20
erythrocyte sedimentation rate, 57
escitalopram, 122, 167, 239, 240, 241, 242, 244, 245, 247, 248, 249, 250, 251, 252, 253, 254, 255, 256
ESI, 146
ESR, 57
ethanol, 272
ethics, 36, 204
ethnic groups, 164
ethnicity, 286, 288, 289, 291
etiology, 56
Europe, 153, 273
European Commission, 273
event-related potential, 17, 18, 19, 26, 27, 28
everyday life, 201
evidence, 12, 19, 25, 27, 28, 37, 39, 41, 46, 47, 48, 50, 52, 56, 61, 62, 76, 116, 127, 143, 162, 166, 168, 172, 212, 213, 223, 296, 299
evidence-based practices, 213
evoked potential, 28
evolution, 105
examinations, 31, 90
excitability, 119, 120
excitation, 116
exclusion, 167, 221, 251, 302
excretion, 69
executive function, 76, 79
exercise, 162
experimental design, 199, 202
expertise, 37
exposure, 41, 283, 284, 285, 286, 288, 296, 297, 300, 301
extrapyramidal effects, 40
eye movement, 21

F

face validity, 76, 145, 146
facial expression, 166, 208, 209, 211
factor analysis, 162
FAD, 283, 288, 292
faith, 201
false teeth, 133, 135, 137, 138, 139, 140
families, 30, 182, 191, 192, 193, 195, 200, 201, 204, 212, 213, 276, 288, 297, 298, 299, 300
family functioning, 283, 288, 296, 299
family history, 20, 42, 90, 98, 99, 100, 106
family life, 299
family members, 276, 288, 307, 308
family relationships, 303
family violence, 306
fasting, 38, 42, 46, 52
fasting glucose, 52
fat, 52
fear, 59, 70, 278
fears, 59
feelings, 57, 69, 180, 201, 299
fever, 56, 59
financial, 127, 128, 130, 142, 143, 151, 158, 267
financial crimes, 128
financial support, 158
first generation, 47
fish, 307
five-factor model, 20
flexibility, 56, 57, 58
fluctuations, 167
fluorescence, 242, 244
fluoxetine, 167, 241, 255
fluvoxamine, 167
fMRI, 34, 166, 172
food, 43, 103
Food and Drug Administration (FDA), 76, 81
force, 158
Ford, 26, 27, 50

forecasting, 69
formation, 166, 273, 284
foundations, 202, 204
fractures, 192
fragments, 222
France, 87, 94
fraud, 305, 307
freedom, 21
frontal cortex, 165, 166, 173
frontal lobe, 26, 165
functional imaging, 18, 165
funding, 297, 298, 299
future orientation, 302

G

Gaza Strip, 284, 285
gel, 222
gender differences, 4, 5, 7, 8, 10, 12
gene expression, 120, 123
General Health Questionnaire, 180, 184, 185, 196
generalized anxiety disorder, 4, 11, 15
genes, 219, 220, 221, 232, 234, 235, 236, 237
genetic factors, 219
genetic predisposition, 223
genetics, 219
genome, 220, 235, 236
genotype, 222, 223, 224, 225, 226, 227, 228, 229, 230, 231, 232, 233, 234, 236
genotyping, 224, 225, 226, 227, 228, 229, 230, 231
Germany, xii, 21, 55, 305
germination, 163
global scale, 79
glucose, 31, 38, 41, 42, 46, 47, 102, 116
glucose tolerance, 41, 46, 47
glucose tolerance test, 46
God, 162
GPS, 32
grades, 58, 60, 95, 286
grading, 37
grants, 82, 158
graph, 263
gray matter, 26
grounding, 21
grouping, 67, 70
growth, 106, 200, 233, 234, 279, 296, 302
growth factor, 234
growth rate, 279
guardian, 148
guidance, 234
guidelines, 38, 43, 45, 47, 52, 61, 62, 87, 88, 113, 122, 143, 147, 167, 204, 244
guilt, 20, 113, 162, 163
guilt feelings, 20, 113
Guinea, 172

H

half-life, 59
hallucinations, 18, 20, 25, 27, 28, 57, 58, 59, 162, 172
handedness, 20
haplotypes, 220
head injury, 20
head trauma, 117
headache, 61, 117
health, 5, 14, 39, 41, 43, 100, 154, 155, 157, 158, 159, 177, 178, 180, 194, 196, 243, 258, 259, 262, 269, 270, 271, 273, 274, 275, 278, 286, 288, 292, 296, 297, 298, 299, 300, 301, 305, 306, 307, 309
health care, 5, 178, 275
health problems, 262, 270, 271, 298, 299
health psychology, 196
health risks, 43
health services, 309
health status, 262
heart transplantation, 164, 172
heavy drinking, 240, 244, 245, 251, 253, 258, 259, 263, 264, 265, 267, 270
height, 20, 41, 46, 60
hemisphere, 19
hemispheric asymmetry, 25
heroin, 7, 9, 13, 57
heterogeneity, 4, 285
high risk patients, 39
high school, 148, 149, 150, 152
higher education, 288
histogram, 181
history, 8, 10, 11, 19, 20, 47, 51, 56, 90, 96, 98, 105, 106, 117, 190, 193, 242, 243, 245, 256, 262, 306
HIV, 7, 236
homes, 284
homogeneity, 118, 245
Hong Kong, 164, 169
hormone, 42, 103
hospitalization, 101, 105
hostility, 20, 286, 287, 288
House, 34, 149, 259
human, 28, 123, 173, 178, 220, 235, 236, 237, 238, 273, 297, 298
human development, 297
human right, 178
human rights, 178

hybrid, 285
hydrophobia, 164
hyperactivity, 106
hypercholesterolemia, 46
hyperlipidemia, 39, 40
hypertension, 38, 39, 40, 57, 103, 237, 266, 272
hypothesis, 20, 25, 163, 165, 166, 220, 235, 241
hypothyroidism, 103

I

ID, 225, 226
identification, 52, 57, 148, 219
identity, 166, 172, 284, 285, 298, 301, 303
ideology, 285
illegal drug use, 4
image, 307
imbalances, 26
imitation, 213
immigrants, 285
immortality, 162, 163
immunoglobulin, 234
impairments, 20, 78, 128, 143
improvements, 76, 79
impulses, 113
impulsivity, 190, 240, 272
in transition, 284
in vitro, 122, 236
incidence, 33, 39, 43, 56, 164, 234, 245, 253, 257, 258, 260, 261, 272, 275
income, 178, 181, 182, 191, 192, 193, 195
independent living, 128
independent variable, 245
India, 170
indirect effect, 66
individual character, 66, 245
individual differences, 120, 214
individuals, 15, 38, 52, 152, 194, 214, 236, 241, 259, 260, 261, 273, 284, 287, 298
induction, 113
infant mortality, 284
infarction, 164
infection, 56, 57
inflammation, 56
inflation, 21
information processing, 66, 68, 76, 166
informed consent, 20, 59, 61, 78, 148, 221, 242, 246
inheritance, 236
inhibition, 17, 24, 28, 116, 235
inhibitor, 95, 240
initiation, 213
insanity, 307, 309
insertion, 237
insomnia, 113
institutions, 45, 70
insulin, 20, 38, 41, 42
insulin resistance, 38, 41, 42
integration, 25, 119, 120
integrity, 19, 241
intelligence, 128
intensive care unit, 59
internal consistency, 79, 146, 287
International Classification of Diseases, 276
international standards, 245
intervention, 117, 128, 199, 200, 201, 202, 203, 204, 205, 207, 210, 211, 212, 213, 214, 255, 275, 298
intoxication, 59, 258
intron, 221, 234, 236
investment, 50, 201, 299
investments, 49
ion-exchange, 222
IPR, 292
ipsilateral, 18, 19, 20, 24, 27, 120
IQ scores, 127
Iran, 115, 199
Iraq, 179
iron, 58
irritability, 113, 240, 252
isolation, 99, 101, 221
Israel, 179, 283, 284, 285, 286, 287, 297, 298, 299, 300, 301, 302, 303
issues, ix, 50, 120, 147, 154, 155, 156, 157, 161, 297
Italy, xii, 17

J

Japan, xii, xiii, 75, 82, 127, 128, 143, 144, 145, 146, 152
Jews, 300
joints, 259
Jordan, xi, 195
junior high school, 148
juvenile delinquency, 296

K

kicks, 192
kidneys, 242
kindergarten, 58
Kuwait, 195

L

lack of control, 120
languages, ix, 146, 153
latency, 18, 21, 24, 25, 27, 28
laterality, 19, 27, 28
LDL, 38, 45
lead, 17, 22, 24, 25, 37, 46, 56, 57, 59, 104, 151, 153, 166, 167, 190, 210, 296
Leahy, 62
learning, 76, 78, 156, 172, 173, 297
Lebanon, 179, 195, 303
left hemisphere, 17, 18, 19, 24, 25, 116, 165
leisure, 298
leukocytosis, 57
leukopenia, 33
level of education, 5, 78, 193, 298
libido, 113
life expectancy, 39, 258
lifestyle changes, 46
lifetime, 116, 178, 194, 259, 261, 264, 265
light, 37, 47, 109, 242, 244
limbic system, 116
lipid metabolism, 47, 48
lipid peroxidation, 67
lithium, 88, 102, 105, 106, 107, 108, 109, 111, 113, 167
Lithuania, 222
liver, 33, 233, 237, 242, 256
liver cirrhosis, 233, 237
liver disease, 256
living conditions, 179, 278
lobbying, 308
locus, 236
longitudinal study, 213
loss of consciousness, 192
lymphocytes, 236

M

magnesium, 34
magnet, 62
magnetic field, 19, 116
magnetic resonance, 26, 28
magnetic resonance imaging, 26
magnetoencephalography, 27
magnitude, 41
major depression, 13, 119, 120, 121, 122, 123, 170, 254
major depressive disorder, 5, 7, 115, 116, 122, 165, 167, 240, 254, 255
majority, 4, 8, 11, 12, 18, 116, 119, 284, 285
maltreatment, 180, 195, 197, 304
man, 169, 171
management, 52, 87, 88, 100, 104, 105, 106, 109, 113, 168, 244, 246, 256, 279, 280
mania, 56, 88, 92, 93, 96, 97, 104, 113, 114, 120, 124
manic, 88, 90, 93, 94, 97, 98, 101, 104, 105, 107, 108, 113, 163, 242, 305, 307
manic episode, 88, 94, 98, 104, 105, 107, 108, 305, 307
manic symptoms, 93, 113
manic-depressive psychosis, 242
MANOVA, 247
marijuana, 259
marital status, 5, 290, 299
married women, 8
Maryland, 76
masking, 20
mass, 38
matter, iv, 26, 39, 308
measurements, 21, 46, 243
media, 178, 179, 213, 307, 308
mediation, 31
Medicaid, 309
medical, 7, 8, 11, 20, 37, 47, 55, 58, 66, 116, 144, 147, 152, 154, 180, 183, 200, 212, 221, 240, 242, 244, 246, 247, 257, 258, 259, 262, 263, 264, 267, 272, 273, 284, 305, 306, 307
medical history, 58
medication, 8, 12, 27, 29, 30, 31, 32, 33, 39, 41, 42, 47, 48, 50, 55, 56, 57, 59, 65, 66, 67, 68, 69, 70, 71, 73, 115, 117, 119, 121, 146, 147, 148, 153, 155, 156, 157, 239, 240, 241, 242, 244, 255
medication compliance, 241
medicine, 3, 30, 57, 130, 132, 134, 137, 139, 181, 182, 183
mellitus, 54
membranes, 58
memory, 58, 60, 62, 65, 67, 68, 72, 75, 76, 78, 79, 128, 130, 131, 142, 155, 156, 157, 272
mental activity, 18
mental capacity, 128
mental disorder, 3, 4, 5, 8, 12, 14, 128, 168, 194, 234, 273, 305, 308, 309
mental health, 5, 14, 179, 192, 194, 196, 259, 263, 270, 283, 286, 288, 296, 297, 298, 299, 301, 302, 303, 308
mental illness, 4, 13, 34, 46, 52, 192, 304, 306, 307
mental retardation, 19, 78, 164, 306, 307
mental state, 143
mentally ill persons, 306

meta analysis, 119, 122
meta-analysis, 18, 26, 61, 122, 123, 235, 236, 253
Metabolic, v, 35, 36, 37, 38, 39, 41, 42, 47, 50, 51, 52, 53, 103
metabolic changes, 40, 41, 47, 48
metabolic disorder, 36, 37, 41, 43, 46
metabolic disorders, 36, 37, 41, 43, 46
metabolic syndrome, 35, 36, 37, 38, 50, 51, 52, 53
metabolism, 38, 220, 235
metals, 117
meter, 203
metformin, 42
methodology, 33, 77, 87, 164, 179
methylation, 233
Miami, 214
mice, 120, 254
Michigan Alcoholism Screening Test (MAST), 221
Microsoft, 259
middle class, 178, 191
Middle East, xi, 178, 179, 195, 284, 302
migration, 285
military, 195, 221, 284, 300
misuse, 12
MMS, 143
models, 122, 298, 303
modifications, 150, 152
mood change, 68, 72
mood disorder, 7, 90, 116, 122, 173
Moon, 164, 171
morbidity, 37, 39, 43, 50, 51, 258, 303
mortality, 35, 39, 40, 50, 51, 52, 53, 59
mortality rate, 39
mortality risk, 59
motivation, 200, 263, 264, 266, 275, 278, 279, 280
motor activity, 56
motor skills, 75, 78
MRI, 26, 58
mRNA, 120, 122
multidimensional, 201, 202, 259
multiple factors, 67
multiple regression, 288, 292
multiple sclerosis, 164
muscle contraction, 31
mutation, 220
mutations, 220
mutilation, 171
myocardial infarction, 39, 51

N

naming, 130, 131
National Health and Nutrition Examination Survey, 38, 41, 51
national identity, 284
National Institute of Mental Health, 76
National Research Council, 214
nationality, 292
natural disasters, 11
nausea, 62, 252
negative attitudes, 285, 302
negative effects, 283
negative emotions, 202
neglect, 178, 180, 181, 183, 190, 191, 193, 195, 197
neocortex, 18
nerve, 33, 62, 116, 120
nervous system, 242
Netherlands, 144, 161
neurobiology, 18, 219
neuroimaging, 116
neuroleptic malignant syndrome, 61
neuroleptics, 56, 60, 62, 69, 72, 309
neurologic complications, 172
neurologist, 161
neuronal systems, 67, 68, 69
neurons, 116, 120, 233
neuropsychiatry, 172, 173
neuropsychological tests, 129, 131
neuropsychology, 172
neurotransmitters, 66, 116, 220, 235
neutral, 67, 172
NHANES, 41, 53
nicotine, 40, 259
nicotinic acid, 46
NIJ, 197
NK cells, 234
NMDA receptors, 120
norepinephrine, 95
normal children, 201, 202, 204
normal distribution, 245
North America, 50
NPR, 222
nucleus, 120, 123
nurses, 68, 70
nursing, 57, 58
nursing care, 57, 58
nutrition, 41, 43

O

obedience, 56
obesity, 38, 39, 40, 42, 43, 50, 51, 52
obsessive-compulsive disorder (OCD), 4, 10, 15
obstacles, ix
occupational therapy, 201, 212
offenders, 305
olanzapine, 40, 43, 91, 92, 94, 95, 98, 99, 111, 167, 173
operations, 205
opiate addiction, 279
opiates, 6, 279, 280
opioids, 69
opportunities, 211
organic disease, 163
organs, 56
osteoarthritis, 39
outpatient, 5, 13, 19, 258, 267, 275, 277, 309
outpatients, 6, 9, 52, 77, 257, 307
overweight, 38, 39, 40, 42, 43, 46, 52
oxygen, 31

P

pain, 68, 116, 162, 259
panic attack, 113
panic disorder, 256
paralysis, 62, 162, 163, 168
paranoia, 165
Paranoid Ideation, 291
paranoid schizophrenia, 307
parents, 57, 58, 59, 61, 62, 191, 192, 193, 203, 204, 205, 211, 212, 213, 214, 288, 297
parietal cortex, 165
parietal lobe, 171
paroxetine, 109, 167
participants, 12, 36, 37, 43, 48, 148, 180, 181, 183, 190, 191, 192, 201, 203, 257, 258, 259, 261, 262, 263, 264, 266, 267, 273, 283, 286, 287, 288, 292, 296
pathogenesis, 161, 234
pathologist, 205
pathology, 4, 43, 55, 108, 242, 288
pathophysiology, 165, 166, 168, 219
pathways, 18, 19, 25
patient care, 87, 88, 89, 106, 109
PCM, 89, 106
PCR, 221, 222, 236, 237
peace, 299, 301
peace process, 299
Pearson correlations, 79, 288
peer group, 287
peer review, 162
peptides, 235
perfusion, 165
peripheral blood, 236
permit, 90
personal hygiene, 57, 59
personal identity, 298
personal problems, 151, 153
personality, 5, 7, 65, 72, 104, 105, 106, 165, 265, 266, 272, 276
personality characteristics, 165
personality disorder, 5, 7, 104, 105, 272
PET, 18, 27, 120
pharmaceutical, 49
pharmacological treatment, 66, 70, 71, 88, 242
pharmacology, 65, 72, 255
pharmacotherapy, 61, 63, 65, 66, 67, 148, 154, 255, 276
phenomenology, 72, 167, 169
phenotype, 15, 220
Philadelphia, 122, 213
phobia, 10
phobic anxiety, 272, 283, 286, 288, 296
phosphate, 120
physical abuse, 11, 179, 181, 183, 190, 191, 192, 193, 196
physical activity, 40, 46, 103
physical aggression, 283, 287, 296
physical exercise, 39, 42, 43, 48
physical fitness, 68
physical health, 190
physicians, 41
pitch, 20, 28
placebo, 37, 53, 69, 71, 72, 116, 123, 204, 239, 240, 241, 242, 244, 245, 246, 247, 248, 249, 250, 251, 252, 253, 254, 255, 256
platform, 233
playing, 200, 201, 202
Poland, vii, xiii, 65, 305, 307
polarity, 97, 99
policy, 273, 283, 298, 299, 302, 304
policy makers, 298, 299
policy responses, 273
political opposition, 179
political parties, 179
politics, 195
polydipsia, 46
polymorphism, 220, 221, 222, 223, 224, 225, 226, 227, 228, 229, 230, 232, 233, 234, 235, 236, 237, 238
polymorphisms, 219, 220, 221, 222, 223, 232, 233, 235, 236

polyuria, 46
population, ix, 5, 8, 9, 10, 12, 13, 14, 39, 40, 41, 47, 53, 128, 164, 196, 197, 199, 223, 229, 233, 234, 238, 240, 241, 258, 284, 285, 287, 297, 299
portfolio, 196
positive emotions, 201, 202, 212
positive relationship, 17, 24
positron, 26, 27
positron emission tomography, 26, 27
posttraumatic stress, 301
post-traumatic stress disorder, 4, 14, 284
poverty, 193, 284, 297, 298, 299
poverty reduction, 298
precedent, 153
preferential treatment, 191
prefrontal cortex, 119, 121, 123
pregnancy, 109, 110, 117, 163, 168, 222, 234
preparation, iv, 59, 214
preschool, 199
prevalence rate, 260
prevention, 104, 146, 240, 253, 254, 255, 302
primacy, 285
primary school, 201
probability, 232, 233
probe, 172
problem behavior, 304
problem drinkers, 8, 255
problem solving, 75, 78, 82
processing deficits, 19
prodrome, 13
professionals, 39, 53, 70, 104, 154, 167, 201, 298
prognosis, 3, 4, 7, 11, 100, 167, 168
project, 147, 201, 221, 236, 245, 253, 259
propagation, 235
prophylactic, 89, 91, 97, 98, 99, 100
prophylaxis, 88, 104
protection, 235, 279
protective factors, 301
proteinuria, 102
PST, 268
psychiatric diagnosis, 6
psychiatric disorders, 12, 14, 20, 58, 61, 99, 122, 162, 164, 258, 306
psychiatric illness, 306
psychiatric morbidity, 13
psychiatric patients, 40, 164, 169, 309
psychiatrist, 37, 42, 43, 48, 79, 90, 117, 128, 221, 277, 308
psychiatry, ix, 3, 37, 57, 59, 65, 66, 68, 69, 71, 121, 122, 144, 161, 169, 219, 255, 275, 309
psychoactive drug, 69, 221
psychological distress, 301
psychological functions, 128
psychological phenomena, 180
psychological problems, 177, 178, 180, 182, 193
psychological tools, 180
psychological variables, 181
psychological well-being, 298
psychologist, 130, 148
psychology, 121, 122, 199, 203, 214
psychometric properties, 76, 145, 146, 153, 158
psychopathology, 5, 13, 17, 20, 27, 121, 166, 168, 287
psychopharmacology, 73
psychoses, 257, 260, 261, 262
psychosis, 4, 7, 12, 13, 14, 26, 28, 37, 40, 43, 61, 62, 65, 66, 67, 71, 72, 90, 128, 162, 259, 267, 272
psychosocial functioning, 296
psychosocial interventions, 276
psychosomatic, 69
psychotherapy, 101, 104, 110, 116, 117, 214, 242, 244, 277
psychotic symptoms, 8, 37, 56, 66, 88, 92, 93, 95, 96, 97, 99, 128
psychoticism, 283, 286, 288, 296
PTSD, 11, 12, 13, 188, 189, 196, 283, 284, 287, 288, 291, 292, 293, 296, 297, 298, 302, 303
public awareness, 194
public health, 36, 179
public interest, 178
publishing, ix, 37, 122, 179
punishment, 191, 192, 195

Q

quality of life, 37, 43, 100, 145, 146, 149, 151, 152, 154, 157, 158, 159, 259
questioning, 90
questionnaire, 118, 130, 145, 146, 147, 148, 149, 150, 151, 152, 153, 154, 159, 180, 193, 196, 201, 221, 247, 264, 267, 283, 286, 287, 294, 300, 309
quetiapine, 40, 167, 173

R

race, 5
racism, 283
random numbers, 244
rating scale, 78, 83, 254, 255, 277
reaction time, 26
reactions, 30, 33, 70, 276, 296, 301
reactivity, 59, 60

reading, 57, 78, 155, 156
reality, 163, 285, 298
reasoning, 75, 78, 156, 172
recall, 150, 190, 192, 204, 272
reception, 67
receptors, 24, 62, 66, 67, 120, 220, 235
recognition, 161, 166, 168, 202
recommendations, iv, 35, 55, 56, 60, 61, 88, 89, 92, 94, 95, 103, 113
reconciliation, 77, 147
recovery, 26, 121, 165, 167, 297
refugees, 284
regulations, 116
rehabilitation, 60, 63, 76, 202, 212, 213, 275, 276, 277, 278, 279
rehabilitation program, 275, 276, 277
rejection, 69, 162
relapses, 98, 99, 251
relatives, 42, 43, 117, 130, 143, 155, 275, 276, 277, 279, 280, 297
relevance, 298
reliability, 81, 83, 117, 146, 153, 159, 191, 204, 256, 286, 287, 288
relief, 146
religion, 285, 286
religiosity, 288, 302
remission, 26, 29, 31, 32, 33, 37, 89, 101, 165, 173, 240, 241, 245, 250, 251, 252, 253, 255, 275, 277, 278, 279
repetitions, 223
replication, 24
requirements, 27
researchers, ix, x, 41, 76, 154, 194, 204, 210, 211, 220, 240, 259, 272
resistance, 38, 56, 73, 91, 116, 210, 211
resolution, 18, 88, 91, 94, 97, 173
resources, 5, 27, 192, 194, 273
respiration, 56
response, 4, 19, 20, 24, 25, 27, 47, 48, 69, 72, 88, 93, 94, 96, 106, 113, 116, 117, 120, 122, 124, 150, 152, 166, 207, 211, 274, 275, 283, 297
responsiveness, 56, 113, 153
restrictions, 200
retail, 200
retardation, 20, 204
retrograde amnesia, 60
rhythm, 101
riboflavin, 239, 241, 242, 244, 247
right hemisphere, 19, 25
risk, 4, 5, 8, 10, 11, 12, 13, 15, 27, 30, 35, 36, 38, 39, 40, 41, 42, 45, 46, 50, 52, 62, 89, 92, 97, 103, 104, 105, 108, 109, 120, 128, 167, 169, 196, 297, 298, 301, 306, 308, 309
risk assessment, 109
risk factors, 15, 41, 42, 105, 298
risk profile, 40
risperidone, 40, 63, 91, 92, 98, 111, 167
rules, 107, 108
Russia, 239, 257, 258, 261, 272, 275, 285

S

safety, 29, 30, 31, 37, 122, 128, 168, 306
Sarajevo, 301
SAS, 247, 248
Saudi Arabia, 177, 179, 193, 196
scattering, 204
schizophrenia, x, 4, 5, 7, 11, 12, 13, 14, 17, 18, 19, 20, 21, 22, 23, 24, 25, 26, 27, 28, 29, 30, 33, 34, 35, 36, 37, 39, 40, 41, 43, 46, 47, 49, 51, 52, 53, 54, 55, 56, 61, 62, 63, 69, 72, 75, 76, 77, 78, 79, 81, 82, 83, 162, 171, 194, 234, 237, 242, 305, 307, 308, 309
schizophrenic patients, 26, 27
scholarship, 296, 298
school, 58, 60, 148, 149, 150, 191, 192, 195, 200, 203, 212, 267, 283, 284, 286, 296, 298, 301, 302
science, 200
scientific publications, 65, 179
scope, x
search terms, 4
second generation, 36, 47, 88
secondary damage, 56
secondary schools, 192
secretion, 42, 234
security, 296
sedative, 7, 94, 104
sedentary lifestyle, 41
seizure, 116, 117, 146, 153, 156, 157, 167, 266
selective attention, 19, 27
selective serotonin reuptake inhibitor, 240, 241
selectivity, 212, 241, 253
self esteem, 181, 183
self-assessment, 247
self-esteem, 40, 180, 190, 191, 196, 284, 285, 298, 301
self-identity, 166
self-mutilation, 105
self-reports, 214
self-sufficiency, 279
sensations, 69
senses, 202
sensitivity, 67, 268, 286, 292
serotonin, 95, 120, 240, 241, 253, 255
sertraline, 122, 167

serum, 38
service provider, 299
SES, 283, 284, 285, 288, 296, 297
settlements, 285
sex, 30, 181, 212, 223, 245, 246
sexual abuse, 8, 10, 178, 180, 181, 183, 190, 191, 194, 195, 197, 202, 214
sexual harassment, 178
sham, 120, 122, 123
shape, 66, 72
shock, 34
showing, 24, 57, 61, 208, 209, 210, 247, 260
siblings, 181, 183, 190, 192, 193, 289
side effects, 31, 33, 35, 36, 48, 59, 61, 101, 103, 243, 245, 253
signals, 67
significance level, 245
signs, 57, 100, 163, 240
simple random sampling, 203
sine wave, 21
single-nucleotide polymorphism, 236
skewness, 181, 191
skin, 31, 162, 166
sleep disturbance, 180
smoking, 38, 39, 40, 41, 221
social activities, 155, 211
social adjustment, 303
social behavior, 207, 208, 209, 210, 264, 265, 267, 270, 271
social behaviour, 284
social capital, 301
social class, 178, 191
social cognition, 78
social competence, 213
social context, 65, 284
social development, 296
social environment, 105
social exclusion, 284, 299
social identity, 285
social network, 70
social phobia, 11
social problems, 146, 157, 257, 273, 288, 297
social relations, 68, 298
social services, 178, 297, 299
social status, 180, 245, 279, 284
social structure, 296
social welfare, 132, 134, 142
socialization, 279
society, 178, 190, 192, 195, 284, 285, 298, 299, 303, 307, 308
socioeconomic status, 180, 283, 284, 286, 299
sociology, 179
software, 21, 79, 223
solution, 162
somatization, 283, 286, 288, 296
South Asia, 302
Spain, xiii, 3, 4, 5, 13
speech, 28, 200, 205, 212
speech sounds, 28
spontaneity, 20
spontaneous recovery, 167
St. Petersburg, 239, 242, 257
stability, 114
stabilization, 240, 253, 255, 276
stabilizers, 92
staff members, 244
stakeholders, 298
standard deviation, 79, 205
starch, 242
starvation, 170
state, 4, 17, 19, 24, 26, 72, 91, 92, 104, 113, 157, 163, 167, 180, 193, 195, 204, 239, 242, 243, 247, 256, 258, 275, 276, 284, 300
statistics, 79, 181, 259
status epilepticus, 62
stereotypes, 191
stigma, 278, 306
stimulation, 17, 19, 20, 24, 25, 27, 31, 33, 34, 62, 115, 116, 117, 119, 120, 121, 122, 123, 124
stimulus, 21, 22, 27, 201, 204, 212
stomach, 162
stress, 8, 14, 100, 143, 180, 193, 194, 213, 287, 291, 292, 293, 297, 302
stressful events, 297
stroke, 50, 51
structural changes, 165
structure, 66, 82, 128, 196, 258, 278, 286, 297
stupor, 56
style, 165, 166, 172
subjective experience, 67, 69, 284
substance abuse, 3, 12, 14, 15, 78, 254, 255, 259, 306, 308
substance use, 4, 10, 11, 12, 13
substitution, 104
substrate, 18, 81
succession, 18
SUD, 4, 5, 6, 7, 8, 9, 10, 11, 12
suicidal ideation, 298
suicide, 8, 10, 12, 39, 89, 90, 105, 167, 196, 286, 301
suicide attempts, 10
Sun, 13
supervision, 191, 193
supplementation, 103
support services, 297
suppression, 120

survival, 236, 245, 250
susceptibility, 39, 219, 236, 237
Sweden, xiii, 214
Switzerland, 121, 122
symptoms, 4, 8, 10, 18, 20, 25, 27, 28, 29, 32, 36, 37, 40, 43, 55, 56, 57, 59, 60, 61, 66, 68, 70, 71, 98, 100, 101, 105, 113, 115, 116, 128, 146, 163, 164, 167, 205, 240, 241, 242, 252, 267, 272, 276, 283, 286, 288, 292, 296, 297, 302
synaptic plasticity, 234
syndrome, 41, 50, 52, 55, 56, 103, 161, 162, 163, 164, 165, 166, 167, 168, 169, 170, 171, 172, 173, 214, 262, 263, 264, 265, 266, 270, 272, 273, 305, 307
synthesis, 51, 235
Syria, 195
systolic blood pressure, 38

T

T lymphocytes, 233
tachycardia, 33, 56, 58, 59, 60
Taiwan, 237
tardive dyskinesia, 36
target, 26, 116, 146
tau, 260
TCC, 222
teachers, 106, 192, 213
techniques, 18, 219
technology, 50, 154, 220, 233
teeth, 133, 135, 137, 138, 139, 140
telephone, 57, 132, 134, 136, 137, 138, 139
temperature, 57, 68
temporal lobe, 17, 18, 26, 28, 164, 165, 171
temporal lobe epilepsy, 164, 171
tension, 20, 56
terrorism, 300, 301
test scores, 128, 143
testing, 56, 77
test-retest reliability, 77, 79, 81, 146, 286, 287, 288
textbook, 122
TGA, 222
thalamus, 165
therapeutic community, 276
therapeutic effects, 32, 33, 115, 116, 119, 120
therapeutic interventions, 200, 201, 202, 207, 212, 214
therapist, 117, 203, 207, 210, 211, 212
therapy, 20, 25, 30, 31, 32, 33, 34, 55, 56, 60, 62, 63, 66, 91, 101, 104, 105, 111, 112, 116, 120, 121, 165, 167, 170, 171, 173, 199, 200, 201, 202, 203, 204, 207, 210, 211, 212, 214, 215, 243, 244, 245, 247, 253, 255, 256
therapy interventions, 207
thoughts, 68
threats, 296
thrombosis, 164, 171
thyroid, 102, 103, 106
time constraints, 204
time series, 117, 120
TNF, 221, 226, 232
tobacco, 13, 234, 242
toddlers, 213, 214
tones, 17, 18, 19, 20, 21, 22, 24, 25
total cholesterol, 42
toxic effect, 272
toys, 200
tracks, 58
training, 33, 200, 201, 204, 213, 215
trait anxiety, 256
Trait Anxiety Scale, 247
traits, 105
trajectory, 298
transactions, 288
transference, 71
translation, x, 75, 77, 129, 144, 146, 147, 151, 152, 153, 158, 180, 190, 194
transmission, 69
transportation, 130, 155
trauma, 180, 258, 283, 285, 296, 297, 298, 299, 300, 301, 302, 303
traumatic brain injury, 169
traumatic events, 11, 283, 288
treatment methods, 62
trial, 53, 72, 121, 122, 240, 241, 242, 243, 244, 245, 246, 247, 251, 252, 253, 255, 256, 305, 306
triglycerides, 38, 42
tumor, 171, 221
tumor necrosis factor, 221
type 2 diabetes, 38, 39, 43, 50, 51
typhoid fever, 164, 171
tyrosine, 122

U

United, 36, 39, 41, 51, 128, 144, 193, 197, 213, 287
United Kingdom (UK), 177, 196, 197, 256
United Nations, 128, 144
United States (USA), 36, 39, 41, 51, 123, 193, 197, 213, 221, 287
universities, 179, 212
UNRWA, 179, 195

unusual experiences, 27
urban, 14, 286
urine, 239, 241, 242, 243, 244, 247, 277
US Department of Health and Human Services, 256

V

validation, 82, 145, 146, 147, 152, 153, 159, 213
valvular heart disease, 170
variables, 5, 6, 21, 22, 67, 181, 183, 188, 190, 245, 250, 260, 288, 289, 292
variations, 11, 12, 24, 66, 67
vascular dementia, 129
vascular system, 62
venlafaxine, 122, 173
ventricle, 164
ventricular fibrillation, 59, 62
ventricular tachycardia, 59, 62
verbal fluency, 76, 79
very low density lipoprotein (VLDL), 38
victimization, 11, 194, 302
victims, 6, 128, 178, 296
violence, 10, 195, 197, 238, 256, 283, 284, 285, 286, 288, 291, 292, 293, 294, 295, 296, 297, 298, 299, 300, 301, 302, 303, 305, 306, 307, 308, 309
violent behavior, 296, 301, 306, 308
violent crime, 308
visceral adiposity, 41

W

war, 179, 296, 297, 301, 303
Washington, 13, 48, 82, 121, 168, 195, 196, 197, 214, 300
water, 222
web, 178, 179, 196
web sites, 179
websites, 178
weight gain, 35, 36, 40, 42, 46, 47, 48, 51, 52, 53, 54, 103, 252
weight loss, 41, 43, 48, 163
welfare, 5, 212, 298
well-being, 149, 285, 298
West Bank, 284, 285, 286, 296, 301, 302
white matter, 28
withdrawal, 20, 57, 104, 203, 238, 262, 263, 264, 265, 266, 267, 270, 271, 272, 273
withdrawal symptoms, 263, 264, 267
witnesses, 296
work activity, 5
working memory, 28, 75, 76, 78, 79
World Health Organization (WHO), 38, 39, 50, 51, 121, 179, 195, 200, 273
worldwide, 116
worry, 146, 149, 157

X

X chromosome, 223

Y

young adults, 169
young people, 309
youth populations, 287

Z

ziprasidone, 40